W9-CNP-475

Regional Anesthesia

Dr. med. M. Zenz
Associate Professor, Chief, The Center for Anesthesiology, The University Medical School, Hannover, Division IV, Oststadt Hospital, Hannover, West Germany

Dr. med. C. Panhans
Chief of the Pain Clinic, Mainz, West Germany

Dr. med. H. Chr. Niesel
Chief, Division of Anesthesiology, St. Marien's Hospital, Ludwigshafen, West Germany

Dr. med H. Kreuscher
Professor and Chief, Institute of Anesthesiology of the City Hospitals, Osnabrück, West Germany

Translated by

Thomas J. DeKornfeld, M.D.
Professor of Anesthesiology, University of Michigan Medical School, Ann Arbor, Michigan

Year Book Medical Publishers, Inc.
Chicago · Boca Raton

Wolfe Medical Publications, Ltd.
London

This book is an authorized translation from the second German edition copyrighted by Astra Chemicals GmbH and published in 1985 by Gustav Fischer Verlag, Stuttgart, Germany. Title of the German edition: *Regionalanästhesie.*

1 2 3 4 5 6 7 8 9 0 KE 92 91 90 89 88

Library of Congress Cataloging-in-Publication Data

Regionalanästhesie. English.
Regional anesthesia.

Translation of: Regionalanästhesie.
Bibliography: p.
Includes index.
1. Conduction anesthesia. I. Zenz, M. (Michael)
II. Title. [DNLM: 1. Anesthesia, Conduction. WO 300
R3355]
RD84.R42413 1988 617′.964 87-18878
ISBN 0-8151-9881-7

Sponsoring Editor: Linda A. Pierpoint

Assistant Director, Manuscript Services: Frances M. Perveiler

Project Manager: Carol A. Reynolds

List of Contributors

Dr. med. H. Albrecht
Professor and Chief, Medical Division of the Women's Clinic, University of Dusseldorf

Dr. med. P. Berle
Professor and Chief, the Women's Clinic, Wiesbaden

Dr. med. D. Čović
Chief of the Pain Clinic–Anesthesiology–City Hospital, Konstanz

Dr. med. Th. Flöter
Anesthesiologist, Frankfurt/M.

Dr. med. U. Hankemeier
Chief of the Anesthesiology Section of the Pain Clinic, St. Mary's Hospital, Herne

Dr. med. H.-J. Hartung
Institute for Anesthesiology and Resuscitation, City Hospital, Mannheim

Dr. med. W. Hoerster
Anesthesiologist, Giessen

Dr. med. H. Kreuscher
Professor and Chief, Institute of Anesthesiology of the City Hospitals, Osnabrück

Dr. med. E. Lanz
Associate Professor, Chief of the Institute for Anesthesiology, Johannes Gutenberg University Hospitals, Mainz

Dr. med. W. Müller-Holve
Associate Professor, Chief of the City Hospital for Women, Hamburg-Barmbek General Hospital

Dr. med. H. Chr. Niesel
Chief of the Division of Anesthesiology, St. Marien's Hospital, Ludwigshafen

Dr. med. C. Panhans
Chief of the Pain Clinic, Mainz

Dr. med. O. Schulte-Steinberg
Anesthesiologist, Söcking

Dr. med. W. L. A. Simgen
Chief, The Section of Anesthesiology, Moabit Hospital, Berlin

Dr. med. R. Schwarz
Chief, Section of Anesthesiology, St. Gertrude's Hospital, Berlin

Dr. med. K. Strasser
Associate Professor, Senior Physician, Department of Anesthesiology and Intensive Care, Alfried Krupp Hospital, Essen

Dr. med. D. Theiss
Chief, Institute of Anesthesiology, Johannes-Gutenberg University Hospitals, Mainz

Dr. med. F. Wagner
Chief, Section of Anesthesiology, District Hospital, Offenburg

Dr. med. M. Zenz
Associate Professor, Chief, The Center for Anesthesiology, The University Medical School, Hannover, Division IV, Oststadt Hospital, Hannover

Translator's Foreword

The original German edition of this book was the cooperative effort of a number of outstanding German anesthesiologists under the editorship of Professors Zenz, Panhans, Niesel, and Kreuscher. It presents the most advanced thinking and technology in the field of regional anesthesia and illustrates the anatomy and the technical problems of nerve blocks with a wealth of drawings and color photographs. The first two chapters discuss the advantages of regional anesthesia and the complications of this approach to surgical and pathologic pain control. The rest of the book discusses the individual nerve blocks. Separate chapters are devoted to the major peripheral plexuses and their terminal branches. Separate chapters deal with spinal, lumbar epidural, thoracic epidural, and caudal anesthesia. A separate section is devoted to obstetrical regional anesthesia. The last section of the book discusses the therapeutic blocks.

Each chapter follows the same path and presents the anatomy, the equipment, the positioning, the technical approach, the drugs to be used, the side effects, the indications, and the contraindications. Thus, each chapter stands by itself and both the novice and the relatively inexperienced anesthesiologist should be able to follow the instructions with ease. Even the expert should find both instruction and enjoyment in perusing the outstanding illustrations.

It is the obvious intent of the authors and the editors to provide the anesthesiology community with a most useful handbook. The translator, having spent his entire professional life in academic anesthesiology, is convinced that they have achieved their purpose fully. This volume should be of the greatest assistance to the trainees in anesthesiology, to the trained anesthesiologist who performs some of these blocks only infrequently, and also to our surgical and obstetrical colleagues who may wish to perform some of these blocks in the emergency room, in the delivery room, or in the operating room.

THOMAS J. DEKORNFELD, M.D.

Contents

Obstetrics

Pain Therapy

The Advantages of Regional Anesthesia over General Anesthesia

O. Schulte-Steinberg

It has become evident that carefully conducted regional anesthesia is, even today, the safest technique for pain control in a large segment of the surgical procedures. The incidence of cardiac arrest is 1:2,500 cases of general anesthesia, but only 1:11,000 cases of regional anesthesia. Regional anesthesia techniques can supplement, replace, or be combined with general anesthesia. By using them, the anesthesiologist has a better opportunity to adapt anesthesia to the requirements of the patient, of the surgeon, and of the surgical procedure. The full spectrum of the anesthesiologic armamentarium can be brought to bear on the safety of the patient only if the anesthesiologist is fully conversant with both general and regional anesthesia. Procedures in the area of the head, neck, and thorax are largely the domain of general, endotracheal anesthesia. Even here, however, superficial procedures can be done under peripheral nerve blocks. For procedures in all other areas, regional anesthesia provides an alternative technique, or one which can be used in combination with general anesthesia. During the last 15 years, the drugs and techniques of general anesthesia have expanded substantially. The same is true for regional anesthesia. We have learned from general anesthesia how important it is for the anesthesiologist to combine a profound theoretical knowledge with the technical mastery of the field. The same is equally true for regional anesthesia. The drugs used currently in conduction anesthesia have fewer side effects when used skillfully. The amide-type local anesthetics, e.g., those which produce practically no allergic responses, do not potentiate digitalis and have no undesirable effects on the myoneural junction.

Skillful use of the newer agents makes it possible to meet the requirements of the given situation and provide both short and very long-lasting blockade. Thus, for example, lidocaine without epinephrine and chlorprocaine are suitable for short procedures in outpatient surgery. The admixture of lidocaine to the long acting, but slow onset bupivacaine, can hasten the onset of anesthesia. The newer agent etidocaine combines rapid onset with long duration and provides excellent relaxation. In spinal anesthesia, lidocaine can be used for short procedures, while bupivacaine and tetracaine are suitable for longer operations.

The Advantages of Conduction Anesthesia Over General Anesthesia

1. Conduction anesthesia, by isolating one area of the body, places less stress on the entire organism than general anesthesia. It produces only minor changes in metabolism and acid-base balance.

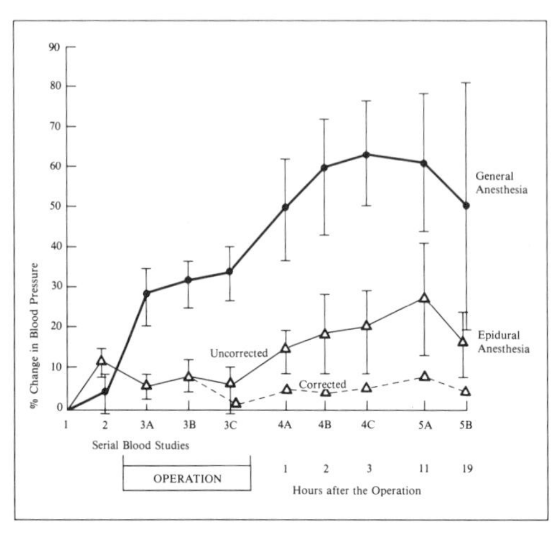

FIG 1.
Changes in blood glucose levels during and after upper abdominal and thoracic surgical procedures under general anesthesia and under epidural anesthesia (44 patients) (after Bromage).

Figure 1, taken from a study by Bromage, shows that when general anesthesia is used for upper abdominal surgery, there is much greater stress on the body. The blood glucose level is increased by 65% (a function of increased epinephrine release) as compared with a 10% increase under epidural anesthesia, which blocks the adrenals. A catheter technique makes it possible to sustain this effect. This is particularly important in diabetic patients, where the postoperative rise in blood sugar can be controlled by the use of an infusion pump and the continued administration of a local anesthetic. In view of the above, geriatric patients, who tolerate physiologic changes poorly, are ideal candidates for conduction anesthesia.

In the past, theoretical concerns were raised that high spinal or epidural anesthesia may trigger bronchospasm or an asthmatic attack. The basis for this theory was the fear that blockade of the bronchodilator sympathetic fibers would permit the unopposed action of the vagus. Lund has demonstrated, on the basis of extensive clinical experience, however, that not only will no bronchospasm ensue even in the bronchospastic patients, but that a status asthmaticus could be made to disappear a few minutes after the establishment of a spinal or epidural block. The drop in blood pressure leads to a decrease in blood volume and to a decreased filling of the pulmonary vessels, with a corresponding increase in alveolar space and an improvement in the vital capacity. From a respiratory point of view, controlled hypotension is a desirable effect, rather than something that has to be corrected rapidly.

Lower blood pressure stimulates the baroreceptors. This causes a reflex bronchodilation and explains the improvements in ventilation. Lower blood pressure also improves the oxygen uptake in the lungs.

Toader reports that postoperative ileus can be avoided by continuous epidural anesthesia. Peristalsis sets in sooner, as can be demonstrated by radiography and auscultation.

The occasionally quoted danger of rupture of the bowel, by unopposed vagal action and elimination of the sympathetic tone, was not supported by the large scale statistical studies of American authors.

Conduction anesthesia permits excellent perfusion of the kidneys and preservation of renal function. In contrast, general anesthesia always reduces renal blood flow and glomerular filtration. Rothauge has shown that creatinine clearance and phenol red excretion are reduced by 40% during general anesthesia, but that both are increased under epidural anesthesia. In the latter situation, the perfusion of the kidney is totally a function of blood pressure. Postoperative anuria can be completely eliminated by proper hydration of the patient. The direct nervous connection between the portal vein area, the mesenteric area, and the kidney, described by Haberich, must also play a significant role in this relationship. Its efferent and afferent limbs are both sympathetic fibers, with a segmental switch in the spinal cord.

In comparing two groups of patients with ileus, we were able to show that the group that had epidural anesthesia had no renal complications.

In patients with eclampsia, lowering the blood pressure by epidural anesthesia removes them from the convulsive range and reestablishes diuresis. With this form of therapy, it is possible to maintain pregnancy until the fetus reaches the age of viability.

2. Regional anesthesia makes it possible for the patient to cooperate during the surgical procedure. Under spinal or epidural anesthesia, the sudden appearance of pain during a transurethral prostatectomy may indicate that the cutting current is getting perilously close to the peritoneum. This is, of course, conditional on the spinal anesthesia level being at or below the tenth thoracic segment from where the sensory innervation of the peritoneum derives. The bladder and the prostate are innervated by S_1 to S_4.

   Blocking the ulnar, median, and radial nerves at the wrist maintains the motor function of the fingers and facilitates the identification of transsected tendons with the cooperation of the patient.
3. Using regional anesthesia for postoperative pain relief and avoiding the use of opiates is clearly sparing the respiration. When the pain originates in the abdomen or the thorax, the vocal chords are reflexly adducted during expiration and the patient exhales against resistance, which produces a moaning type of respiration. The muscles of the torso are tense and pulmonary ventilation is decreased by 50–75%. Expiratory flow rate is decreased by the same amount, and this results in the inability to cough up the mucus. The moaning type of respiration also produces a constant Valsalva effect, which raises

the central venous pressure. The use of centrally acting analgetics (primarily opiates) will cause a slight improvement in vital capacity without changing any of the other defects. These agents, however, cause nausea and vomiting, depress consciousness, and suppress the appetite. Blocking the afferent nerve fibers will eliminate practically all the undesirable reflex effects of pain and will reestablish expiratory flow rates. Figure 2 shows a comparison of pain management with demerol and epidural anesthesia. The latter produces a significant improvement in vital capacity and in inspiratory negative pressure.

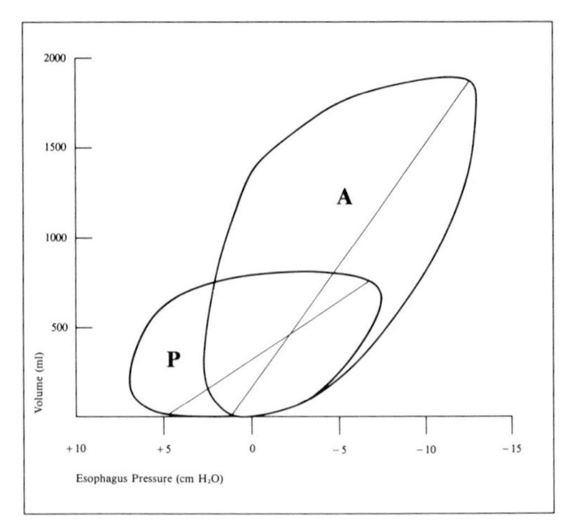

FIG 2.
Changes in respiratory patterns in postoperative upper abdominal pain and analgesia (after Bromage.)
Loop P: Deep inspiration while in pain after analgesia with meperidine
Loop A: Deep inspiration under epidural anesthesia to T_4

4. Patients with coronary insufficiency and hypertension are ideal candidates for regional anesthesia. High-risk patients, e.g., patients who have recently experienced myocardial infarction, tolerate even major abdominal surgery well under intercostal block, perhaps with intubation and the administration of nitrous oxide and oxygen. The stability of the circulation under this technique is truly remarkable. Furthermore, respirations are not depressed postoperatively by pain.
5. Regional anesthesia has made major inroads in obstetrics in recent years. It offers the unique opportunity to adapt anesthesia to any specific aspect of the birthing process. This is accomplished by an epidural block of the T_{11-12} segments which eliminates the uterine pain during dilatation. During the expulsive stage, the pelvic floor can be anesthetized through a second, larger dose of the anesthetic agent administered in the sitting position, through the previously inserted catheter. This will render the perineum both pain-free and relaxed. The same approach also makes an emergency section possible. In addition to the relatively problem-free anesthesia for the mother lasting, if necessary, several hours, this technique also assures that the fetus suffers from less acidosis, not only in comparison with general anesthesia, but even when compared to delivery without any anesthesia. Epidural anesthesia has made cervical dystocia a rarity.

Regional anesthesia has particular advantages over general anesthesia in relaxing the pelvic floor in breech deliveries, premature deliveries, and multiple births. In the latter case, the second twin will have no more anesthesia than the first one. For mothers with cardiac problems it is very important to decrease the effort they have to make in overcoming the resistance of the pelvic floor to the advancing head of the fetus. Here again, this technique has a clear advantage over general anesthesia. The introduction of epidural anesthesia in obstetrics has reduced maternal mortality by 50%.

Aspiration of gastric contents—the most important complication of general anesthesia in obstetrics—is practically eliminated in the mother who is awake and free of pain by virtue of a good block.

The caudal approach to the epidural space is also used frequently in obstetrics, and with similar results.

6. The intraoperative and postoperative blood loss is distinctly less in patients under block anesthesia. In major procedures, the estimates for a reduction in blood loss vary from 30 to 50%.
7. According to recent findings, the frequency of thromboembolic phenomena is markedly reduced after epidural anesthesia when compared to straight general anesthesia. After hip replacement, the incidence of thrombosis is four times as high when general anesthesia is used. The reduction in the frequency of thromboembolism is due to earlier mobilization of the patient after epidural anesthesia, and to the improved arterial and venous perfusion during the procedure. Apparently, the fibrinolytic system is also less depressed postoperatively.
8. Anesthesia and therapy can be combined, e.g., in epidural anesthesia for vascular occlusion in the lower extremity. Here the anesthetic allows diagnostic and therapeutic (surgical) manipulation, while it also contributes to the opening of collateral channels. Another example is given by the skin lesions in compound fractures, where the improved perfusion and increased oxygen delivery under epidural anesthesia contribute to an improved healing process. This technique can also provide pure therapy in perfusion disturbances, pain problems (dystrophies, phantom pain, cancer, pancreatitis, etc.), and in the diagnosis and prognosis of neurosurgical interventions.

Complications of General Anesthesia Which Can Be Avoided by Conduction Blocks

1. In order to avoid complications which may affect the myoneural junctions, spinal or epidural anesthesia can be used in patients with a low serum potassium or in patients with myasthenia gravis, and provides good relaxation without worries concerning postoperative ventilation.
2. The airways are not compromised by positioning (prone position).

3. In patients with multiple injuries, conduction anesthesia offers a simple alternative to the use of general anesthesia for the complicated surgical procedures and for the occasionally impossible endotracheal intubation.
4. The danger of cardiac arrest due to hyperkalemia after succinylcholine can be avoided entirely by regional anesthesia.
5. Patients with airway diseases are ideal candidates for regional anesthesia, since the drying of the airways by anesthetic gases can be avoided. Furthermore, there is no danger of contaminating the anesthetic equipment by patients with tuberculosis.
6. Previous anesthesia with halothane and other halogenated hydrocarbons are contraindications for the use of the same agents within a period of 4 weeks, because of the danger of hepatic toxicity. In this situation, regional anesthesia offers an alternative.
7. During regional anesthesia, there is no danger of trace gas exposure to the anesthesia and operating room personnel.
8. The combination of succinylcholine and inhalation anesthetics may lead to malignant hyperthermia in some cases. This danger can also be avoided when local anesthetics of the ester type (procaine, tetracaine) or even the amide type (lidocaine) are used.
9. In a hot climate, general anesthesia may be affected by CO_2 retention and hyperthermia. Some agents are also flammable and explosive. Because of a reduction in partial pressures, general anesthesia becomes difficult at altitudes over 3000 meters. Conduction anesthesia again offers a welcome alternative.

Contraindications for Conduction Anesthesia

1. Hysteria.
2. Patients with a tendency for exaggerated complaints.
3. Neurologic complications, e.g., headaches, residuals of previous strokes, spinal cord pathology, multiple sclerosis, peripheral nerve disease, and pernicious anemia are all relative contraindications.
4. Skin infection near the site of the injection.
5. Septicemia and the possible seeding of an abscess with the needle.

Bleeding tendencies and hypovolemia due to bleeding or to other causes are also contraindications for spinal and epidural anesthesia.

Prerequisites for regional anesthesia are a satisfied patient and a satisfied surgeon. These can be achieved by a preoperative visit and thorough explanation of the procedure, by a skillful performance of the block with ongoing explanations to the patient, by intraoperative monitoring, and by good postoperative care. It is only at the time of the postoperative visit that one can find out whether the patient is satisfied and whether perhaps some improvement in technique could be made. Usually the patient sleeps during the procedure and remembers little. This can be achieved by good premedication, by additional sedation while the block is being administered, and by intraoperative sedation. In cases where paresthesias must be obtained and the patient's cooperation is necessary, sedation can be provided after the block is established. It is important not to delay the surgeon. This can be accomplished easily by appropriate timing and by the establishment of the block while the previous surgical procedure is still underway. When diaphragmatic respiration interferes with the surgical procedure, additional sedation, general anesthesia, intubation, ventilation, and small amounts of muscle relaxants may be used. In primary general anesthesia, the anesthesiologist is always prepared to use additional agents or techniques. It is obvious that general anesthesia and regional anesthesia interdigitate and overlap in this area.

The Complications of Regional Anesthesia

H. Chr. Niesel

Because of their specific properties, local anesthetics can produce systemic complications, which depending on timing, dose, and application, may be highly dramatic or may have a delayed course. The central nervous system (CNS) and the cardiovascular system (CVS) are of particular importance as specially reactive target organs.

The CNS complications consist of two distinct phases. The *milder* intoxication produces a central stimulation; *more severe* intoxication results in the depression of all CNS cells and a total paralysis. In the CVS, intoxication is always manifested as a dose-dependent depression.

All complications are treatable, provided that appropriate preparations had been made.

Preparation

Prerequisites for the treatment of complications:

1. Venous access
2. Anesthesia machine—tested and functioning
   In minor regional anesthetic procedures, a simple, self-inflating bag and mask with oxygen connection and outlet are sufficient.
   Suction equipment
3. Intubation equipment—complete, just as for general anesthesia
4. ECG (defibrillator), particularly in spinal and epidural anesthesia or if epinephrine-containing local anesthetics are used.
5. Drugs*

   Ready to be injected:
   a. A sedative (e.g., diazepam)
   b. A vasopressor (e.g., ephedrine)
   c. A vagolytic (e.g., atropine)

   Immediately available:
   Succinylcholine, metaproterenol, epinephrine, metaraminol, dopamine, diphenhydramine, methylprednisolone, phentolamine, lidocaine, metoprolol

Severe, Early Complications

1. Accidental IV or IA injection
2. Accidental subarachnoid injection of epidural dose (total spinal)
3. Massive hypotension in high spinal or epidural anesthesia

These complications require immediate therapy. All other complications occurring during local anesthesia can be treated in a stepwise fashion. They are triggered by relative or absolute overdose (excessive dose, enhanced absorption related to the site of administration).

Note: The **IV toxicity,** particularly the cardiac toxicity of the **long-acting local anesthetics,** is greater than that of the intermediate- or short-acting local anesthetics. This increased toxicity is further aggravated by hypoproteinemia, respiratory or metabolic acidosis, and electrolyte imbalance. For this reason particular care must be taken with these drugs. Following accidental IV administration successful cardiac resuscitation may take 30 min or more.

*The effect of vasoconstrictors on uterine blood flow must be considered. In severe hypotension ephedrine is the drug of choice.

Clinical Symptoms

CNS

Stimulation

Cortex
Restlessness, muscle twitches, disorientation, convulsions, hypotension, tachycardia

Medulla
Deep breathing, arrhythmias, vomiting

Depression

Cortex
Speech disturbances, unconsciousness

Medulla
Hypotension, syncope, respiratory arrest, mydriasis

CVS

Heart
Bradycardia, QRS widening, myocardial depression

Circulation
Vasodilatation, hypotension

Reaction to vasoconstrictors:
Apprehension, restlessness, sweating, arrhythmias, tachycardia, fibrillation

Allergic reactions:
Anaphylactic shock, urticaria

Psychologic reactions:
Restlessness, apprehension, tremors (similar to the early signs of toxicity)

Vasovagal reactions:
Bradycardia, hypotension, sweating (these may occur prior to the administration of the local anesthetic)

Management

	SYMPTOMS	THERAPY	CAUSE, PREVENTION, PECULIARITIES
CNS stimulation, moderate intoxication	Restlessness, agitation, tremors, ringing in the ears, muscle twitches, dizziness, metallic taste	O_2 mask Sedation: Diazepam 2.5–5 mg IV Thiopenthal 25–50 mg IV, repeat, PRN	Watch the dose; aspirate before injection, repeat if needle is moved; use local anesthetic with vasopressor if larger dose is used
	Deep, irregular respiration		
	Nausea, vomiting	Droperidol	Stay in verbal contact with the patient, ask for warning signs
	Convulsions	As above; ventilation-intubation correction of acidosis (150 mEq $NaHOC_3$), further correction after blood gas determination	Keep the circulation stable
CNS and CVS depression, severe intoxication	Speech disturbances, disorientation, unconsciousness, sphincter paralysis, apnea	O_2 mask, intubation, ventilation	Avoid IV injection. Vasoconstrictors in the local anesthetic may aggravate the toxic symptoms when given IV
	Bradycardia, hypotension	Atropine and/or metaproterenol Vascoconstrictor Metaraminol drip*	Trendelenburg position elevate legs, start therapy promptly
	Asystole	CPR	

*In obstetrics: Life threatening hypotension should be treated with ephedrine

Management (Continued)

	SYMPTOMS	THERAPY	CAUSE, PREVENTION, PECULIARITIES
Reaction to vasopressor	Apprehension, cold sweat, tachycardia, arrhythmias, ventricular fibrillation	O_2, sedation Beta blocker carefully, IV Phentolamine or nitroprusside IV Defibrillation CPR	Epinephrine 1:200,000. Max. dose 0.25 mg Special precaution: when vasopressor is used in LA in patients with coronary artery insufficiency, no vasopressor or reduced dose ECG monitoring (recognize the prodrome)
Allergic reactions	Erythema, urticaria, hypotension, tachycardia, bronchospasm, abdominal pain, vomiting, anaphylactic shock	Epinephrine (0.05–0.1 mg), antihistamine, corticosteroid	Rare after amide LA, more common after ester LA or due to additives
Vasovagal reactions (also before or during the administration of the regional anesthesia)	Pallor, sweating, nausea Bradycardia, hypotension	Supine position In obstetrics: lateral position Atropine, ephedrine, diazepam	Administer regional anesthesia with the patient in the lateral position ECG monitoring

Regional Anesthesia in Surgery

Brachial Plexus Blocks

Anatomy

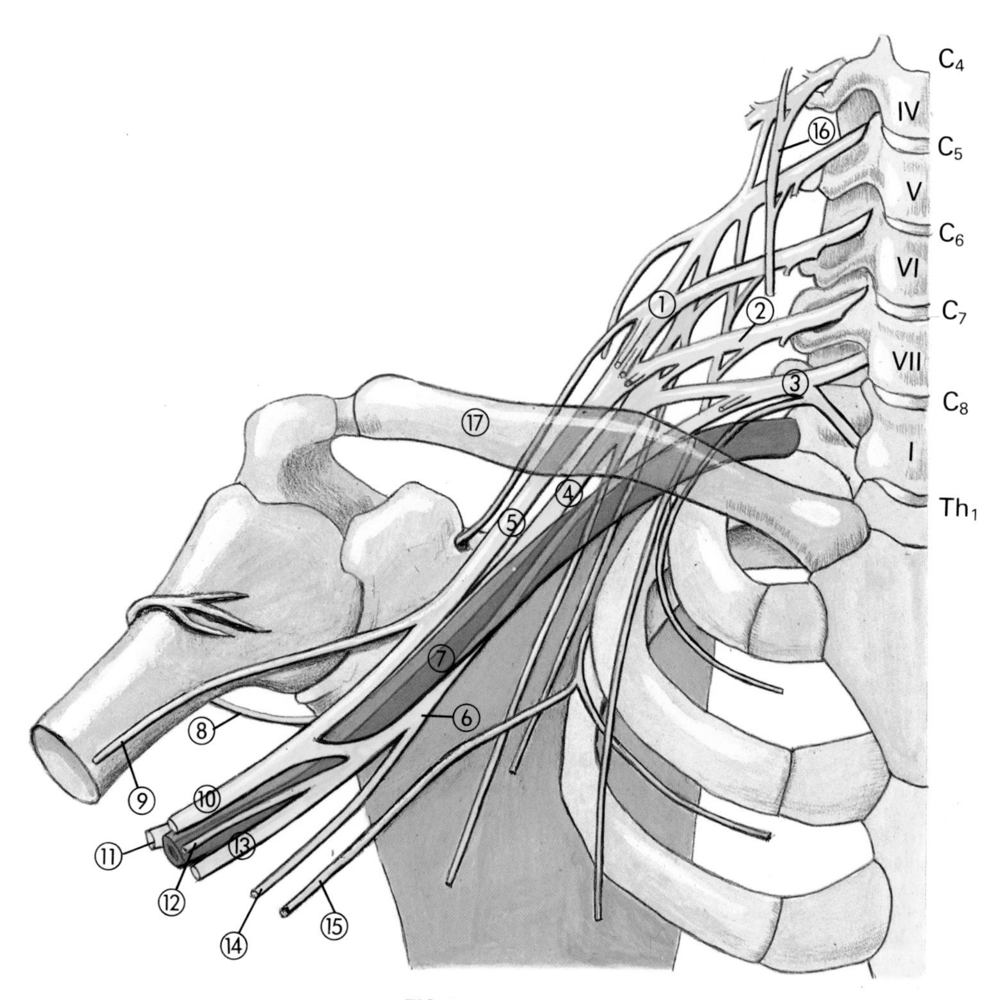

FIG 3.
(after v. Lanz/Wachsmut)

1. Superior trunk
2. Medial trunk
3. Inferior trunk
4. Posterior cord
5. Lateral cord
6. Medial cord
7. Axillary a.
8. Axillary n.
9. Musculocutaneous n.
10. Median n.
11. Radial n.
12. Med. antebrachial cutaneous n.
13. Ulnar n.
14. Med. brachial cutaneous n.
15. Intercostobrachial n.
16. Phrenic n.
17. Clavicle

The brachial plexus is composed of the ventral rami of the spinal nerves C_5–C_8 and T_1, which proceed laterally and caudally and emerge between the origins of the scalene muscles. They unite at the posterior scalene hiatus. The upper roots C_5 and C_6 each form a trunk, while C_7 constitutes a trunk by itself. Each trunk divides into an anterior and posterior branch. The dorsal branches fuse to form the posterior cord, the ventral branches of the upper and middle trunk form the lateral cord, and the inferior trunk forms the medial cord (Fig 3).

The three cords surround the subclavian artery and proceed caudal of the clavicle, cross the first rib and enter the axilla. The three cords and the artery are surrounded by a connective tissue sheath, which originates from the prevertebral fascia and which also invests the scalene muscles.

The three cords of the brachial plexus form the following nerves:

1. The posterior cord: the axillary nerve and the radial nerve
2. The lateral cord: the musculocutaneous nerve, and the lateral part of the median nerve
3. The medial cord: the medial root of the median nerve, the ulnar n., the medial brachiocutaneous n., and the medial antebrachial cutaneous n.

I. The interscalene approach to the brachial plexus block—the Winnie technique

E. Lanz, D. Theiss

1. Definition

Blockade of the cervico-brachial plexus by injection into the fascia-enveloped, perineural, connective tissue space, between the anterior and middle scalene muscles at the level of C_6 (4).

2. Topographic Anatomy

The ventral rami of the spinal nerves which form the cervico-brachial plexus enter the "*interscalene space*" between the anterior and posterior tubercles of the lateral processes. The branches coming from C_5 to T_1 form the primary cords of the brachial plexus at this point, converge in a lateral-caudal direction, and emerge jointly from the posterior scalene hiatus where they assume an anterolateral position in relation to the subclavian artery (Fig 4). The interscalene space is formed ventrally and dorsally by the fascia of the anterior and medial scalene muscles, laterally by a continuation of the prevertebral cervical fascia, and medially by the transverse processes.

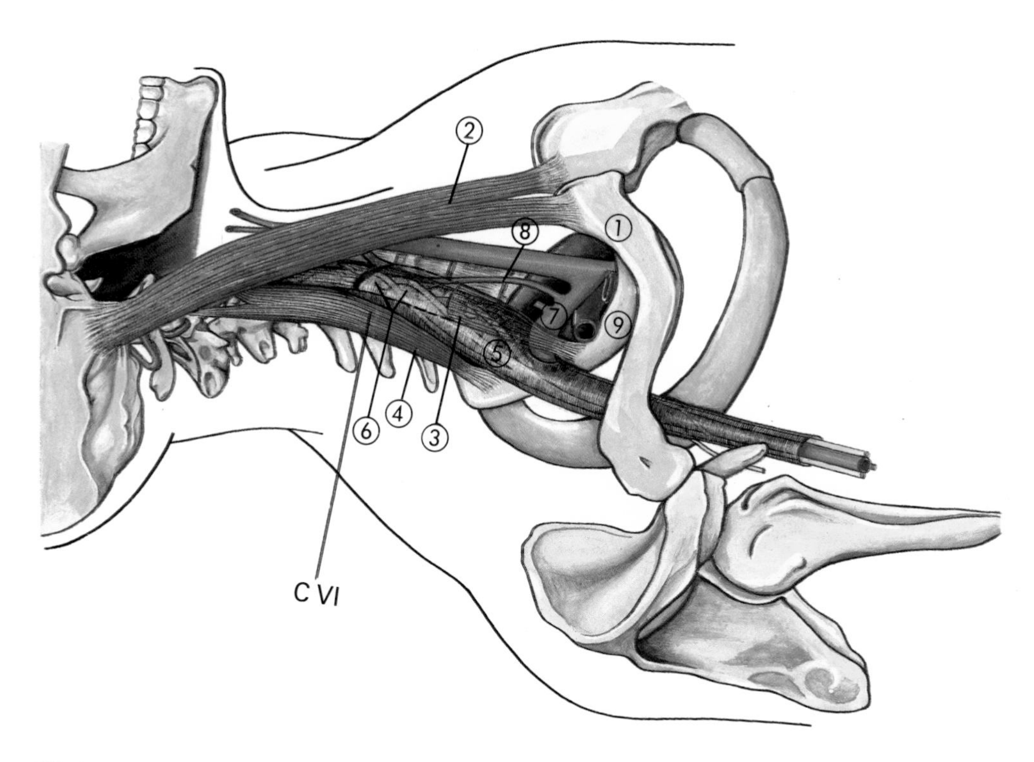

FIG 4.
1. Clavicle
2. Sternocleidomastoid m.
3. Scalenus anterior m.
4. Scalenus medius m.
5. Scalene hiatus, brachial plexus
6. Perineural connective tissue space
7. Subclavian a.
8. Vertebral a.
9. 1st rib

3. Technique

The local anesthetic is injected into the continuous perineural connective tissue space from a single needle position (Fig 4). Winnie compares this space to the epidural space: the potential space for the spread of the local anesthetic is given; the different parts of the plexus are "found" by the local anesthetic solution and not by the needle; the extent of the block is determined by the volume of the local anesthetic solution.

3.1. Anesthesiologic Assessment

Careful anesthesiologic assessment including the identification of any contraindication.

3.2. Preparation

Intravenous cannula, intubation set-up, ventilation equipment with O_2 connection, atropine, sedative, succinylcholine, vasopressor, catecholamine.

3.3. Equipment

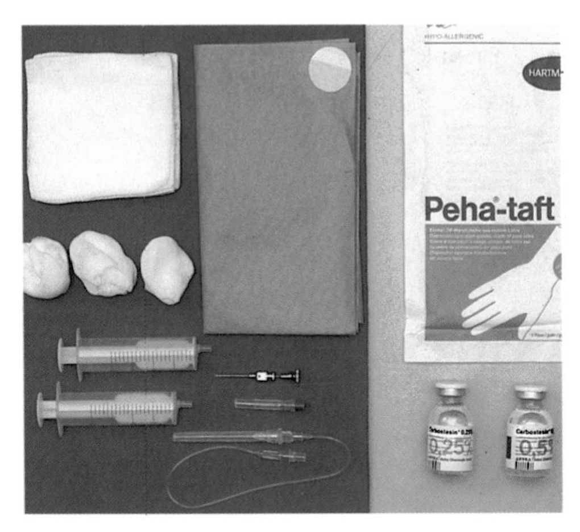

FIG 5.

Antiseptic solution
Sponges
Drape with a hole
Sterile gloves
24 g needle for the injection
Two 20 ml syringes

Optional extras:
"Winnie immobile needle": needle with extension tubing; NaCl 0.9% in the refrigerator
Equipment for electrical nerve stimulation

3.4. Positioning

The head is positioned horizontally and turned to the contralateral side. The arms require no particular positioning. The anesthesiologist is standing at the head.

3.5. Landmarks

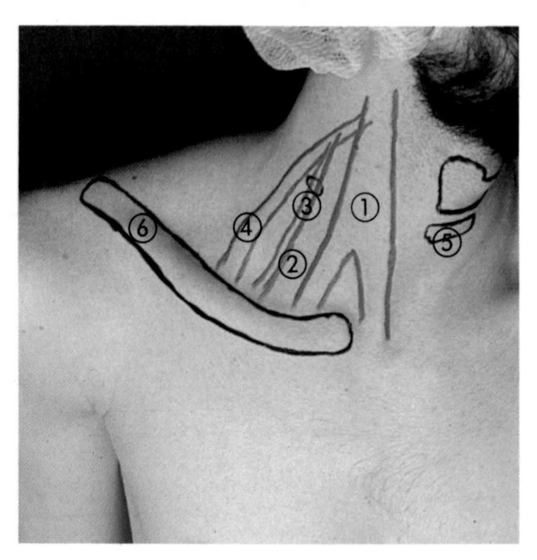

FIG 6.
1. Sternocleidomastoid m.
2. Scalenus anterior m.
3. Interscalene groove
4. External jugular v.
5. Cricoid cartilage
6. Clavicle

The sternocleidomastoid muscle, the interscalene groove between the anterior and medial scalene muscles, the cricoid cartilage, the external jugular vein.

3.6. The Technical Procedure

Cleansing the skin with an appropriate antiseptic solution. Turning the head makes the sternocleidomastoid muscle clearly visible. Just dorsal to this muscle, the fingertips rest on the anterior scalene muscle. Pulling laterally with the fingers for a distance of 0.5–1.5 cm, the interscalene groove between the anterior and medial scalene muscles becomes palpable. The groove becomes more obvious on deep inspiraton due to the increased tension of the scalene muscles. The following findings prove that the depression palpated is indeed the interscalene groove: the transverse processes provide the palpating finger with a solid resistance; increased pressure by the fingertips frequently produces paresthesias in the shoulder and arm; at the caudal end of the interscalene groove the subclavian artery should be palpable.

Injection site

It is at the level of the cricoid (Fig 7). The external jugular vein frequently crosses the interscalene groove at this point. One fingertip remains craniad and one fingertip remains caudad of the injection site in the interscalene groove. At this point a skin wheal is raised.

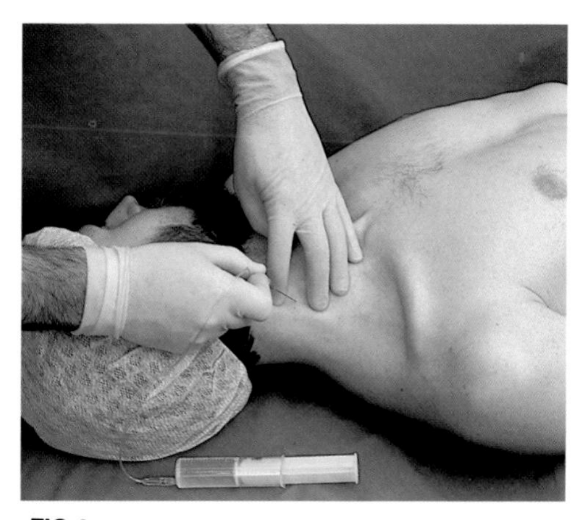

FIG 8.

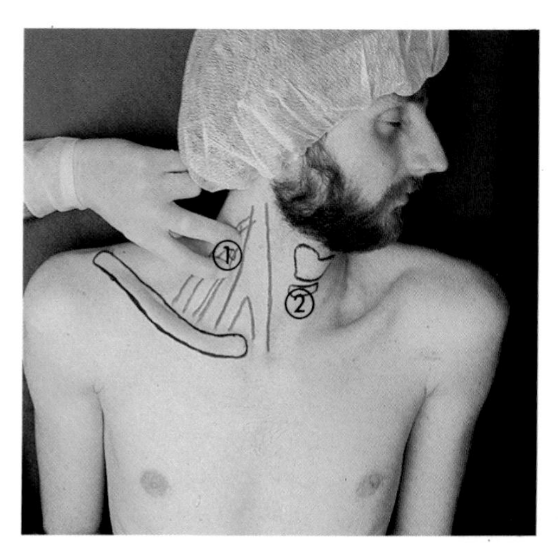

FIG 7.
1. Entry point
2. Cricoid cartilage

Direction of the needle

The needle aims at the transverse process of C_6, i.e., medially, caudally (approximately 30° to the sagittal plain), and slightly dorsally (Fig 8). The needle is advanced until paresthesia is elicited, usually in the shoulder or the arm. Touching the transverse process with the tip of the needle helps in the orientation; the anterior and posterior tubercle can frequently be identified.

Checking the correct placement of the needle

Aspirate in two planes; neither blood nor CSF should be aspirated.
If no paresthesias were obtained, 5 ml chilled 0.9% NaCl can be injected rapidly. If paresthesias are triggered in the shoulder area, a correct placement of the needle can be assumed.

Injection

The fingertips remain in the interscalene groove during the injection. The patient is advised that the injection of the first ml of solution may be painful and is asked not to move. Verbal contact with the patient will give an early warning about possible complications (CNS intoxication, total spinal anesthesia). By pressure with the finger above the injection site, the spread of the local anesthetic can be directed caudad and by pressure below the injection site it can be directed craniad.
When the "immobile needle" is used, an assistant can inject the local anesthetic (Fig 8).

Spread

The caudal portion of the cervical plexus and the cranial portion of the brachial plexus (2). The median and ulnar nerves which divide from the brachial plexus more caudally are affected more rarely. The same is true for the sensory cutaneous branches on the inner aspect of the arm.

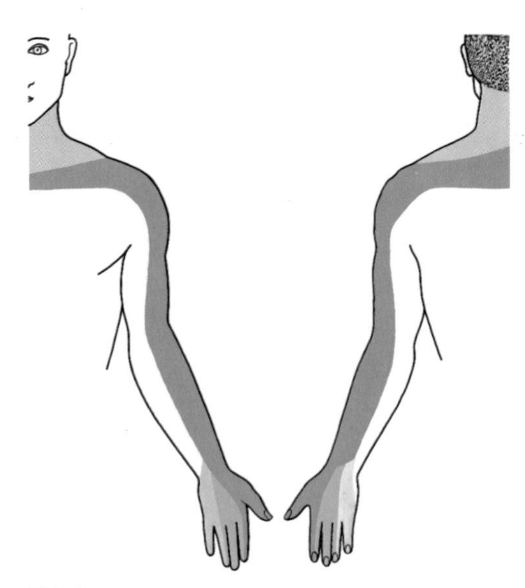

FIG. 9.
Area of analgesia.

Failure of the block becomes evident in about 5 min. If at this time there is no clear evidence of a sensory and motor block, no surgical anesthesia can be expected. No time should be wasted and some other method of anesthesia should be used.

Success rate

90–95% (3)

3.7. Dosage

For surgical procedures

20–40 ml local anesthetic solution, e.g., lidocaine or mepivacaine 1%; bupivacaine 0.375%, etidocaine 1%.

For pain therapy

20–40 ml of the local anesthetic solution, e.g., bupivacaine 0.125–0.25%; lidocaine, mepivacaine 0.5–1.0%.

4. Special Side Effects and Complications

Side effects

Horner's syndrome
Block of the phrenic nerve (unilateral diaphragmatic paralysis)
Recurrent laryngeal nerve block (hoarseness)
Compression of the lumen of the carotid artery

Complications

Intravascular injection into a vessel in the neck, particularly the vertebral artery and diffusion of the local anesthetic solution through the wall of the vertebral artery (CNS intoxication)
Subarachnoid injection (total spinal anesthesia)
Epidural injection (high epidural anesthesia)
(The above complications can be avoided if the tip of the needle is directed caudad.)

5. Indications

For surgical procedures

Surgical procedures on the clavicle, shoulder, and arm with the exception of the medial aspect of the arm (1).

Reduction of a subluxated shoulder joint. It is the method of choice if other approaches to the brachial plexus are made difficult or undesirable by anatomic or pathologic problems, e.g., obesity or severe emphysema.

In pain therapy

Pain conditions in the shoulder-arm area, e.g., reflex dystrophy, shoulder joint arthrosis, pain due to neoplasm, vessel pathology or injury, etc.

6. Special Contraindications

Absolute

Contralateral recurrent laryngeal nerve or phrenic nerve palsy.

Relative

Preexisting nerve injury or pathology in the distribution of the brachial plexus.

References

1. Balas, GI: Regional anesthesia for surgery on the shoulder. *Anesth. Analg.* 1971; 50:1036–1042.
2. Lanz E, Theiss D, Jankovic D: The extent of blockade following various techniques of brachial plexus block. *Anesth. Analg*. 1983; 62:55–58.
3. Ward ME: The interscalene approach to the brachial plexus. *Anesthesia* 1974; 29:147-157.
4. Winnie, AP: Interscalene brachial plexus block. *Anesth. Analg*. 1970; 49:455-466.

II. Brachial plexus block—the supraclavicular approach

H.-J. Hartung

1. Definition

Blockade of the brachial plexus in the lateral neck region in the supraclavicular fossa.

2. Topographic Anatomy

After the primary trunks of the brachial plexus emerge from the scalene hiatus as a bundle, they pass over the first rib and enter the axilla dorsally to the clavicle. When crossing the first rib, the three cords of the plexus are dorsolateral to the subclavian artery and are surrounded, together with the artery, by a common connective tissue sheet. The main distribution of the plexus is stepwise in a craniocaudal direction.

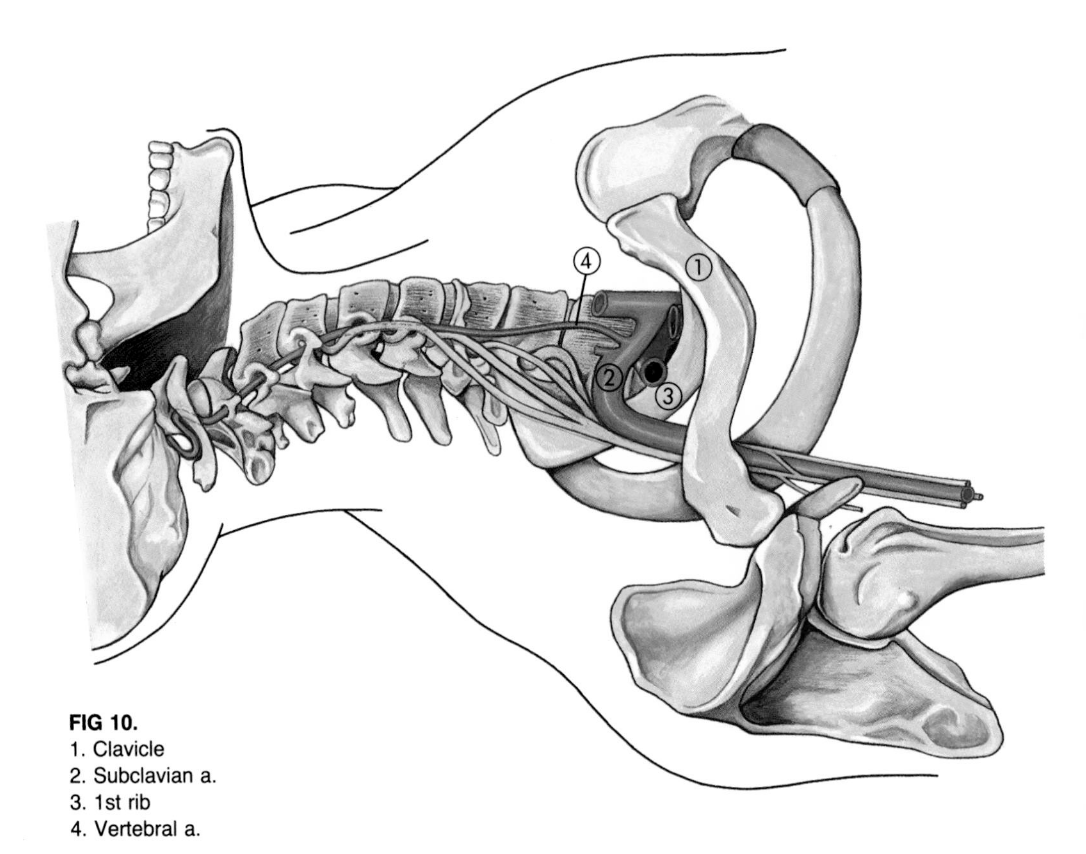

FIG 10.
1. Clavicle
2. Subclavian a.
3. 1st rib
4. Vertebral a.

3. Technique

3.1. Anesthesiologic Assessment

Careful anesthesiologic assessment, including the identification of any contraindication.

3.2. Preparation

IV indwelling catheter, intubation equipment, ventilation equipment with oxygen connection. Atropine, sedative, succinylcholine, vasopressor, catecholamine.

3.3. Equipment

Antiseptic solution
Sponges
Drape with hole
Sterile gloves
10 ml syringes
24 g needles

3.4. Positioning

The patient is supine with the head turned to the contralateral side (Fig 11). The arm is pulled slightly caudad in parallel to the long axis of the body (assistant). A small roll may be placed between the shoulder blades. This position places the brachial plexus under tension, so that the distance between the skin and the plexus is minimized.

3.5. Landmarks

The topographic guides are the clavicle, the external jugular vein, and the subclavian artery, which can be palpated immediately lateral to the vein, just above the clavicle (Fig 11).

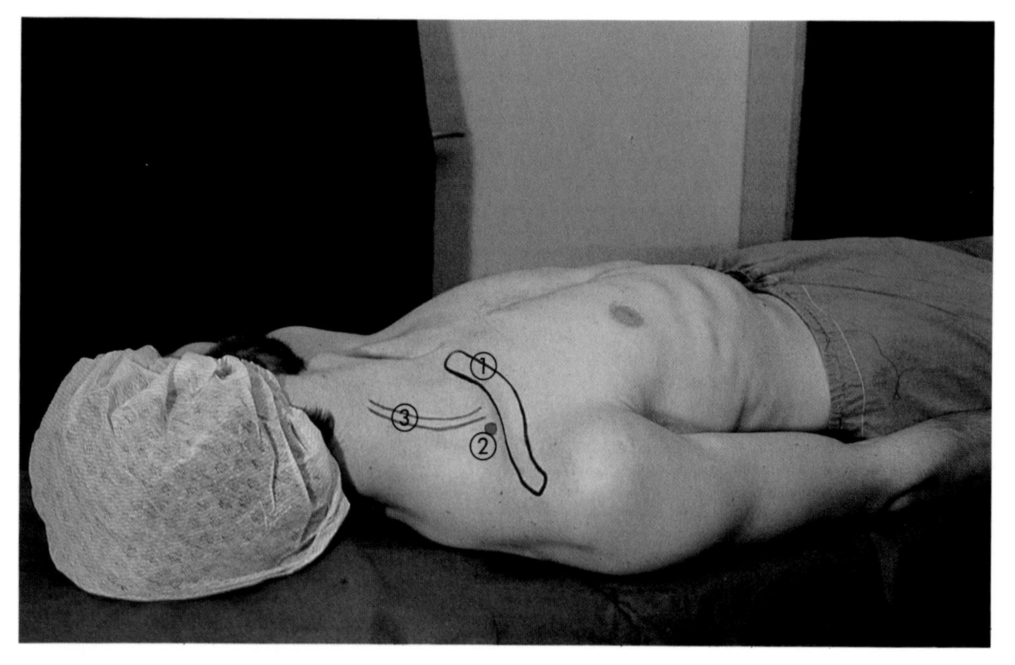

FIG 11.
1. Clavicle
2. Pulsations of the subclavian a.
3. External jugular v.

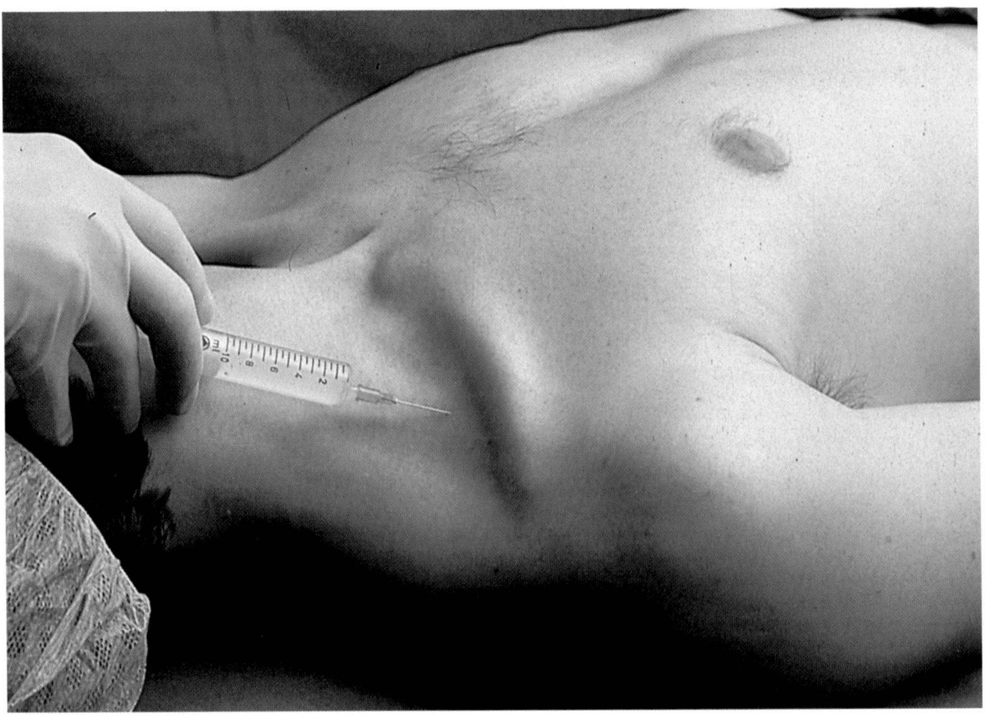

FIG 12.
Direction of the needle in the perivascular technique: parallel to the direction of the scalene muscles.

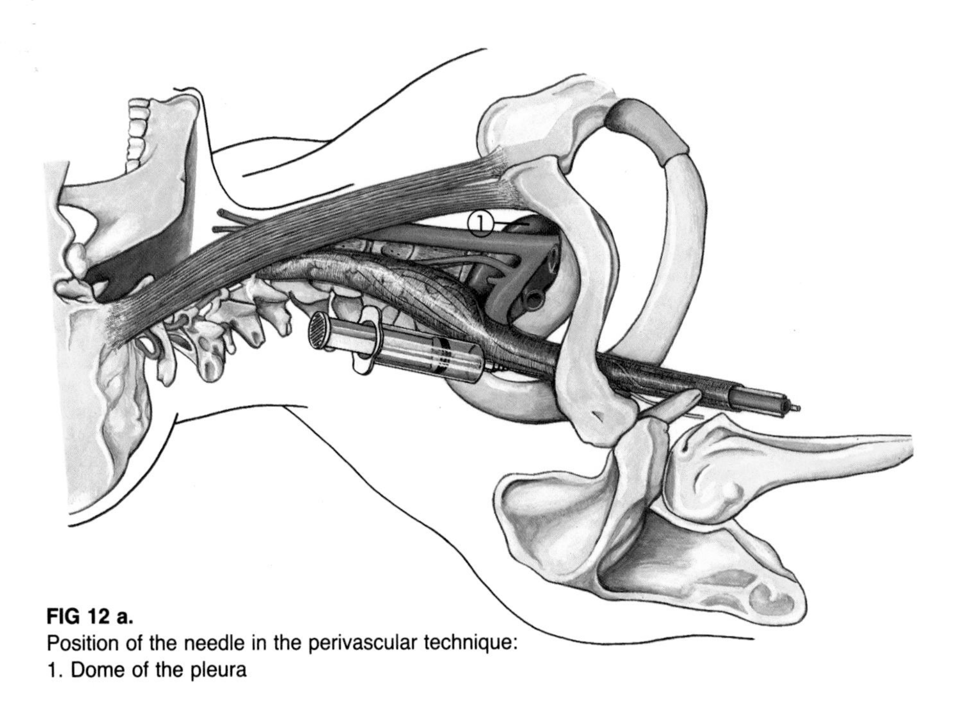

FIG 12 a.
Position of the needle in the perivascular technique:
1. Dome of the pleura

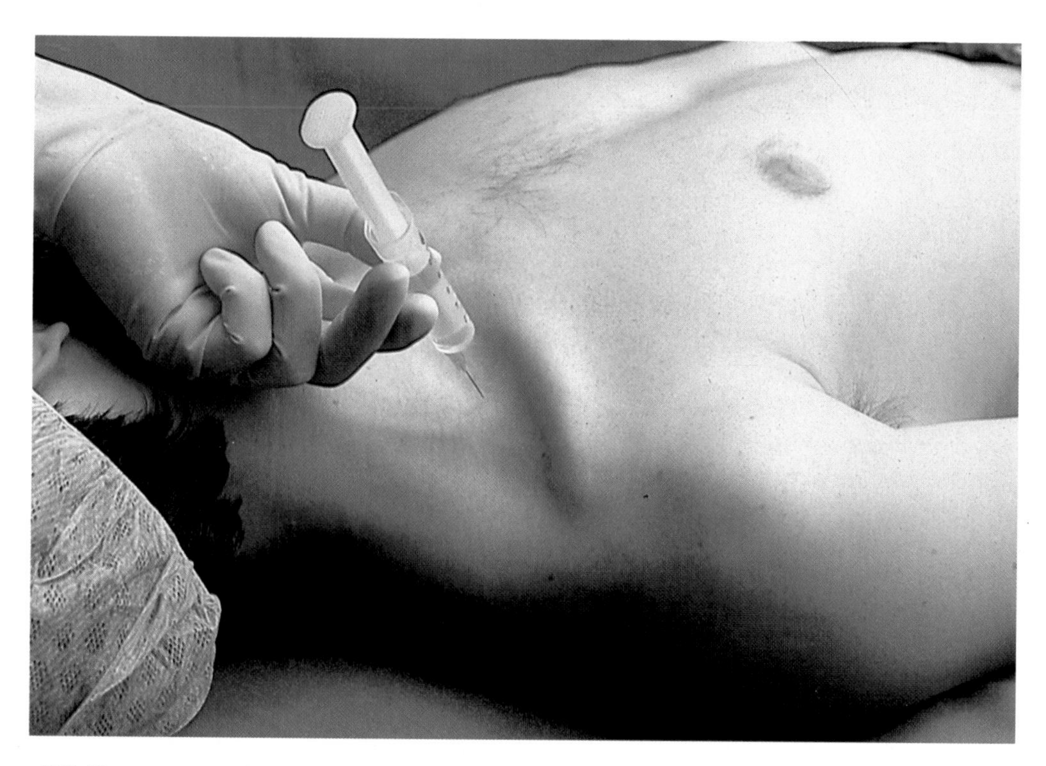

FIG 13.
Direction of the needle in the Kulenkampff technique: vertical to the skin in the direction of the first rib.

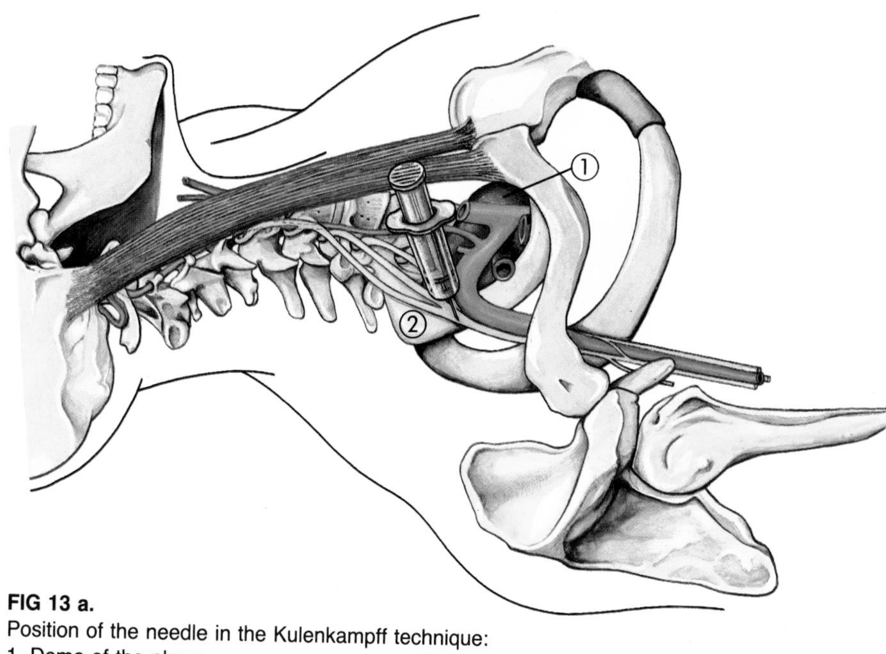

FIG 13 a.
Position of the needle in the Kulenkampff technique:
1. Dome of the pleura
2. 1st rib

3.6. Technical procedure

Cleansing the skin with suitable antiseptic solution.

Perivascular technique (after Winnie)

The pulsation of the subclavian artery is located and a skin wheal is raised immediately dorsolateral to it.

The needle is slowly advanced in a caudal direction and somewhat laterally, i.e., parallel to the direction of the scalene muscles (Fig 12).

After paresthesias have been elicited and after negative aspiration in two planes, one part of the local anesthetic solution is injected.

The distribution of the paresthesias can indicate which part of the plexus has been touched and if the position of the needle should be changed in order to reach other parts of the plexus.

The Kulenkampff technique

The lateral edge of the clavicular insertion of the stenocleidomastoid muscle and the clavicle provides the guideposts. The site of injection is 1 cm craniad above the clavicle and 1.5 cm laterally from the edge of the muscle. The needle is advanced vertically to the skin and in the direction of the first rib (Fig 13). After bony resistance is felt, the needle is carefully "walked along" the first rib until paresthesias are triggered. Before every change of direction, the needle must be withdrawn into the subcutaneous area.

After negative aspiration, the solution is injected slowly. Before the start of the operation, the anesthesia effect must be tested by cold or pain stimulus.

The latency period is 5–30 minutes.

The success rate, i.e., the ability to perform surgery free of pain just with the blockade, is 90–95%.

In case of a partial success the individual nerves can be blocked peripherally (see "Block of the peripheral nerves in the region of the elbow," p. 47, and "Block of the peripheral nerves in the area of the wrist," p. 55).

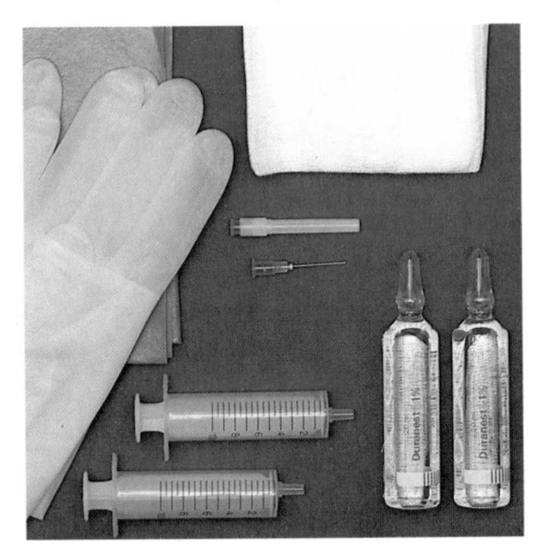

FIG 14.

3.7. Dosage

Depending on body weight, 10 ml (children)–40 ml (adults) local anesthetic solution, e.g., mepivacaine 0.5–1.0%; bupivacaine 0.5%, etidocaine 1.0%.

4. Special Side Effects and Complications

Side effects

Horner's syndrome
Phrenic paralysis
Recurrent laryngeal nerve paralysis

Complications

Pneumothorax
Plexus injury
Hematoma formation
High spinal or epidural anesthesia

5. Indications

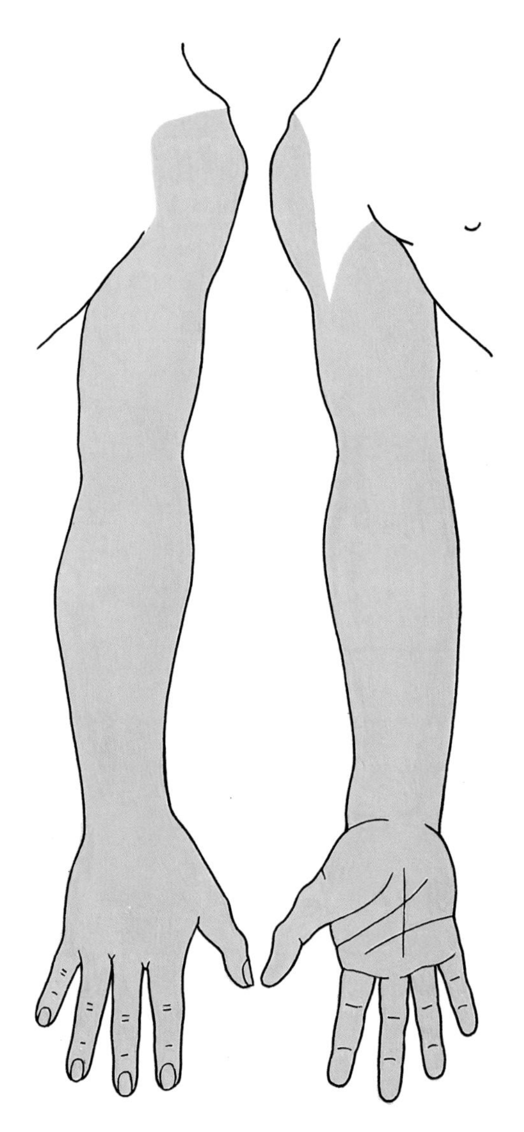

FIG 15.
Area of analgesia.

Surgical procedures on the arm, forearm and hand.

6. Special Contraindications

Hemorrhagic diatheses
Contralateral phrenic or recurrent nerve paralysis
Contralateral pneumothorax (in outpatients)

References

1. Kulenkampff D: Die Anästhesierung des Plexus brachialis. *Beitr Klin Chir* 1912; 79:550.
2. Winnie AP, Collins VJ: The subclavian perivascular technique of brachial plexus anaesthesia. *Anesthesiology* 1964; 25:353.

III. Brachial plexus block—the axillary approach

M. Zenz

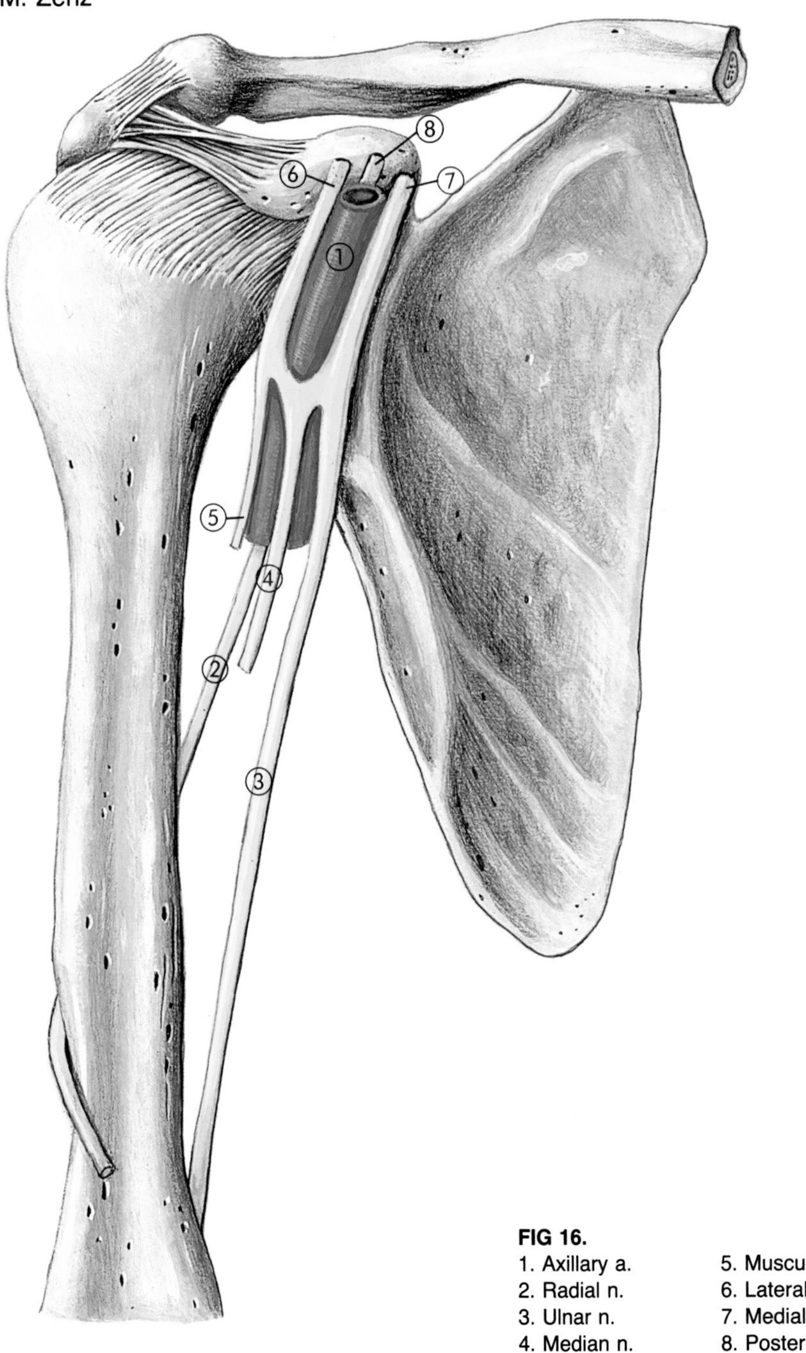

FIG 16.
1. Axillary a.
2. Radial n.
3. Ulnar n.
4. Median n.
5. Musculocutaneous n.
6. Lateral fascia
7. Medial fascia
8. Posterior fascia

1. Definition

Unilateral block of the brachial plexus in the axillary region.

2. Topographic Anatomy

After its passage under the clavicle, the brachial plexus follows the course of the subclavian artery and vein. Beneath the pectoralis major muscle the axillary nerve and the thoracodorsal nerve leave the plexus. At the level of the axilla, the cords of the brachial plexus divide into their individual nerves. They are located caudad of the coracobrachialis muscle and surround the axillary artery.

The origin of the musculocutaneous nerve from the lateral cord is variable and may lie far proximally. Usually this nerve is craniad from the artery. The radial nerve also leaves the plexus in its proximal portion. In 90° abduction of the arm, the radial nerve lies behind and craniad to the axillary artery. The ulnar nerve lies dorsally and caudad to the artery. The median nerve is directly on the artery (Fig 16).

The neurovascular bundle is surrounded by a firm fascial sheath, just as in the neck. The intercostobrachialis nerve and the median brachiocutaneous nerve are external to the sheath and lie between the skin and the fascia (Fig 17).

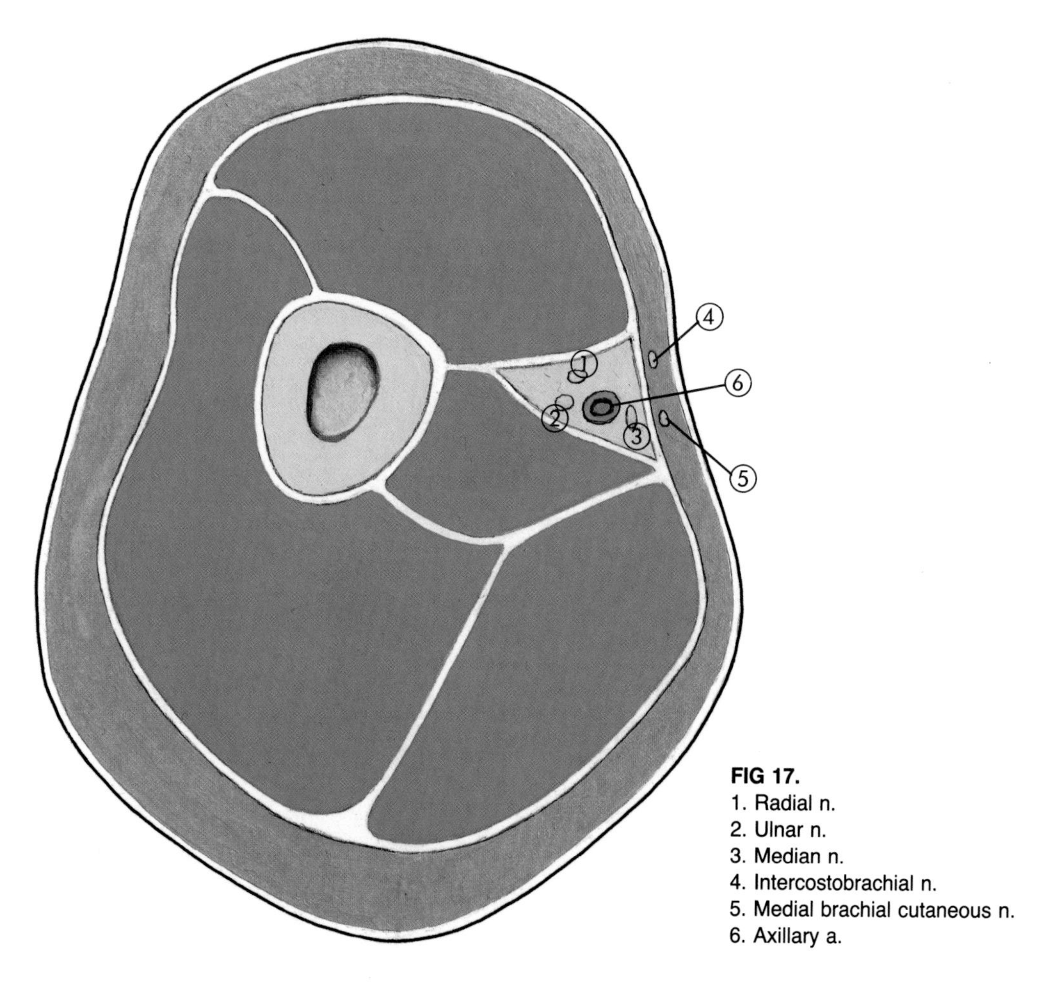

FIG 17.
1. Radial n.
2. Ulnar n.
3. Median n.
4. Intercostobrachial n.
5. Medial brachial cutaneous n.
6. Axillary a.

3. Technique

3.1 Anesthesiologic Assessment

Careful anesthesiologic assessment, including the identification of any contraindication.

3.2. Preparation

Indwelling IV catheter, intubation equipment, ventilation equipment with O_2 connection, atropine, sedative, succinylcholine, vasopressor, catecholamine.

The axilla should be carefully shaved.

3.3 Equipment

Sterile gloves
A needle to draw up solution
24 g needle for the skin wheal
10 ml syringe
18 g needle for skin puncture
Sponges
Drape with hole
Antiseptic solution

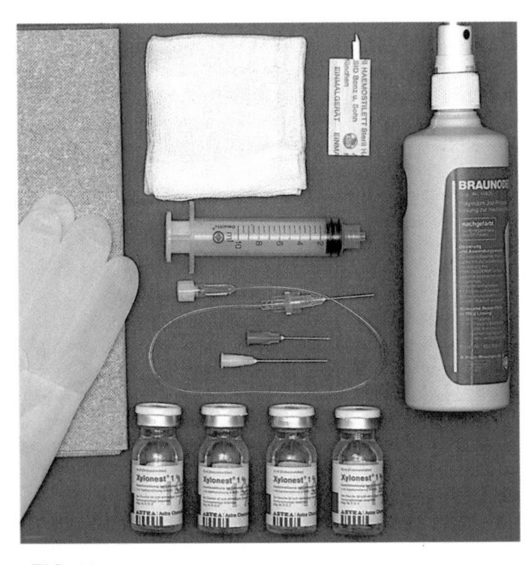

FIG 18.

24 g, short bevel needle
Short extension tubing

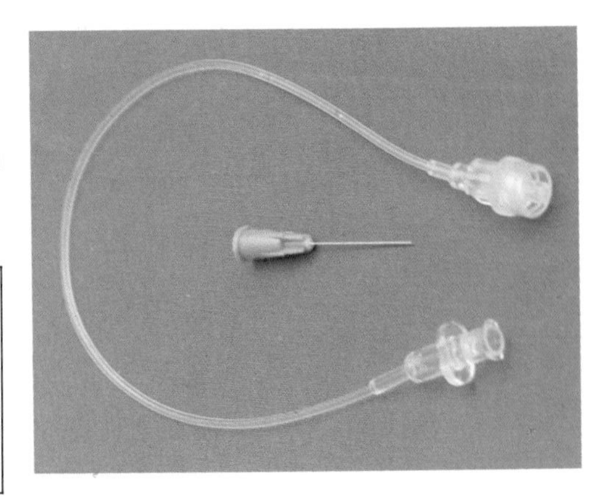

FIG 19.
Plexufix®, Fa. B. Braun Melsungen AG.

3.4. Positioning

The patient is supine. To gain access to the axilla the arm is abducted 100° on the affected side. The forearm is flexed 90°. This position places the plexus under tension and fixes it more securely in the sulcus under the coracobrachialis muscle.
A tourniquet is not required.

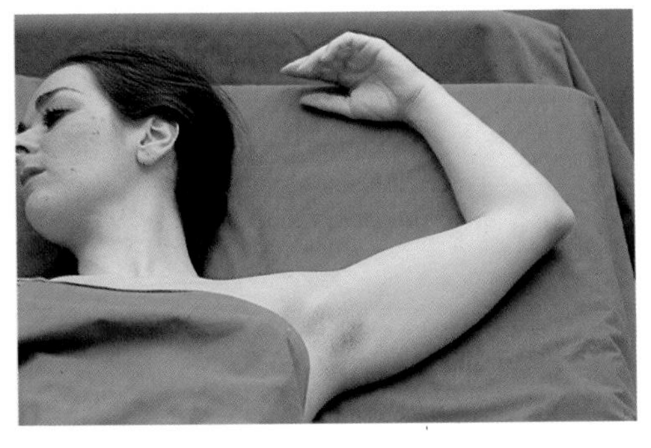

FIG 20.

3.5. Landmarks

The topographic guideposts consist of the pectoralis major muscle as the ventral border of the axilla, and the coracobrachialis muscle as the muscle accompanying the axillary artery. The pulsation of the axillary artery in the axillary groove between the pectoralis major and latissimus dorsi muscles is the final guide point.

3.6. Technical procedure

Careful skin antisepsis in the entire axilla and the inner aspects of the proximal portion of the arm. With the arm in abduction, the pulsations of the axillary artery are palpated at the level of anterior axillary wall. The nerves can be palpated as firm cords alongside the vessel. When the finger is pressed firmly into the tissues and is moved up and down along the artery, paresthesias can frequently be elicited.

Directly over the arterial pulsation a skin wheal is raised. The skin is perforated with an 18 g needle. A short bevel needle is introduced through this opening into the subcutaneous tissues. By palpating the artery the needle can be advanced into the vicinity of the neural bundle (Fig 21). When the short bevel needle reaches the fascial sheath, a distinct springy resistance can be felt. The needle should be pushed through the fascial covering craniad of the arterial pulsations. Thus, the radial nerve will be approximated since this nerve lies behind and craniad to the artery.

When passing through the dense fascial layer, a distinct "pop" can be felt. The needle is advanced a few mm. Without trying to elicit paresthesias 10–15 ml of local anesthetic solution are injected. Before injection, aspiration should be performed in two planes. When injecting, attention must be paid to the pressure required. The fascial sheath always exerts some resistance to the injection. If the injection requires very little pressure, it is likely that the tip of the needle went past the neurovascular bundle in a dorsal direction.

After repeated palpation the second injection is administered directly caudad to the artery. The needle is advanced with a slow vibrating motion until it makes contact with the fascial sheath. Perforation of the sheath will again result in a distinct

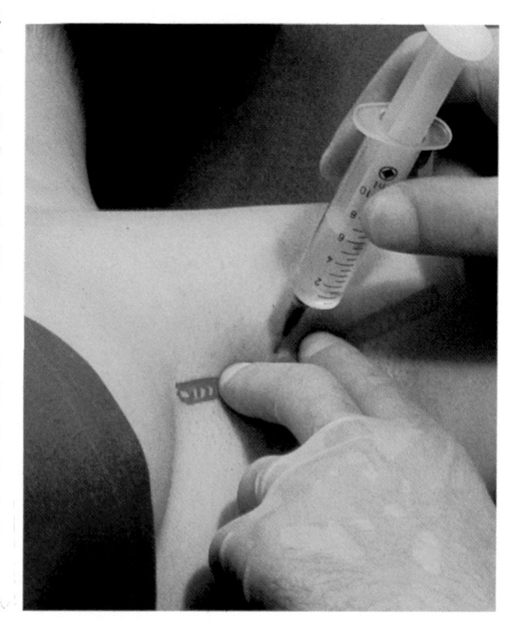

FIG 21.

"pop." An injection of 10–15 ml local anesthetic solution is administered caudally and dorsally to the artery in the region where the ulnar nerve lies. Injection is, of course, again preceded by aspiration in two planes. Paresthesias should not be elicited prior to injection.

To block the median nerve, the tip of the needle must remain inside the fascial sheath, but must be advanced proximally, tangential to the artery. Without trying to elicit paresthesias, 10 ml of the local anesthetic solution are injected. If the resistance is very slight, this could be an indication that the needle has slipped out of the fascial sheath. In this case the needle should be advanced gently, and if the resistance to injection is increased, additional solution should be injected after careful aspiration.

To block the intercostobrachialis and medial brachial cutaneous nerves which innervate the inner aspects of the arm (tourniquet!), a circular field block must be performed on the medial surface of the arm.

The musculocutaneous nerve may have such a high origin from the plexus that the block, as described, may not provide anesthesia for it. In this case the sheath should be punctured one more time, cranial to the artery and tangential to it. A far proximally deposited bolus of 5 ml usually provides complete analgesia in the area of the musculocutaneous nerve.

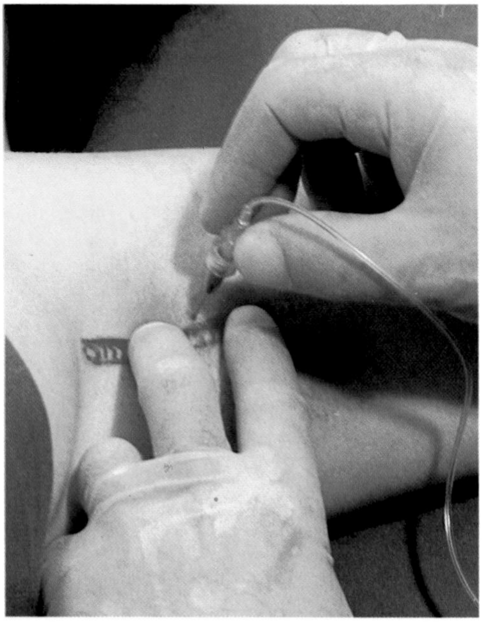

The above technique can also be performed with an extension tube being attached to the needle. The injection can be administered by an assistant, so that both hands remain available for palpation and for positioning the needle (Fig 22). Even without an assistant the "immobile needle" permits a solid fixation of the needle during the change of syringes, during aspiration, and during injection.

It is also possible to inject a bolus of 30–40 ml of local anesthetic solution in a single site within the fascial sheath. In this technique it is important to compress the vascular space immediately distal to the injection site, to prevent the local anesthetic solution from dissipating distally (Fig 23). This technique does not always capture all components of the plexus so that some of the nerves may not be blocked with any certainty.

Advantages of the method using a short bevel needle and an extension tube:

The puncture of the neurovascular sheath can be clearly recognized by the characteristic "pop." The dull tip of the needle makes neural injury or vascular puncture much less likely.

The attached extension tube allows a solid fixation of the needle even during manipulations of the syringe.

FIG 22.

NOTE:

Wide abduction of the arm may prevent proximal spread of the local anesthetic solution by the pressure brought on the plexus by the head of the humerus.

Pulsation of the needle is no guarantee of a correct position for injecting. This sign gives no indication of the position of the tip of the needle, since in spite of visible

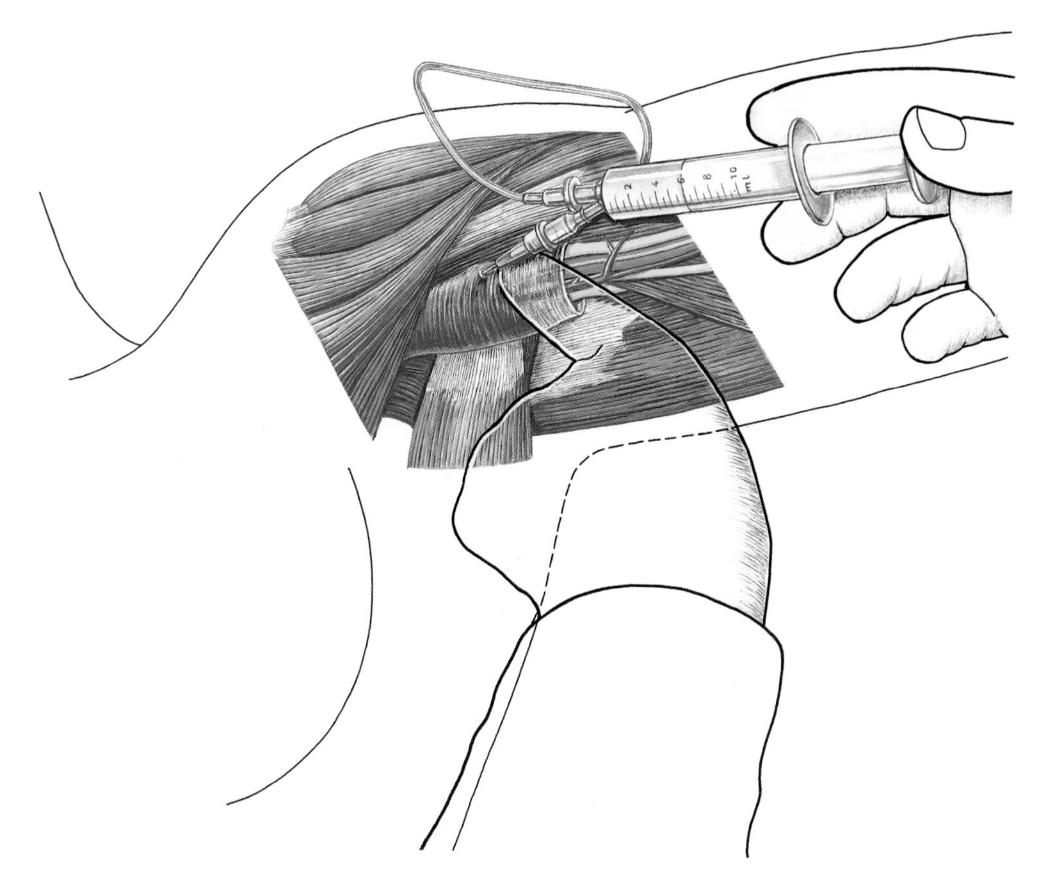

FIG 23.

pulsations the tip of the needle may have passed out of the sheath dorsally.
The latency period is about 10 min. After this time anesthesia should be checked with a cold stimulus. No needle sticks should be used for testing in the projected surgical field.
The success rate is approximately 95%.

3.7. Dosage

30–40 ml local anesthetic solution.
In children: 10–20 ml

4. Special Complications

Hematoma, due to puncture of the artery (pressure injury to the nerves)—prevention: pressure for 5 min

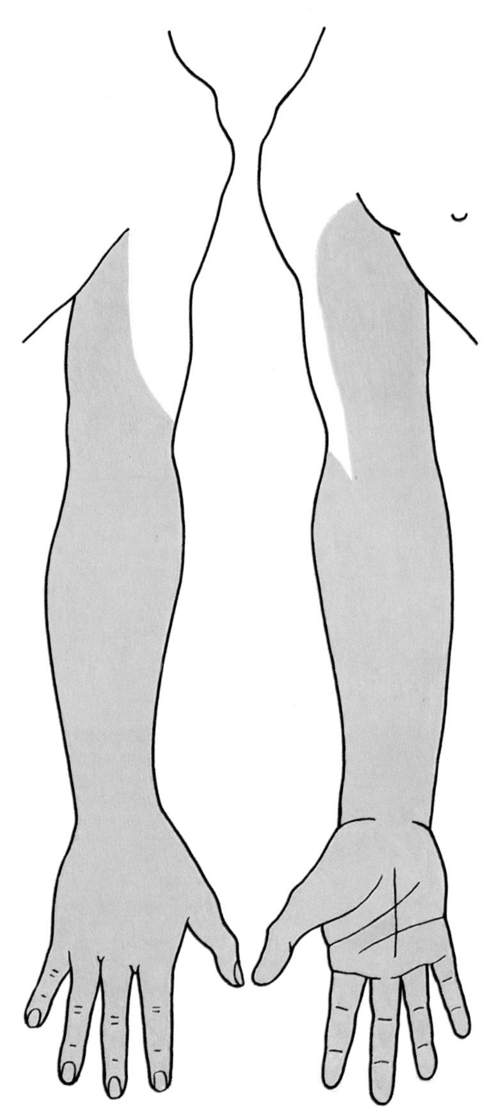

FIG 24.
Area of analgesia.

5. Indications

For surgical procedures

Operations on the forearm and hand.

For pain therapy

An alternative to stellate ganglion block in painful conditions in the area of the arm and hand, e.g., sympathetic reflex dystrophy, Sudeck's disease, arterial occlusive disease.

6. Special Contraindications

Absolute

Lymphangitis

Relative

Preoperative nerve injury

References

1. Hirschel G: *Lehrbuch der Lokalanästhesie.* München, Bergmann, 1923.
2. De Jong RH: Axillary block of the brachial plexus. *Anesthesiology* 1961; 22:215–225.
3. Winnie AP, Radonjic R, Akkineni SR, Durrani Z: Factors influencing distribution of local anesthetic injected into the brachial plexus sheath. *Anesth Analg* 1979; 58:225–234.
4. Zenz M, Glocker R: Eine neue "immobile Nadel" zur Plexusanästhesie. *Regional-Anästhesie* 1981; 4:29.

IV. Continuous brachial plexus block—axillary approach

K. Strasser

1. Definition

Non-time-limited axillary block of the brachial plexus through an indwelling plastic catheter placed into the neurovascular space.

2. Topographic Anatomy

See "Brachial plexus block—axillary approach," p. 32.

3. Technique

3.1. Anesthesiologic Assessment

> Careful anesthesiologic assessment including the identification of any contraindication.

3.2. Preparation

> Indwelling IV catheter, intubation equipment, ventilation equipment with O_2 connection, atropine, sedative, succinylcholine, vasopressor, catecholamine.

The axilla is carefully shaved.

3.3 Equipment

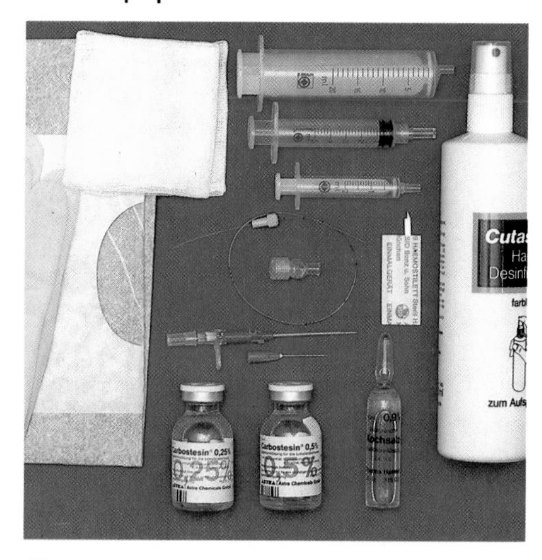

FIG 25.

18 g plastic needle with 45° bevel and Teflon stylet
30 cm plastic catheter of 0.85 mm diameter
Special catheter connector with Luer-lock hub to accept an injection filter (Plexufix® catheter set, Fa. B. Braun Melsungen AG)
24 g needle for local infiltration
2 ml syringe
5 ml syringe with loose plunger
20 ml syringe
Vaccination needle or 18 g needle for skin puncture
Clear plastic drape with hole
Sterile dressing
Sterile gloves
Refrigerated physiologic saline solution

3.4. Positioning

Comfortable supine position. The arm abducted somewhat over 90° so that the axilla is easily accessible and the axillary artery is readily palpable.

3.5. Landmarks

Edge of the pectoralis major muscle, axillary artery.

3.6. Technical procedure

Preparing the skin with a suitable antiseptic solution. Local infiltration about 1 cm distally from the point where the edge of the pectoralis major muscle and the axillary artery cross on the cranial side of the artery. Puncture the skin with the vaccination needle or an 18 g needle. The artery is below the palpating index and middle fingers (Fig 26). At an angle of approximately 30–40° to the artery, with a saline-filled 5 ml syringe attached, the

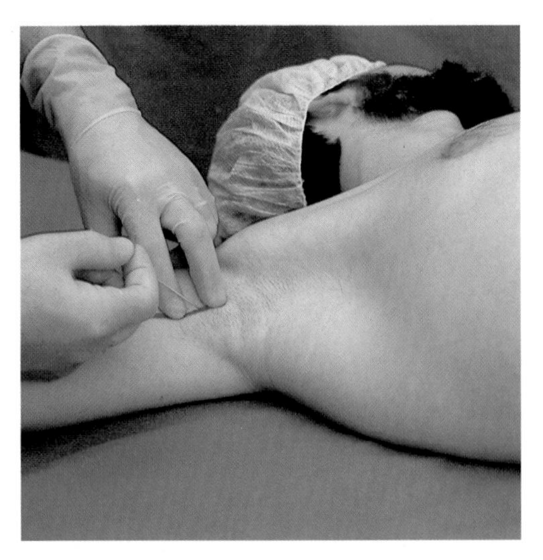

FIG 26.

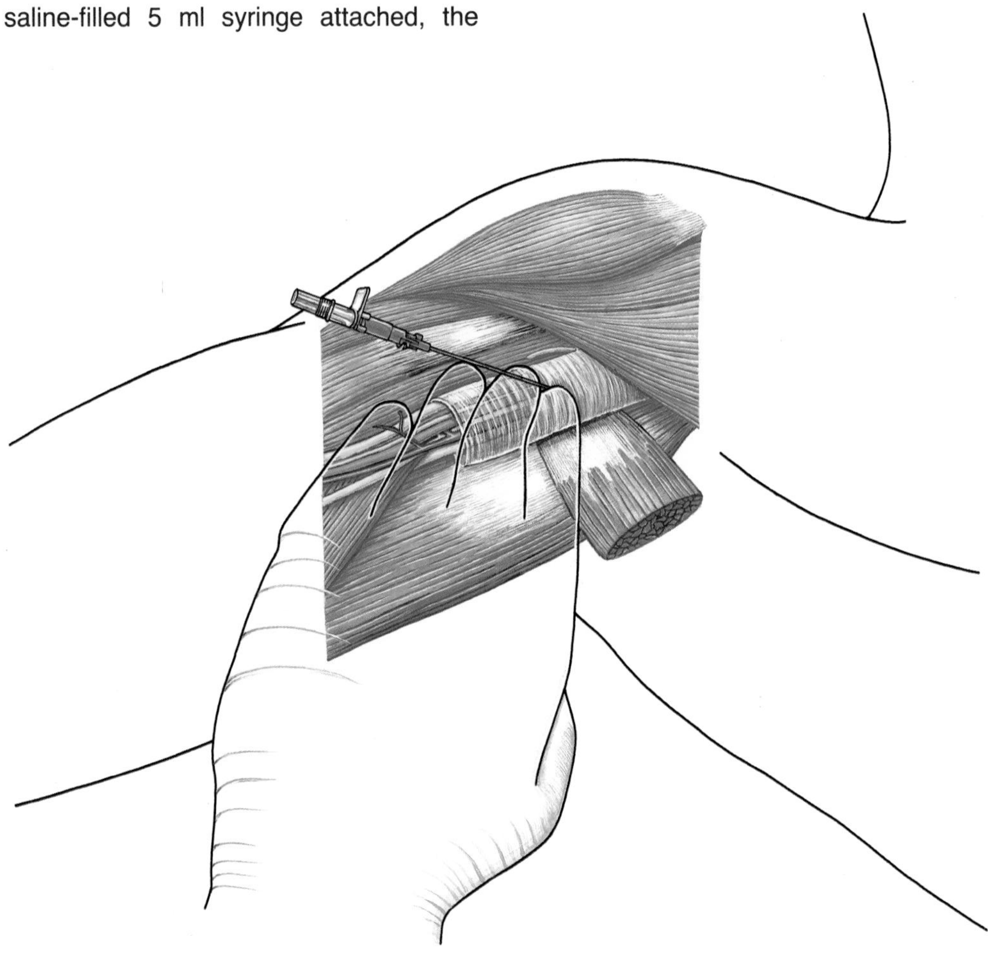

FIG 27.

needle is slowly advanced in the direction of the artery. Passing the connective tissue neurovascular sheath is indicated by a marked decrease in resistance. Paresthesias may be elicited, but need not be. When the neurovascular space is reached, the plastic needle is advanced over the steel stylet. After removal of the metal stylet and the 5 ml syringe, 5 ml of cold saline solution is injected. If paresthesias are elicited, this is a good indication that the needle had been placed correctly. Next, the catheter is advanced about 3–4 cm into the neurovascular space (Fig 28).

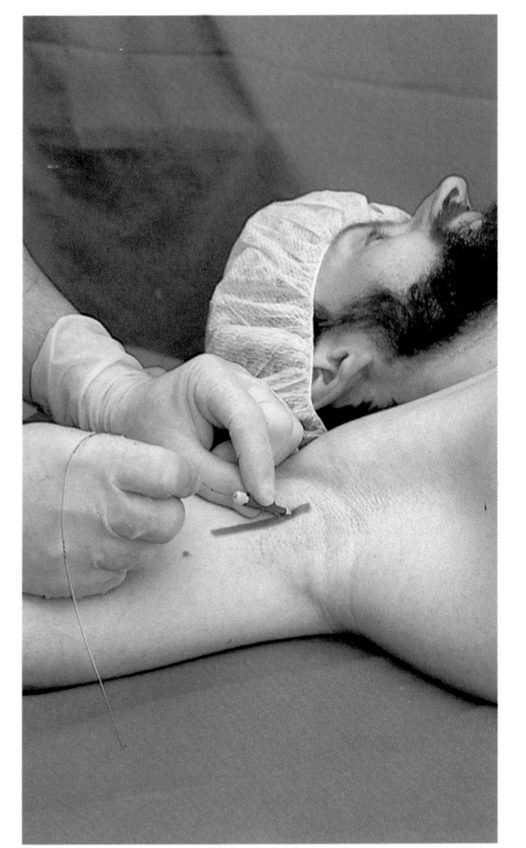

FIG 28.

The plastic needle is removed and the connector is attached to the catheter. Next, the catheter is taped in place, under a sterile dressing (Fig 29).

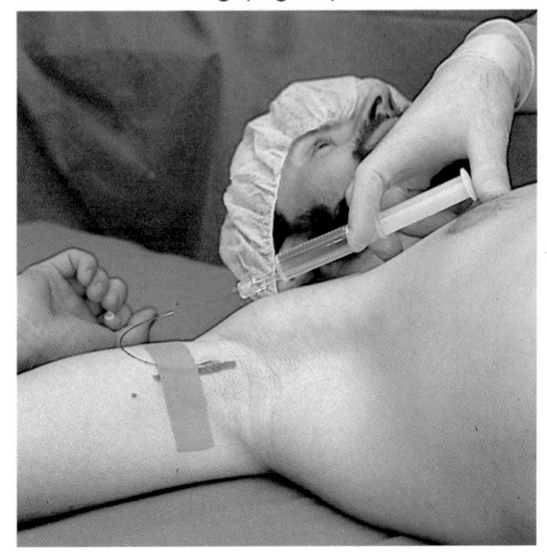

FIG 29.

NOTE:
Slow injection after negative aspiration; manual compression of neurovascular sheath distal to the entry point of the catheter.

In addition to the technique described above, it is also possible to introduce the plastic needle with the aid of a nerve stimulator. The indwelling catheter can be introduced according to the Seldinger technique (3).

3.7. Dosage

For surgical procedures

30–40 ml local anesthetic solution, e.g., bupivacaine 0.5% or 0.375%, etidocaine 1% or 0.75%.

For pain therapy

Bupivacaine 0.125% (mixture of equal amounts of 0.25% bupivacaine and physiologic saline solution). Administered 10–15 ml/hr by precision infusion device.
Advantage: Freedom from pain and sympathetic block with the motor function preserved.

References

1. Selander D: Catheter technique in axillary plexus block. *Acta Anaesth Scand* 1977; 21:324.
2. Mehler D, Otten B: Ein neues Katheterset zur kontinuierlichen axillären plexus anästhesie. *Regional-Anästhesie* 1983; 6:43–46.
3. Postel J, März P: Plexusanästhesie: Elektrische Nervenlokalisation und Kathetertechnik. *Regional-Anästhesie,* 1984.

4. Special Complications

Hematoma due to vascular puncture
(Prevention: manual compression for 3–5 min)
Nerve injury
(Prevention: atraumatic, aseptic technique, short bevel needle)

5. Indications

For surgical procedures

Reconstructive procedures after trauma
A–V fistula for hemodialysis
Other vascular procedures

For pain therapy

Sympathetic reflex dystrophy
Postoperatively, after reimplantation

Intravenous Regional Anesthesia

W. L. A. Simgen

1. Definition

The injection of a vasopressor-free local anesthetic solution into the vein of a desanguinated extremity.

2. Topographic Anatomy

Not applicable

3. Technique

3.1. Anesthesiologic Assessment

> Careful anesthesiologic assessment including the identification of any contraindication.

3.2. Preparation

> Indwelling IV catheter, intubation equipment, ventilation equipment with O_2 connection, atropine, sedative, succinylcholine, vasopressor, catecholamine.

The patient is prepared as for a general anesthetic. As a minimum we must have recent electrolyte values, and in patients older than 40 years an ECG must be obtained.

3.3. Equipment

Esmarch bandage
2 tourniquets or a double tourniquet
20 g plastic IV catheter
20 ml syringe
Rubber tourniquet

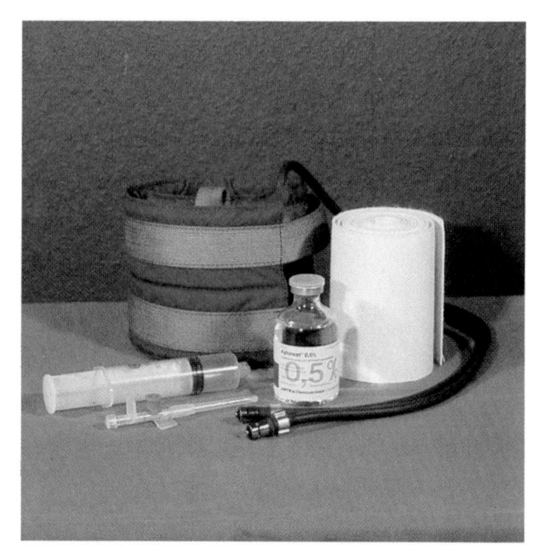

FIG 30.

3.4. Positioning

Supine with arm or leg abducted.

3.5. Landmark

Peripheral vein

3.6. Technical procedure

Placement of indwelling venous catheter. Placement of two blood pressure cuffs, wrapping the extremity with an Esmarch bandage, inflation of the proximal cuff. The pressure in the cuff must be 100 mm Hg higher than the patient's systolic blood pressure.

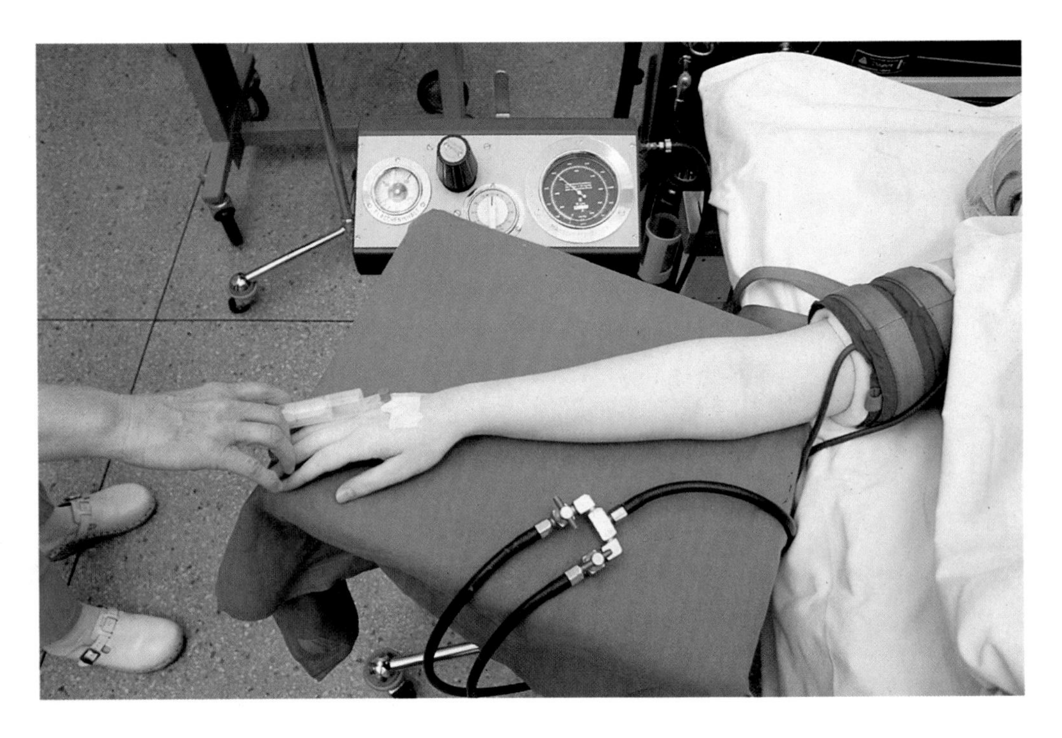

FIG 31.

Removal of the bandage and injection of the low concentration local anesthetic solution through the indwelling venous needle (Fig 31). Distribution of the local anesthetic solution by gentle, stroking massage (removal of the needle).

After good analgesia has been achieved (10–15 min), the distal cuff is inflated. This cuff lies over the anesthetized area and thus should produce no discomfort.

The proximal cuff is now deflated. As soon as the injection has taken place and the needle has been removed, preparation for surgery may begin.

At the end of the operation:

Intermittent full deflation and full re-inflation of the cuff over a period of 3–4 min (e.g., 5 sec "down," 30 sec "up").

Because of the danger of a toxic reaction, the minimum time between injection and the first deflation of the cuff should be no less than 20 min.

In hand surgery the following procedure has been found very satisfactory:

–placement of drain
–closure
–dressing
–pressure dressing

Only at this time is the cuff deflated according to the scheme described above. The pressure dressing should be removed only after 1 hr.

If the surgeon wishes to achieve hemostasis with the cuff deflated, a different technique should be used. After the arm has been desanguinated and prior to the injection of the local anesthetic solution, a third "ligature" is placed on the arm just

proximal to the surgical field (usually a simple rubber tourniquet is used, similar to those used in phlebotomy).
A higher concentration of local anesthetic is injected. The rubber tourniquet is left in place for 2–3 min and is then removed. After full analgesia has been attained: Inflation of the distal and deflation of the proximal tourniquet. To achieve surgical hemostasis, the cuff is intermittently deflated and then completely opened. Usually, it takes 10–15 min for hemostasis and closure.
Pressure problems, which may occur if the cuff is inflated for more than 30–40 min, limit the length of the surgical procedure.

3.7. Dosage

Arm: *Less concentrated solution:*
Up to 40 ml lidocaine 0.5%, or mepivacaine 0.5%, prilocaine 0.5%

More concentrated solution:
15–25 prilocaine 1.5% (≈4 mg/kg)

Leg: *Less concentrated solution:*
Up to 60 ml lidocaine 0.5%, or prilocaine 0.5%

More concentrated solution:
15–40 ml prilocaine 1.5% (≈6 mg/kg)

4. Special Side Effects and Complications

Side effects

After release of the cuff: flooding of local anesthetic solution into the circulation.
This can be recognized by a mild tingling sensation on the tongue and the lips, or by a transient bradycardia.
Therapy: Immediate reinflation of the cuff and O_2 administration.

Complications

Accidental premature release of the anesthetic solution into the circulation. Sudden, dramatic flooding of the circulation. Arrhythmias, usually bradycardia, restlessness, tachypnea, dizziness, nausea; in extreme cases centrally triggered convulsions and apnea.
Therapy: Immediate isolation of the extremity (reinflation of the cuff), intubation and ventilation with O_2.
Since a premature entry of the local anesthetic solution into the circulation can never be predicted or totally eliminated, careful monitoring of the patient is mandatory. This is particularly important during the first few minutes after the release of the cuff.

5. Indications

For surgical procedures

Operations on the arm or leg in procedures lasting up to 30 min.

For pain therapy

Sympathetic block with guanethidine is possible: the information available about this is insufficient at the present time.

6. Special Contraindications

Bi- and trifascicular block on the ECG.
Patients with a history of syncope.
Infected extremity.

References

1. Atkinson DI: The mode of action of intravenous regional anesthetics. *Acta Anaesth Scand* 1969; 36 (suppl):131–134.
2. Auberger HG: Die intravenöse Regionalanästhesie, in Nolte, Meyer, Wurster (Hrsg), *Die peripheren Leitungsanästhesien* (3. int. Symposion, 26.1.74). Stuttgart, Thieme, 1974.
3. Dick W, Teuteberg H, Wessinghage D, Willibrand H: Klinische und experimentelle Untersuchungen zur intravenösen Regionalanästhesie. *Der Anästheist* 1972; 21:104–112.
4. Thorn-Alquist AM: Intravenous regional anesthesia: A seven year survey. *Acta Anaesth Scand* 1971; 15:23–32.
5. Tryba M, Zenz M, Hausmann E: Kontrollierte Untersuchung zur intravenösen Regionalanästhesie mit hoch und niedrig konzentriertem Prilocain. *Regional-Anästhesie* 1983; 6:27–29.

Block of the Peripheral Nerves in the Region of the Elbow

D. Čović

I. The ulnar nerve

1. Definition

Block of the ulnar nerve (C_8–T_1) at the medial epicondyle of the humerus.

2. Topographic Anatomy

The ulnar nerve originates as a mixed nerve from the medial cord of the brachial plexus. The nerve runs along the medial area of the lower arm in the area of the extensor muscle space. In the area of the elbow, the ulnar nerve is located in the ulnar nerve groove on the dorsal aspect of the medial epicondyle of the humerus. Caudally, it runs between the heads of the flexor carpi ulnaris, on the flexor surface of the forearm (Fig 33).

3. Technique

3.1. Anesthesiologic Assessment

> Careful anesthesiologic assessment including the identification of any contraindication.

3.2. Preparation

> Intravenous cannula, intubation set-up, ventilation equipment with O_2 connection, atropine, sedative, succinylcholine, vasopressor, catecholamine.

3.3. Equipment

Drape with a hole
Antiseptic solution and sponges
5 ml syringe
Needle, 2–3 cm long (21 g or 23 g), ideally a butterfly needle with flexible extension tubing between the needle and the syringe ("immobile needle" of Winnie)

3.4. Positioning

Patient in the supine position. Arm internally rotated with the elbow flexed. Forearm in pronation.

3.5. Landmarks

The medial epicondyle of the humerus.
The coronoidal process of the ulna.

3.6. Technical Procedure

Preparing the skin with a suitable antiseptic solution. The ulnar nerve should be palpated, if possible, in the ulnar groove. The needle is introduced through a skin wheal, just proximally from the groove, and the tip of the needle is directed along the longitudinal axis of the humerus. After paresthesias have been elicited, the needle is fixed and, following negative aspiration, 2–5 ml of anesthetic solution are injected.

3.7. Dosage

2–5 ml local anesthetic solution, e.g., lidocaine 1%, mepivacaine 1%: bupivacaine 0.5%, etidocaine 1%.

4. Special Complications

None

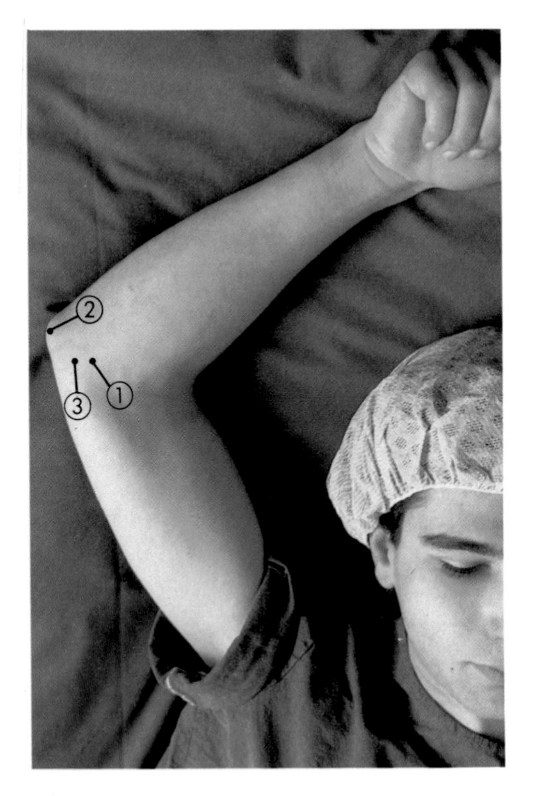

FIG 32.
1. Medial epicondyle of the humerus
2. Olecranon process
3. Entry point

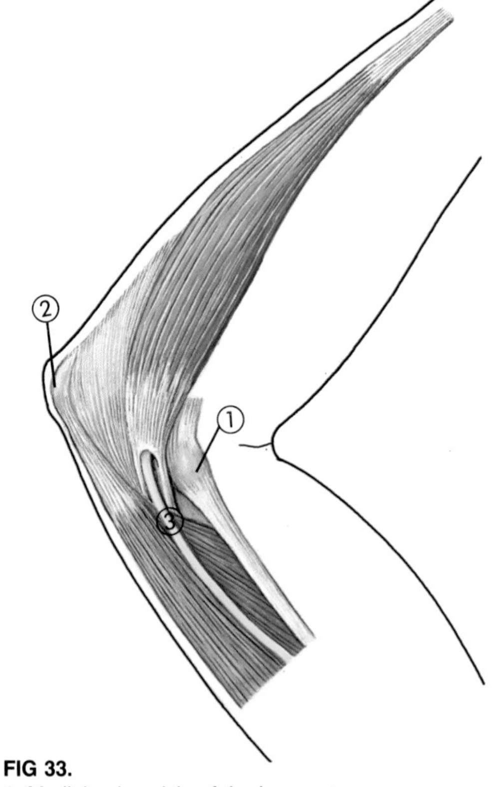

FIG 33.
1. Medial epicondyle of the humerus
2. Olecranon process
3. Ulnar n.

5. Indications

Supplementation of incomplete brachial plexus block.

Diagnostic, therapeutic, and surgical procedure in the area of sensory innervation.

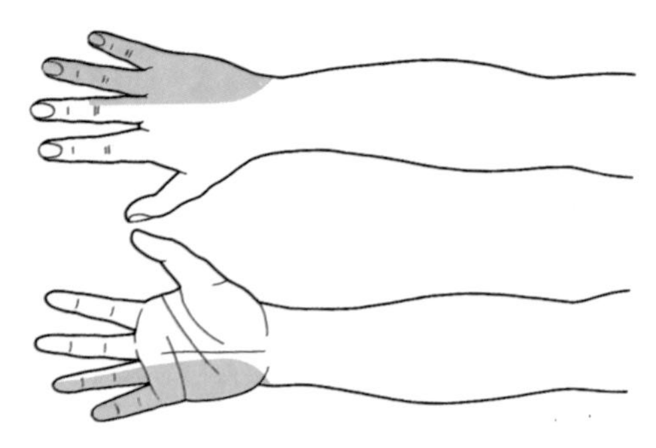

FIG 34.
Area of cutaneous sensory innervation.

6. Special Contraindications

None

II. The median nerve

1. Definition

Block of the median nerve (C_5–T_1) in the area of the elbow.

2. Topographic Anatomy

The median nerve originates from a fork-shaped fusion from branches of the lateral and medial cords of the brachial plexus. On the distal third of the humerus, the nerve lies medially to the brachial artery and follows it, covered by the aponeurosis of the biceps muscle, through the anticubital fossa, and onto the anterior aspect of the forearm (Fig 36).

3. Technique

3.1. Anesthesiologic Assessment

> Careful anesthesiologic assessment including the identification of any contraindication.

3.2. Preparation

> Intravenous cannula, intubation setup, ventilation equipment with O_2 connection, atropine, sedative, succinylcholine, vasopressor, catecholamine.

3.3. Equipment

Drape with a hole
Antiseptic solution and sponges
5 ml syringe
Needle, 2–3 cm long (21 g or 23 g), ideally a butterfly needle with flexible extension tubing between the needle and the syringe ("immobile needle" of Winnie)

3.4. Positioning

Patient in the supine position.
Elbow extended, arm partly abducted.

3.5. Landmarks

The medial and lateral epicondyles of the humerus, the brachial artery (Fig 35).

3.6. Technical procedure

Preparing the skin with a suitable antiseptic solution. The medial and lateral epicondyles of the humerus are connected by a straight line. The needle is introduced immediately medially to the brachial artery, through a skin wheal. At a depth of about 5 cm paresthesias are elicited. After negative aspiration, the local anesthetic solution is injected. If no paresthesias could be elicited, the local anesthetic solution is infiltrated over a fan-shaped area.

3.7. Dosage

With paresthesias

5 ml local anesthetic solution, e.g., lidocaine 1%, mepivacaine 1%; bupivacaine 0.5%, etidocaine 1%

Without paresthesias

8 ml local anesthetic solution

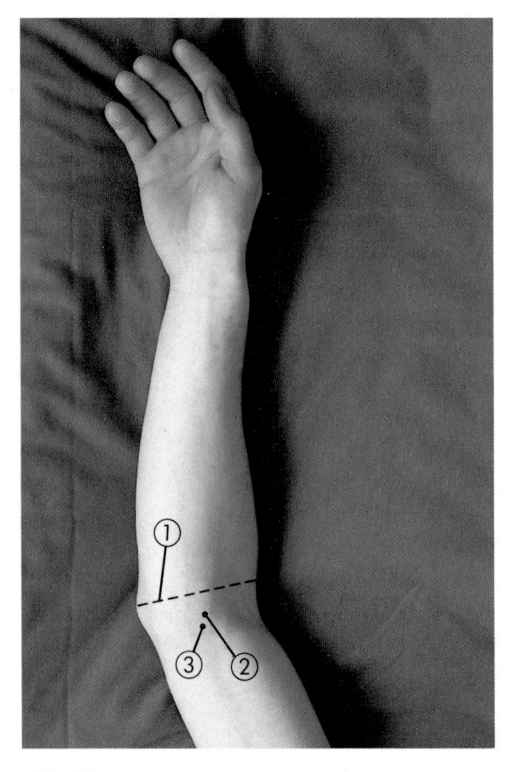

FIG 35.
1. Connecting line between the lateral and medial epicondyle
2. Brachial a.
3. Entry point

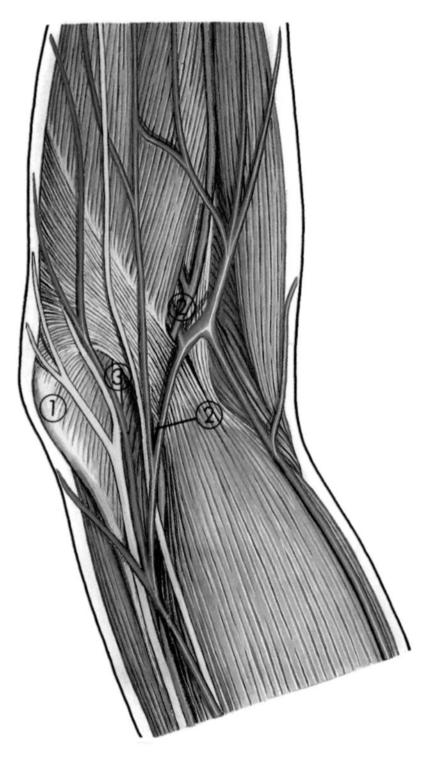

FIG 36.
1. Medial epicondyle of the humerus
2. Brachial a.
3. Median n.

4. Special Complications

None

5. Indications

Supplementation of incomplete brachial plexus block.

Diagnostic, therapeutic, and surgical procedures in the area of sensory innervation.

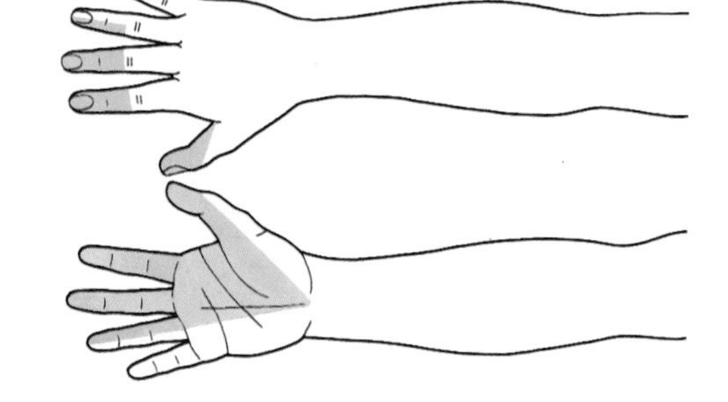

FIG 37.
Area of cutaneous sensory innervation.

6. Special Contraindications

None

III. The radial nerve

1. Definition

Block of the radial nerve (C_5–C_8 T_1) in the area of the elbow, in its course between the biceps and brachioradialis muscles.

2. Topographic Anatomy

The radial nerve originates from the dorsal cord of the brachial plexus. It courses along the radial groove on the dorsal aspect of the humerus. Accompanied by the collateral radial artery, it follows the groove around the dorsal aspect of the arm, into the groove between the biceps and brachioradialis muscles. At this point, it divides into its two terminal branches, the deep and the superficial branch of the radial nerve (Fig 39).

3. Technique

3.1. Anesthesiologic Assessment

Careful anesthesiologic assessment including the identification of any contraindication.

3.2. Preparation

Intravenous cannula, intubation set-up, ventilation equipment with O_2 connection, atropine, sedative, succinylcholine, vasopressor, catecholamine.

3.3. Equipment

Drape with a hole
10 ml syringe
Needle, 2–3 cm long (21 g or 23 g), ideally a butterfly needle with flexible extension tubing between the needle and the syringe ("immobile needle" of Winnie)

3.4. Positioning

Patient in the supine position.
Elbow extended, arm partly abducted.

3.5. Landmarks

The lateral epicondyle of the humerus
The brachioradialis muscle
The tendon of the biceps
(Fig 38)

3.6. Technical Procedure

Preparing the skin with a suitable antiseptic solution. At the level of the elbow joint, the groove between the brachioradialis muscle and the tendon of the biceps is identified. The needle is introduced through a skin wheal, proximally and laterally in the direction of the lateral epicondyle of the humerus. Following the first bony contact, the needle is advanced cranially for about 1–3 cm along the long axis of the humerus, and 2–4 ml of the anesthetic solution are injected. Following this, bony contact is again sought, and when attained, the needle is withdrawn 2–5 mm and fixed. (Paresthesias are occasionally elicited.) In this position 5 ml of the anesthetic solution are injected. Another 5–10 ml are injected while repeating the above performance and while the needle is being withdrawn into the subcutaneous area. Paresthesias in the thumb and the dorsum of the hand are possible but not always present.

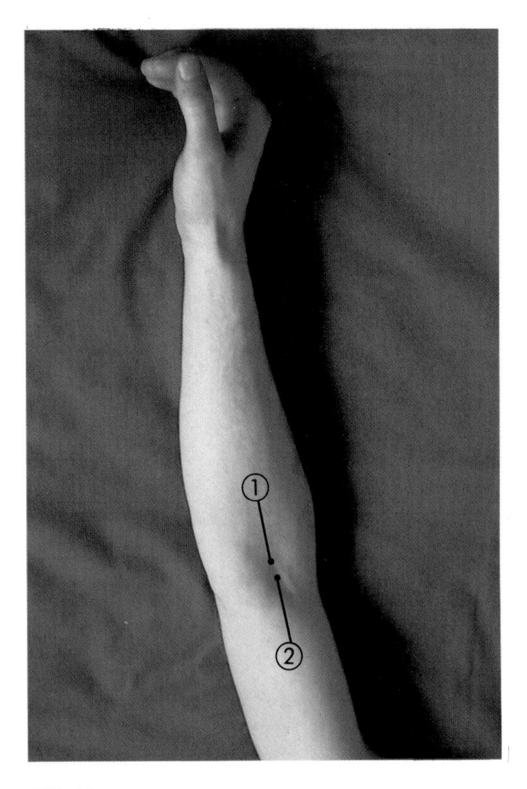

FIG 38.
1. Depression between the brachioradialis m. and the tendon of the biceps
2. Point of entry

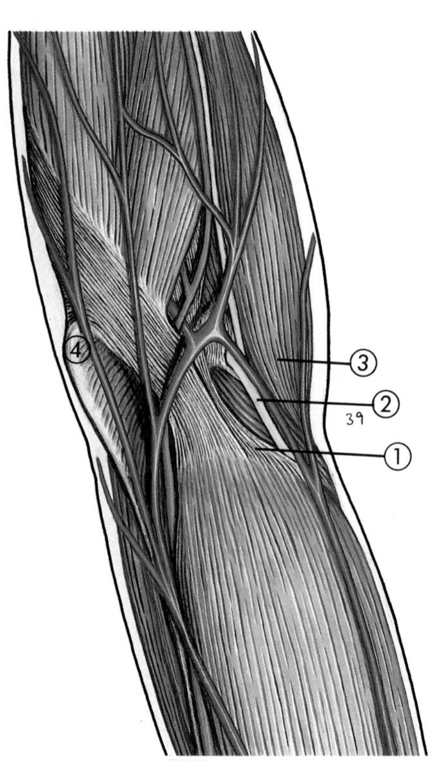

FIG 39.
1. Tendon of the biceps
2. Radial n.
3. Brachioradialis m.
4. Medial epicondyle of the humerus

The technical procedure is very much easier if a butterfly needle with a flexible extension tubing is used since this makes the precise fixation of the needle possible ("immobile needle" principle).

3.7. Dosage

10–15 ml local anesthetic solution, e.g., lidocaine 1%, mepivacaine 1%, bupivacaine 0.5%, etidocaine 1%.

4. Special Complications

None

5. Indications

Supplementation of incomplete brachial plexus block.

Diagnostic, therapeutic, and surgical procedures in the area of sensory innervation.

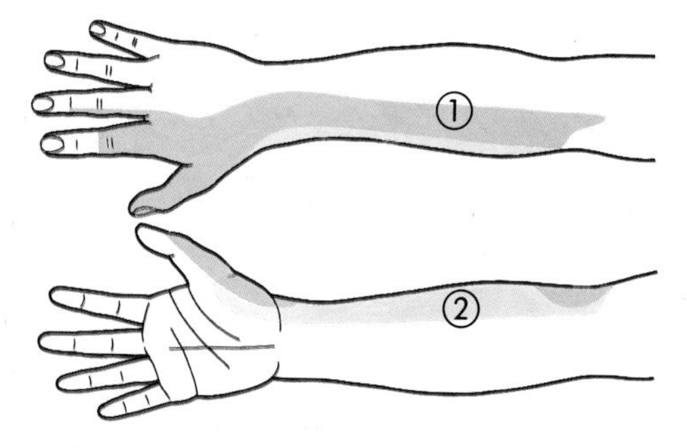

FIG 40.
Area of cutaneous sensory innervation:
1. Radial n.
2. Lateral antebrachial cutaneous n.

6. Special Contraindications

None

IV. Lateral antebrachial cutaneous nerve

1. Definition

Block of the lateral antebrachial cutaneous nerve (C_5–C_7) between the brachioradialis muscle and the tendon of the biceps.

2. Topographic Anatomy

The lateral antebrachial cutaneous nerve is the sensory terminal branch of the musculocutaneous nerve. It perforates the fascia proximally to the elbow joint and laterally to the biceps tendon. The nerve runs in the skin on the lateral aspect of the forearm as far as the wrist.

3. Technique

3.1. Anesthesiologic Assessment

> Careful anesthesiologic assessment including the identification of any contraindication.

3.2. Preparation

> Intravenous cannula, intubation setup, ventilation equipment with O_2 connection, atropine, sedative, succinylcholine, vasopressor, catecholamine.

3.3. Equipment

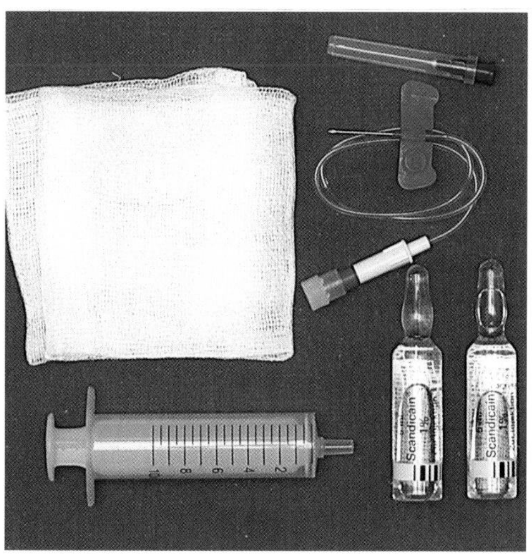

FIG 41.

Drape with a hole
10 ml syringe
Needle, 2–3 cm long (21 g or 23 g), ideally a butterfly needle with flexible extension tubing between the needle and the syringe ("immobile needle" of Winnie)

3.4. Positioning

Patient in supine position. The elbow joint is extended and the arm is slightly abducted.

3.5. Landmarks

The lateral epicondyle of the humerus. The groove between brachioradialis muscle and the tendon of the biceps.

3.6. Technical Procedure

A subcutaneous infiltration of a local anesthetic solution in the antecubital fossa between the brachioradialis muscle and the tendon of the biceps makes the block of lateral antebrachial cutaneous nerve possible.

3.7. Dosage

10–15 ml local anesthetic solution, e.g., lidocaine 1%, mepivacaine 1%; bupivacaine 0.5%, etidocaine 1%.

4. Special Complications

None

5. Indications

Supplementation of incomplete brachial plexus block.
Diagnostic, therapeutic, and surgical procedures in the area of sensory innervation (Fig 40).

6. Special Contraindications

None

Block of the Peripheral Nerves in the Area of the Wrist

D. Čović

I. The ulnar nerve

1. Definition

Block of the ulnar nerve at the wrist next to the tendon of the flexor carpi ulnaris.

2. Topographic Anatomy

The ulnar nerve divides into its two terminal branches, the dorsal branch and the palmar branch, about 5 cm proximal to the wrist on the flexor side of the forearm.

3. Technique

3.1. Anesthesiologic Assessment

Careful anesthesiologic assessment including the identification of any contraindication.

3.2. Preparation

Intravenous cannula, intubation setup, ventilation equipment with O_2 connection, atropine, sedative, succinylcholine, vasopressor, catecholamine.

3.3. Equipment

Drape with a hole
Skin preparation equipment
10 ml syringe
Thin (21 or 23 g) needle, 3–4 cm long, preferably a butterfly needle with flexible tubing between the needle and the syringe

3.4. Positioning

Patient in supine position. The hand supinated at the wrist and slightly flexed.

3.5. Landmarks

The styloid process of the ulna
The ulnar artery
The tendon of the flexor carpi ulnaris m.
The tendon of the palmoris longus m.

A. Block of palmar branch of the ulnar n.

3.6. Technical Procedure

Preparing the skin with a suitable antiseptic solution. Hand slightly flexed. The needle is introduced through a skin wheal, immediately radial to the flexor carpi ulnaris muscle, vertically in the direction of the pisiform bone.
At a depth of 1–2 cm, paresthesias are usually elicited. After negative aspiration and fixation of the needle, the local anesthetic solution is injected.
If no paresthesias are elicited, the needle is advanced until bone is contacted. The local anesthetic solution is injected while the needle is slowly withdrawn.

3.7. Dosage

If paresthesias were elicited

3–5 ml local anesthetic solution, e.g., lidocaine 1%, mepivacaine 1%; bupivacaine 0.5%, etidocaine 1%.

Without paresthesias

5–10 ml local anesthetic solution.

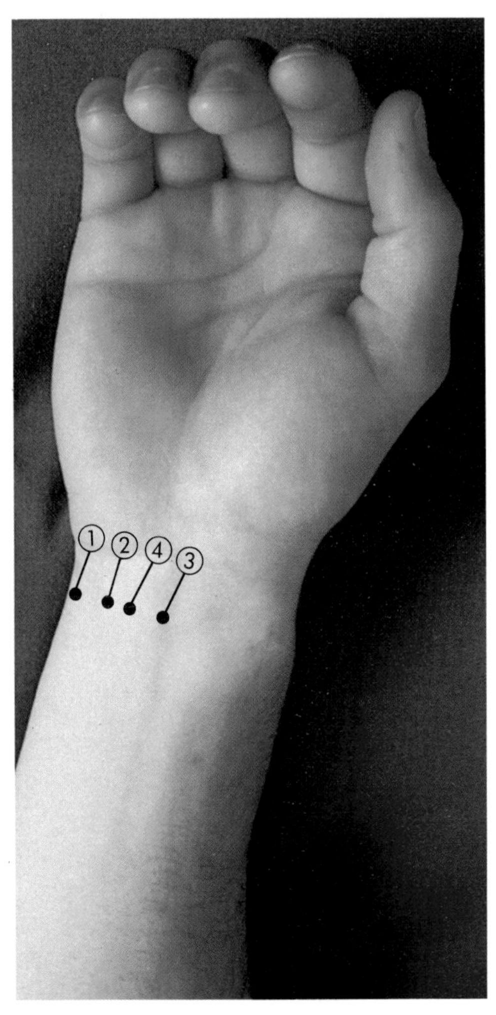

FIG 42.
1. Styloid process of the ulna
2. Tendon of the flexor carpi ulnaris m.
3. Tendon of the palmaris longus m.
4. Point of entry

B. Block of the dorsal branch of the ulnar n.

3.6. Technical Procedure

Preparing the skin with a suitable antiseptic solution. Infiltration of the area medial to the tendon of the flexor carpi ulnaris in the direction of the styloid process of the ulna.

3.7. Dosage

3–5 ml local anesthetic solution, e.g., lidocaine 1%, mepivacaine 1%; bupivacaine 0.5%, etidocaine 1%.

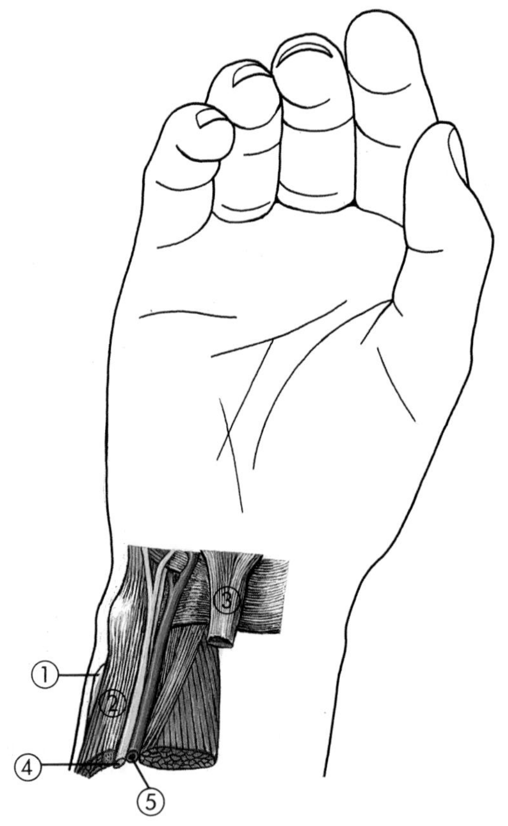

FIG 43.
1. Styloid process of the ulna
2. Tendon of the flexor carpi ulnaris m.
3. Tendon of the palmaris longus m.
4. Ulnar n.
5. Ulnar a.

4. Special Complications

None

5. Indications

Supplementation of incomplete brachial plexus block.

Diagnostic, therapeutic and surgical procedures in the area of sensory innervation (Fig 40).

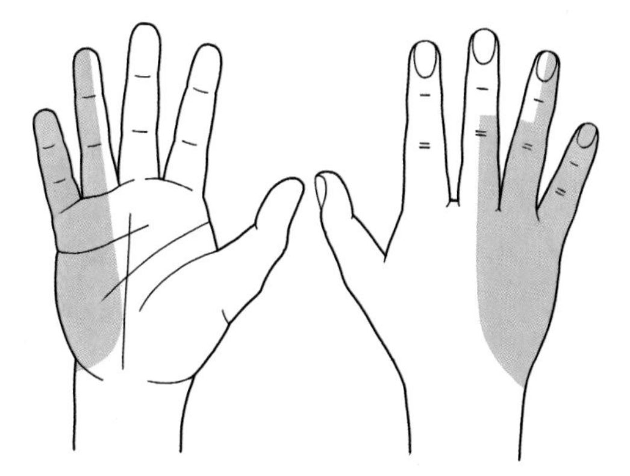

FIG 44.
Area of cutaneous sensory innervation.

6. Special Contraindications

None

II. The median nerve

1. Definition

Block of the median nerve at the wrist medially to the tendon of the palmaris longus muscle.

2. Topographic Anatomy

The median nerve is located very superficially at the proximal level of the wrist laterally to the tendon of the pulmaris longus m. (Fig 46).

3. Technique

3.1. Anesthesiologic Assessment

Careful anesthesiologic assessment including the identification of any contraindication.

3.2. Preparation

Intravenous cannula, intubation setup, ventilation equipment with O_2 connection, atropine, sedative, succinylcholine, vasopressor, catecholamine.

3.3. Equipment

Drape with a hole
Cleansing equipment
5 ml syringe
Thin (21 or 23 g) needle, 2–3 cm long, preferably a butterfly needle with flexible tubing between the needle and the syringe

3.4. Positioning

Patient in supine position.
Hand in supination, slight extension at the elbow.

3.5. Landmarks

The styloid process of the ulna
The tendon of the pulmaris longus m.
The tendon of the flexor carpi radialis m.

3.6. Technical Procedure

Preparing the skin with a suitable antiseptic solution. Palpation of the tendon of the palmaris longus m. and the flexor carpi radialis m. (This is facilitated by the patient making a fist.) The entry point is lateral to the tendon of the palmaris longus m. The needle is introduced vertically through a skin wheal for 0.5–1 cm, and a fan-shaped pattern of infiltration is performed. If paresthesias are elicited, the needle is fixed and, after negative aspiration, the local anesthetic solution is injected.

3.7. Dosage

3–5 ml local anesthetic solution, e.g., lidocaine 1%, mepivacaine 1%; bupivacaine 0.5%, etidocaine 1%.

4. Special Complications

None

5. Indications

Supplementation of incomplete brachial plexus block.

Diagnostic, therapeutic, and surgical procedures in the area of sensory innervation (Fig 40).

6. Special Contraindications

None

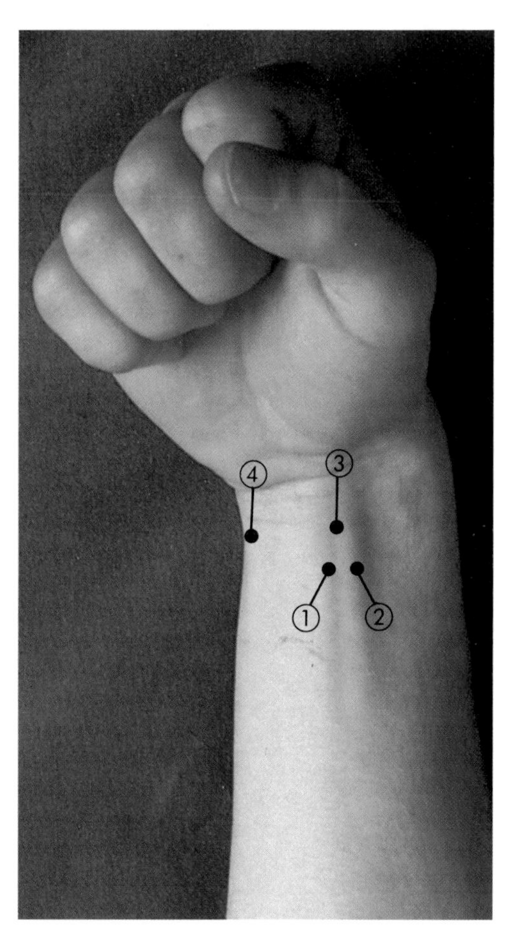

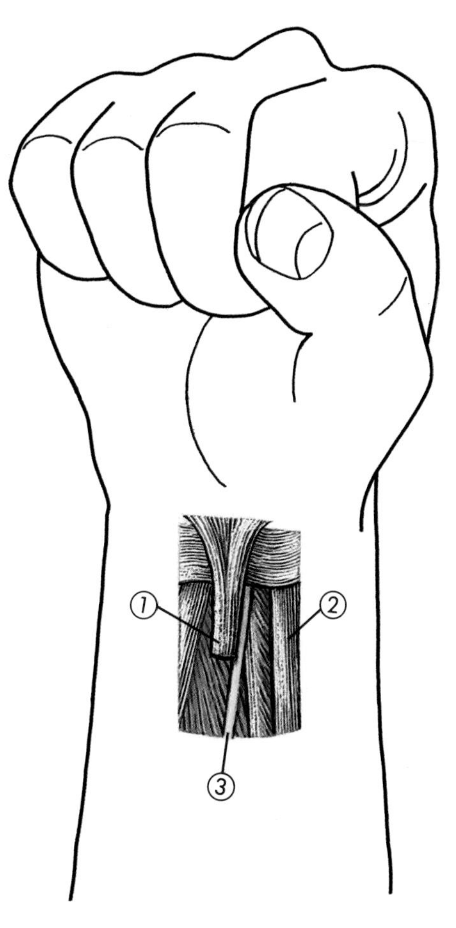

FIG 45.
1. Tendon of the palmaris longus n.
2. Tendon of the flexor carpi radialis m.
3. Point of entry
4. Styloid process of the ulna

FIG 46.
1. Tendon of the palmaris longus m.
2. Tendon of the flexor carpi radialis m.
3. Median n.

FIG 47.
Area of cutaneous sensory innervation.

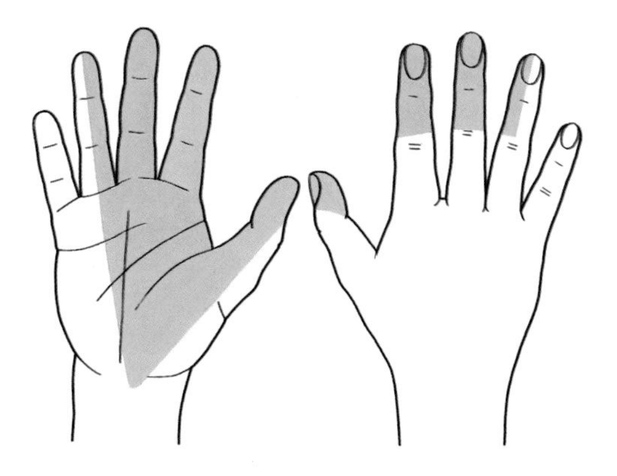

III. The radial nerve

1. Definition

Block of the superficial and radial branch at the wrist laterally to the radial artery.

2. Topographic Anatomy

The superficial branch is a pure sensory terminal branch of the radial n. It is located on the medial side of brachioradialis m. and follows the radial a. in the proximal portion of the forearm. Approximately 8 cm proximal to the wrist, the nerve crosses under the tendon of the brachioradialis m. and proceeds to the extensor side of the forearm. At the level of the wrist it divides into its terminal branches (Fig 50).

3. Technique

3.1. Anesthesiologic Assessment

Careful anesthesiologic assessment including the identification of any contraindication.

3.2. Preparation

Intravenous cannula, intubation setup, ventilation equipment with O_2 connection, atropine, sedative, succinylcholine, vasopressor, catecholamine.

3.3. Equipment

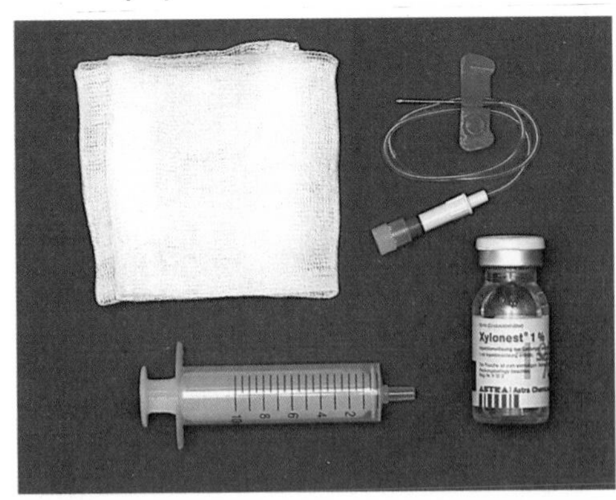

FIG 48.

Drape with a hole
Skin preparation equipment
5 ml syringe
Thin (21 or 23 g) needle, 2–3 cm long, preferably a butterfly needle with flexible tubing between the needle and the syringe

3.4. Positioning

Patient in supine position
Hand in supination

3.5. Landmarks

The styloid process of the ulna
The radial a. (Fig 49)

3.6. Technical Procedure

Preparing the skin with a suitable antiseptic solution. At the level of the styloid process of the ulna, a circular line is drawn around the wrist. At this level the radial artery is palpated. With the hand in supination, the needle is introduced lateral to the radial artery, until paresthesias are elicited. The needle is fixed and, after negative aspiration, the local anesthetic solution is injected.

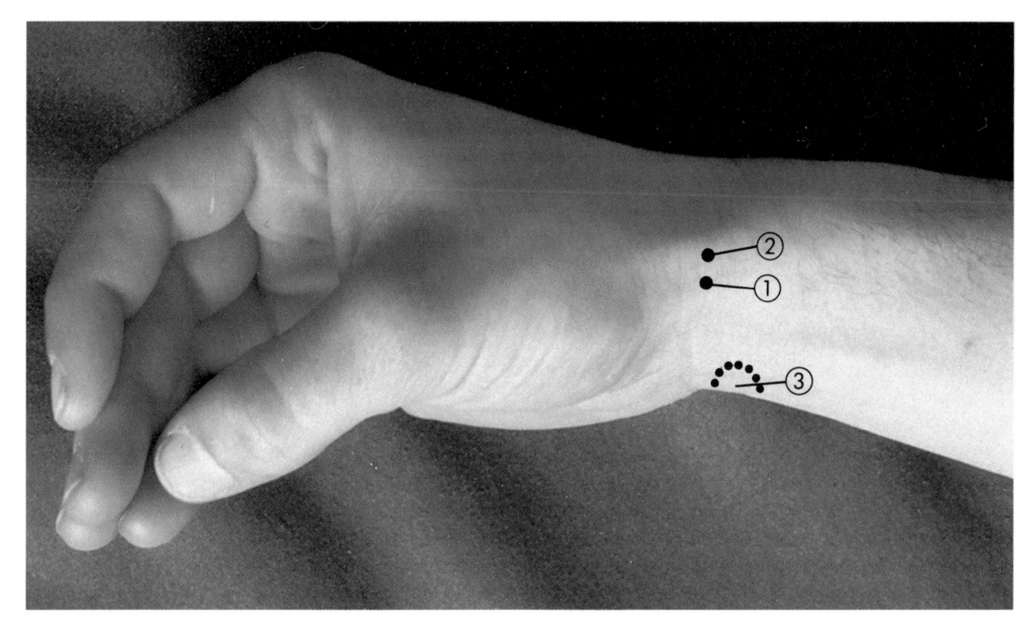

FIG 49.
1. Radial a.
2. Point of entry
3. Styloid process of the ulna

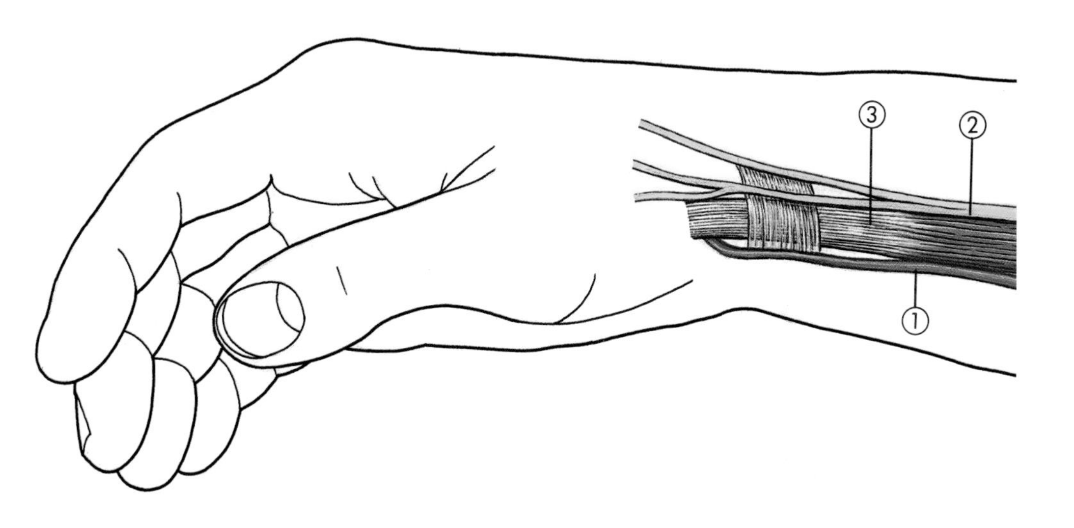

FIG 50.
1. Radial a.
2. Radial n.
3. Brachioradialis m.

3.7. Dosage

3 ml local anesthetic solution, e.g., lidocaine 1%, mepivacaine 1%; bupivacaine 0.5%, etidocaine 1%.

4. Special Complications

None

5. Indications

Supplementation of incomplete brachial plexus block.

Diagnostic, therapeutic, and surgical procedures in the area of sensory innervation (Fig 51).

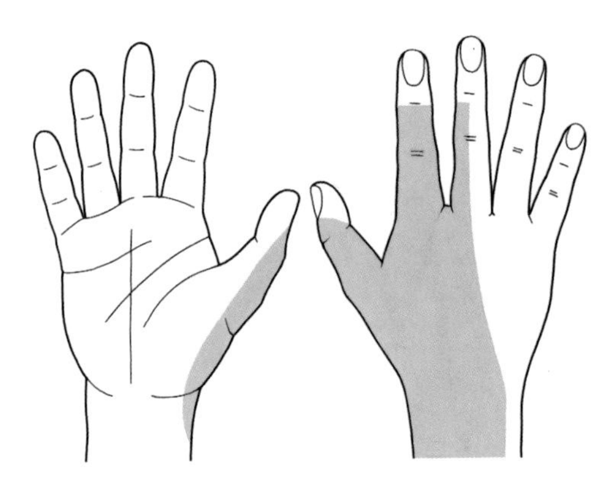

FIG 51.
Area of cutaneous sensory innervation.

6. Special Contraindications

None

References:

1. Albert J, Löfstrom B: Bilateral Ulnar Nerve Block. *Acta Anaesth Scand* 1961; 5:9, 1965; 9:1.
2. Eriksson E (Hrsgl): *Atlas der Lokalanästhesie*. Stuttgart, Thieme, 1970.
3. McDonald JJ, Chusid JG: *Correlative Neuroanatomy and Functional Neurology*. Los Altos, Lange, 1952.

Blocks of the Lumbosacral Plexus

C. Panhans, R. Schwarz

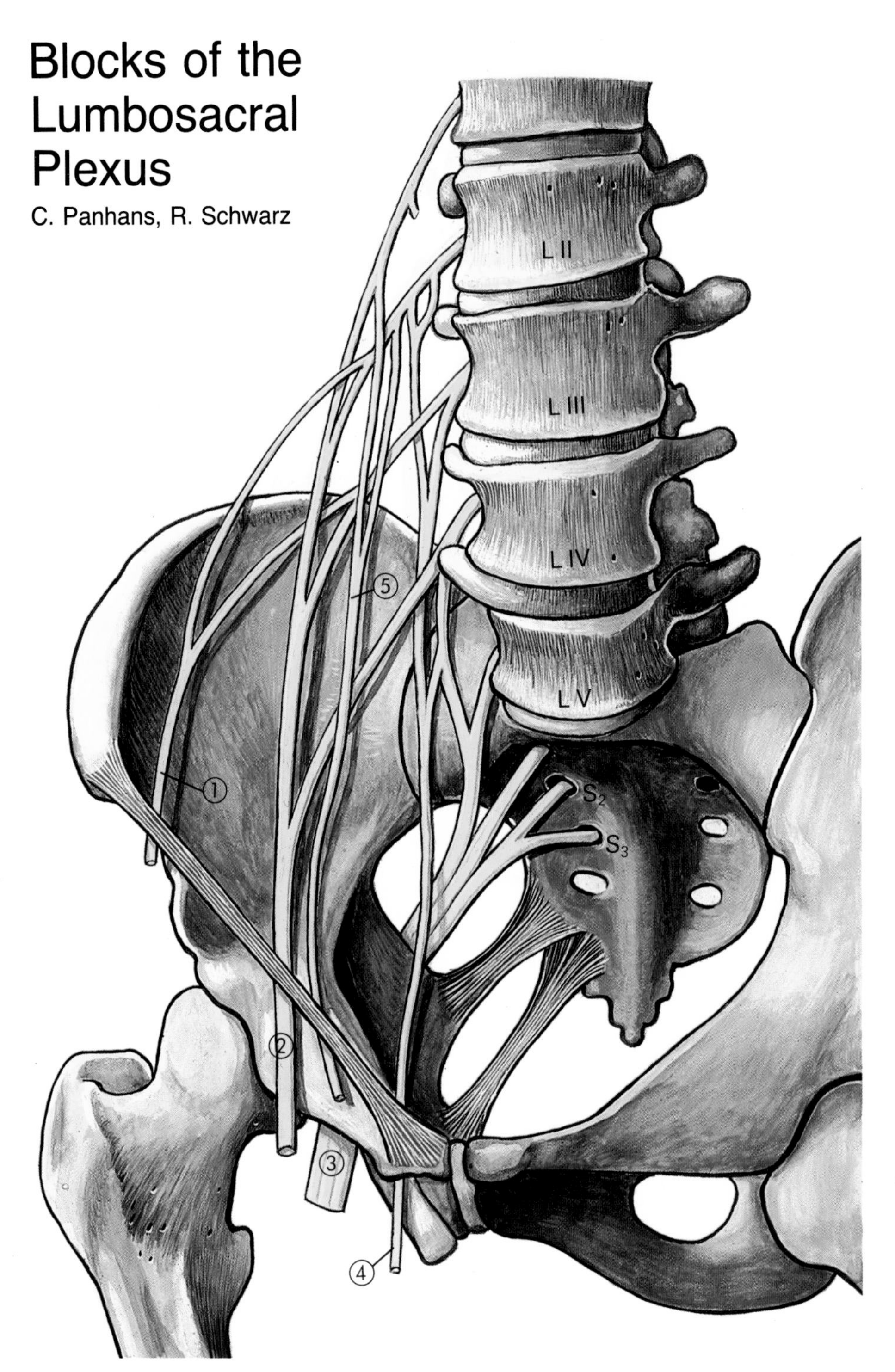

FIG 52.
1. Lateral femoral cutaneous n.
2. Femoral n.
3. Sciatic n.
4. Obturator n.
5. Genitofemoral n.

The lumbosacral plexus is formed by the ventral branches of the lumbar and sacral nerves (L_1–S_3–S_4).
The component nerves of the plexus are arranged as follows:

Genitofemoral n. (L_1–L_2)
Lateral femoral cutaneous n. (L_2–L_3)
Femoral n. (L_2–L_4)
Obturator n. (L_2–L_4)
Sciatic n. (L_4–S_3)

In order to perform an adequate block for surgical procedures on the lower extremity, combinations of blocks are frequently mandated by the overlapping areas of innervation. A certain limitation is imposed by the maximal dose of the various local anesthetic agents which can be safely administered.
The individual blocks and their combinations are discussed below.

I. Psoas compartment block

1. Definition

The psoas compartment block, according to Chayen and coworkers, is a complete peripheral block of the entire lumbosacral plexus. It includes the following nerves:

Femoral n.
Lateral femoral cutaneous n.
Obturator n.
Genitofemoral n.
Parts of the sciatic n.

2. Topographic Anatomy

The components of the lumbosacral plexus, after emerging from the intervertebral foramina, run in a so-called fascial space formed ventrally by the psoas major m., dorsally by the quadratus lumborum m., and medially by the vertebral bodies.

3. Technique

3.1. Anesthesiologic Assessment

Careful anesthesiologic assessment including the identification of any contraindication.

3.2. Preparation

Intravenous cannula, intubation setup, ventilation equipment with O_2 connection, atropine, sedative, succinylcholine, vasopressor, catecholamine.

3.3. Equipment

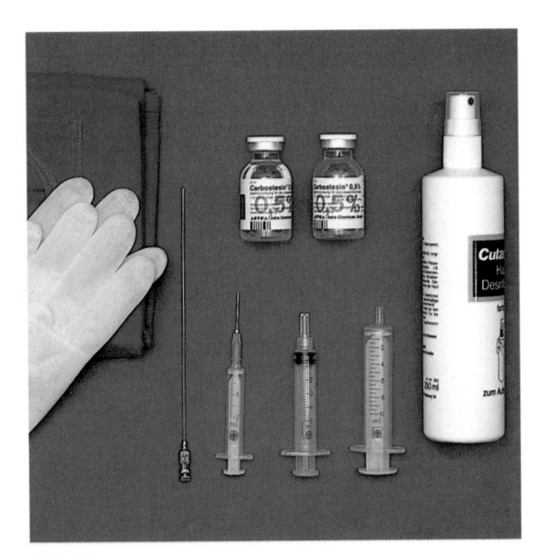

FIG 53.

Drape with hole
Gloves
Skin prep equipment
2 ml syringe with small needle for the skin wheal
22 g needle, 15 cm long
5 ml plastic syringe to test "loss of resistance"
10 ml syringe
"Immobile needle" (Winnie)

3.4. Positioning

Lateral position, resting on side that is not to be anesthetized, hips and knees flexed.

3.5. Landmarks

Spinous process of L_4 (line connecting the two iliac crests)
5 cm laterally
3 cm caudally

3.6. Technical Procedure

Preparing the skin with suitable antiseptic solution. The spinous process of L_4 is identified (line between the iliac crests). A line is drawn 3 cm caudad. At right angles to the end of this line another line is drawn for 5 cm (Fig 54).

Through a skin wheal, a 15 cm-long needle is advanced vertically from the end of the second line, close to the iliac crest, until contact is made with the lateral process of the fifth lumbar vertebra. The direction of the needle is then adjusted, so that the needle can be advanced craniad to the transverse process into the body of the quadratus lumborum m. After negative aspiration in two planes, an air-filled syringe is attached to the needle. A slight pressure on the plunger will reveal a springy resistance. The needle is advanced until this springy resistance can no longer be demonstrated. The tip of the needle is then in the fascial space between the quadratus lumborum m. and the psoas major m.

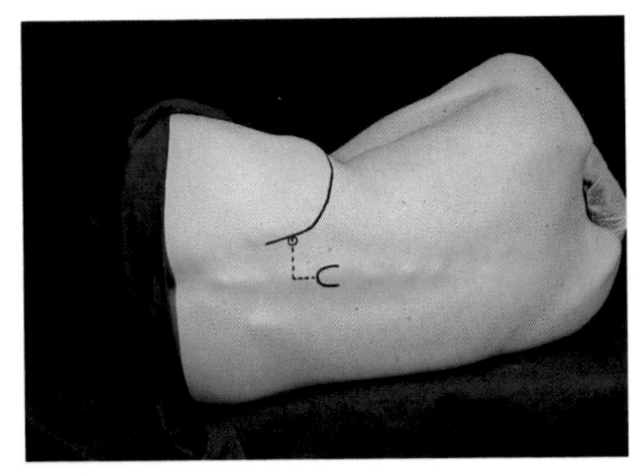

FIG 54.

3.7. Dosage

For surgical procedures

20–30 ml local anesthetic solution, e.g., prilocaine 1%, bupivacaine 0.5%.

For pain therapy

20–30 ml local anesthetic solution, e.g., bupivacaine 0.125%–0.25%.

4. Special Complications

Intrathecal injection through incorrect needle placement.

5. Indications

Surgical procedures on the lower extremity including those in which a tourniquet is used, e.g.:

Open reduction and internal fixation of fractures (thigh and leg)
Meniscectomies
Bursectomies
Ligament repair
Management of ankle fractures
Removal of metal
Wound care
Skin transplants

Painful *diagnostic procedures*, e.g.,
Arthroscopies
Radiography to document ligament tears

6. Special Contraindications

None

7. Advantages–Disadvantages

Advantages

Suitable for outpatient surgery

Disadvantages

Higher local anesthetic level in the serum than after spinal anesthesia

II. Lumbar plexus block—inguinal paravascular approach

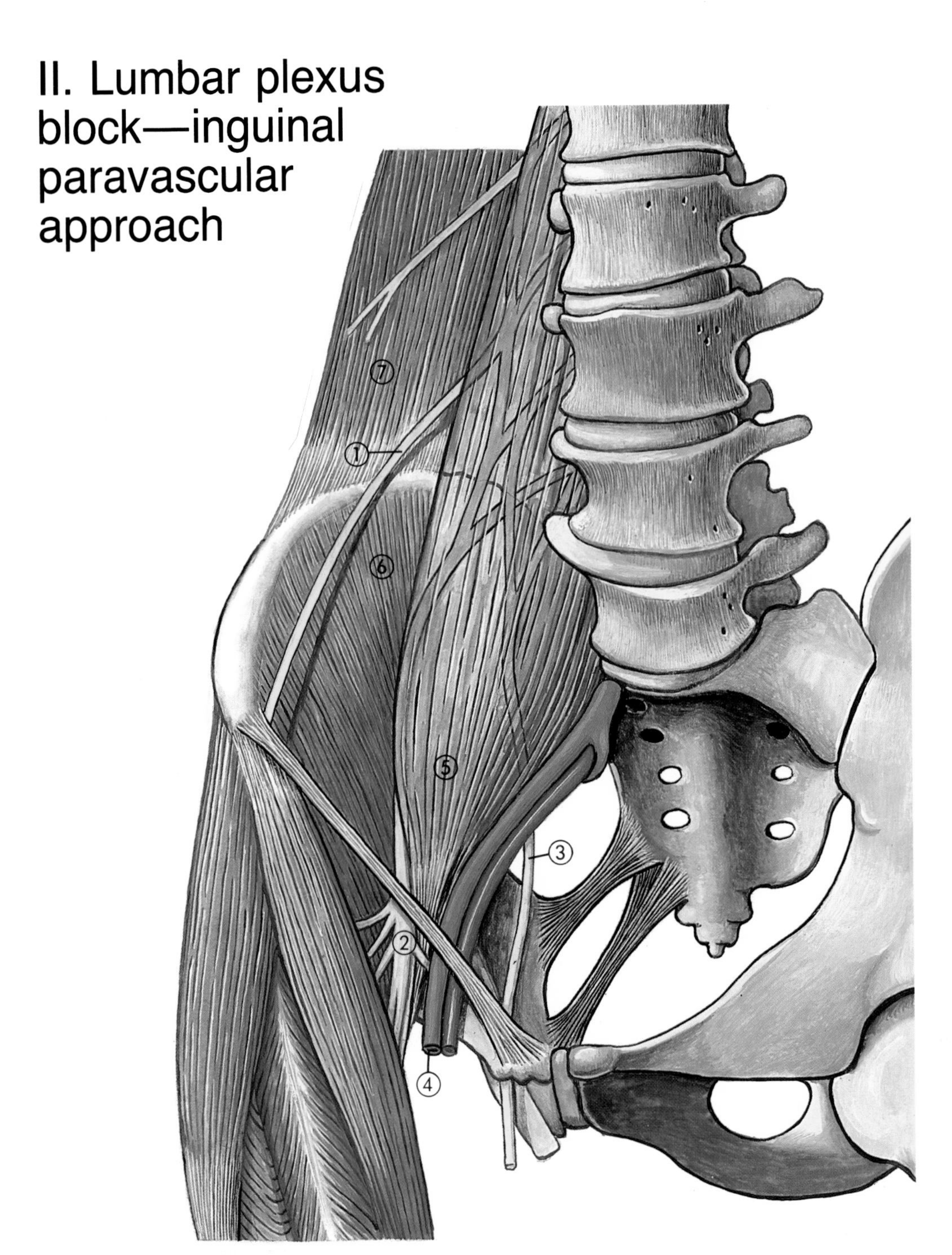

FIG 55.

The lumbar plexus is "sandwiched" (Winnie) between the psoas major m., the quadratus femoris m., and the iliac m. It is enclosed by the fascia of these muscles.

1. Lateral femoral cutaneous n.
2. Femoral n.
3. Obturator n.
4. Femoral a.
5. Psoas major m.
6. Iliac m.
7. Quadratus lumborum m.

1. Definition

The inguinal paravascular block of the lumbar plexus, described by Winnie, results in the block of the following nerves:

Femoral nerve (L_2–L_4)
Lateral femoral cutaneous nerve (L_2–L_3)
Obturator nerve (L_2–L_4)

2. Topographic Anatomy

The lumbar plexus is composed of the ventral branches of L_1–L_4 and runs in a "fascial space" between the psoas major m. and the quadratus lumborum m.

3. Technique

3.1. Anesthesiologic Assessment

Careful anesthesiologic assessment including the identification of any contraindication.

3.2. Preparation

Intravenous cannula, intubation setup, ventilation equipment with O_2 connection, atropine, sedative, succinylcholine, vasopressor, catecholamine.

3.3. Equipment

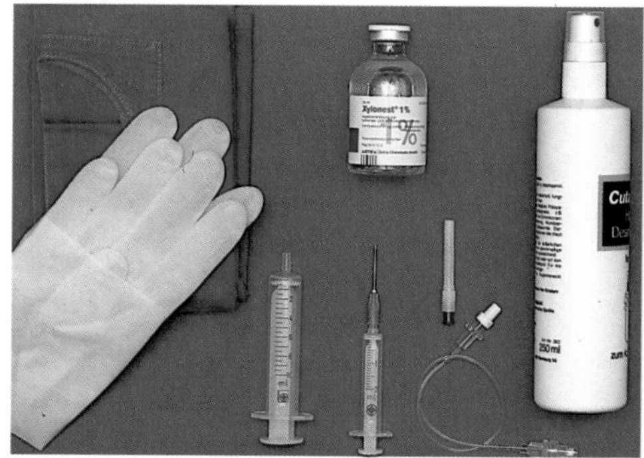

FIG 56.

Gloves
Drape with hole
Skin prep equipment
2 ml syringe with small needle for the skin wheal
22 g needle, 3–5 cm long
"Immobile needle" of Winnie

3.4. Positioning

The patient is in the supine position. Regardless of the side to be blocked, the right-handed anesthesiologist stands on the right side of the patient and the left-handed anesthesiologist stands on the left side.

3.5. Landmarks

The inguinal ligament (line between the anterior superior iliac spine and the pubic tubercle), the femoral artery (Figs 57 and 57a).

3.6. Technical Procedure

Preparing the skin with a suitable antiseptic solution. The area below the inguinal ligament is shaved and the femoral artery is identified by palpation. Approximately 1–1.5 cm laterally to the artery, a 22 g needle is introduced and advanced until paresthesias of the femoral nerve are elicited. After negative aspiration, the local anesthetic solution is injected. The needle can be directed slightly craniad during the injection. Finger pressure just below the needle will prevent a distal spread of the local anesthetic solution.
To establish a continuous 3-in-1 block, a catheter is introduced into the fascial space of the lumbar plexus by using an indwelling plastic needle.

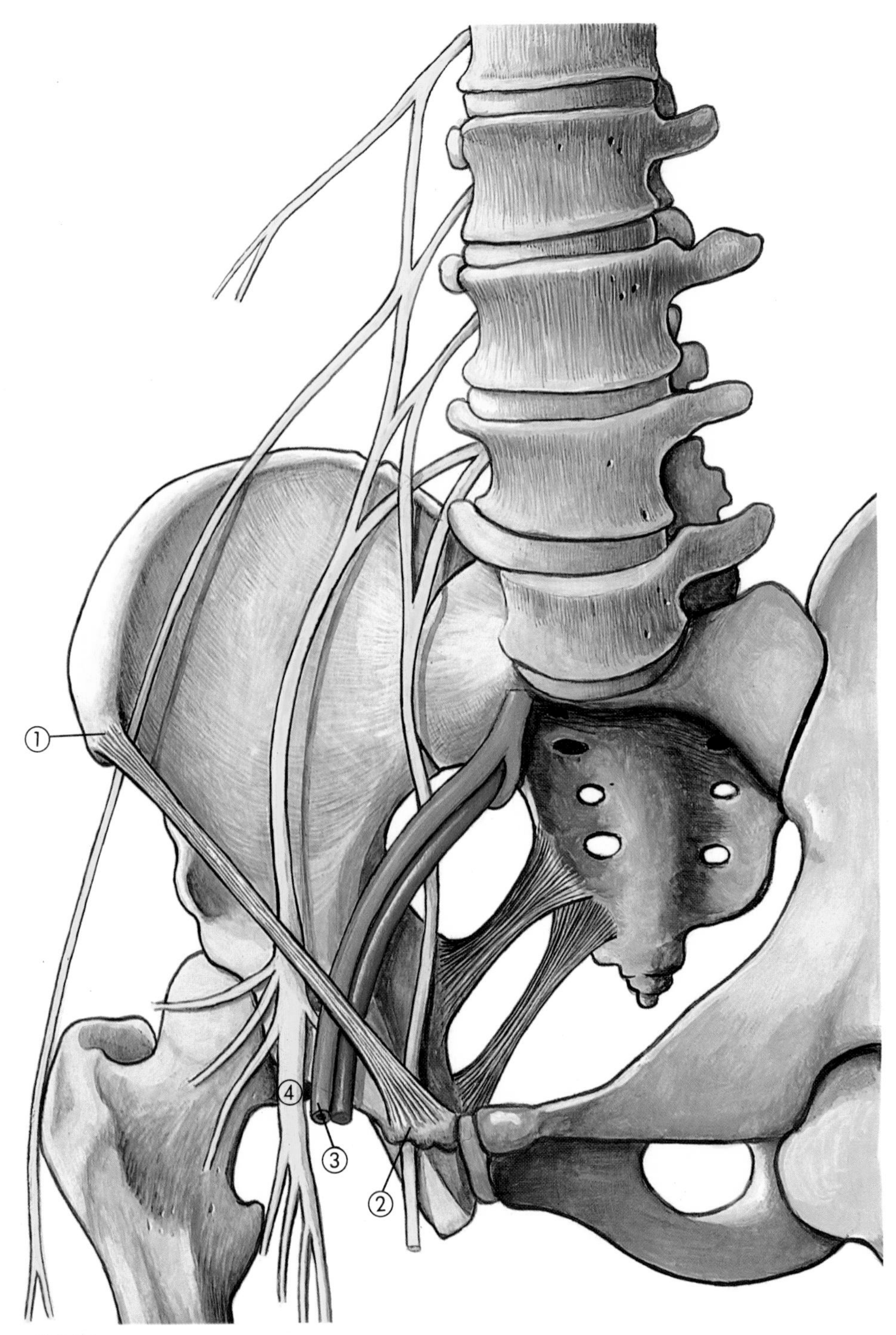

FIG 57.
1. Anterior-superior iliac spine
2. Pubic tubercle
3. Femoral a.
4. Femoral n.

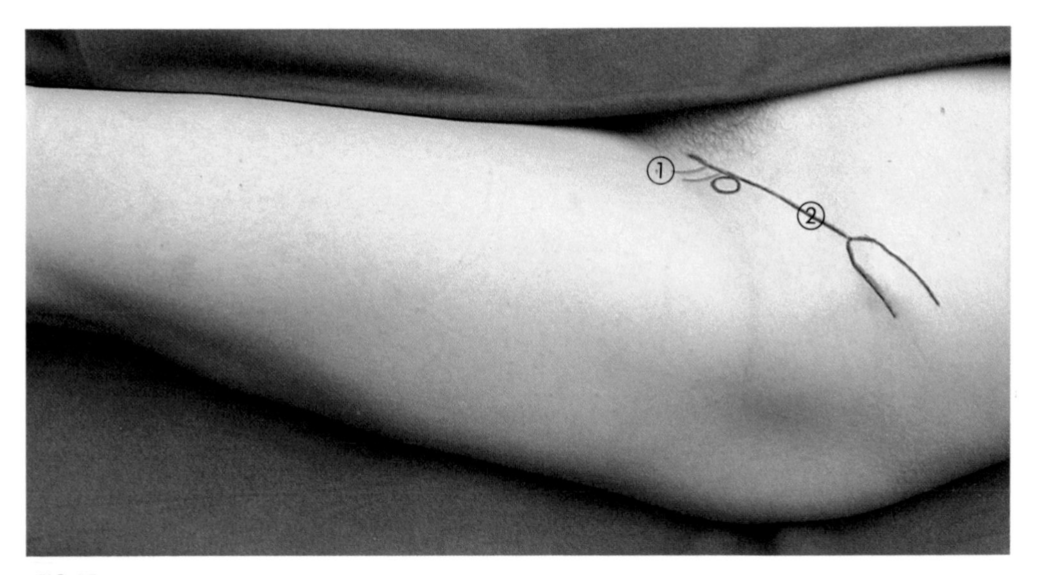

FIG 57 a.
1. Femoral a.
2. Inguinal ligament

3.7. Dosage

For surgical procedures

25–30 ml local anesthetic solution, e.g., prilocaine 1%, bupivacaine 0.5%.

For pain therapy

25–30 ml of the local anesthetic solution, e.g., bupivacaine 0.125%–0.25%.
The large volume is needed to accomplish a block of all three nerves. To block the femoral n. alone, only 5 ml are required.

4. Special Complications

None

5. Indications

For surgical procedures

To eliminate the obturator reflex in transurethral resections.
For wound care on the anterior surface of the thigh
In combination with a sciatic block for the performance of any surgical procedure in the region of the lower extremity
See "Psoas compartment block" (p. 67)

For pain therapy

In the area of the hip, thigh and knee
In pelvic fractures
Prior to the placement of an artificial joint

6. Special Contraindications

None

7. Advantages–Disadvantages

Advantages

Combining the 3-in-1 block with a sciatic n. block is a suitable procedure for outpatient surgery.

Disadvantages

Combining the 3-in-1 block with a sciatic n. block leads to a high concentration of the local anesthetic in the serum.

III. Sciatic nerve block

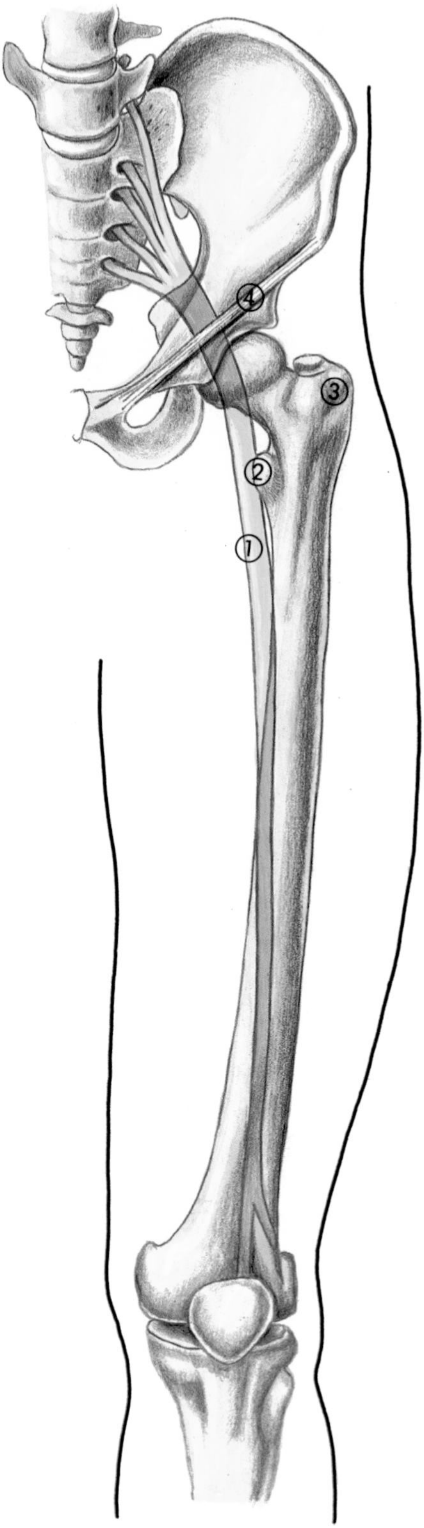

FIG 58.
(after Beck)
1. Sciatic n.
2. Lesser trochanter
3. Greater trochanter
4. Inguinal ligament

1. Definition

The sciatic block is the peripheral blockade of the nerves originating from the ventral branches of the lumbosacral plexus (L_4–S_3).

2. Topographic Anatomy

The sciatic nerve is a mixed nerve. It leaves the pelvis through the greater sciatic foramen and runs between the sciatic tuberosity and the greater trochanter on the posterior aspect of the thigh. In the popliteal fossa the nerve divides into its two terminal branches, the tibial n. and the common peroneal n. (Fig 58).

3. Technique

3.1. Anesthesiologic Assessment

Careful anesthesiologic assessment including the identification of any contraindication.

3.2. Preparation

Intravenous cannula, intubation setup, ventilation equipment with O_2 connection, atropine, sedative, succinylcholine, vasopressor, catecholamine.

3.3 Equipment

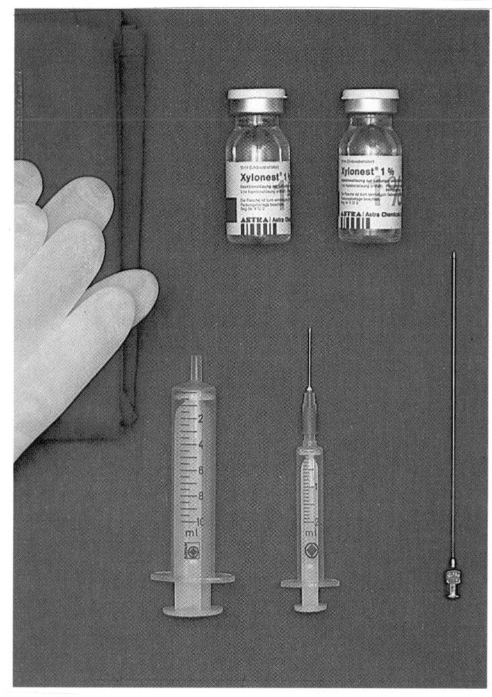

FIG 59.

Sterile gloves
Drape with hole
Skin prep equipment
2 ml syringe with small needle for the skin wheal
10–12 cm long needle
10 ml syringe
"Immobile needle" (Winnie)

There are two approaches to perform a sciatic n. block:

a. The *posterior sciatic n.* block (standard approach)
b. The *anterior sciatic n.* block

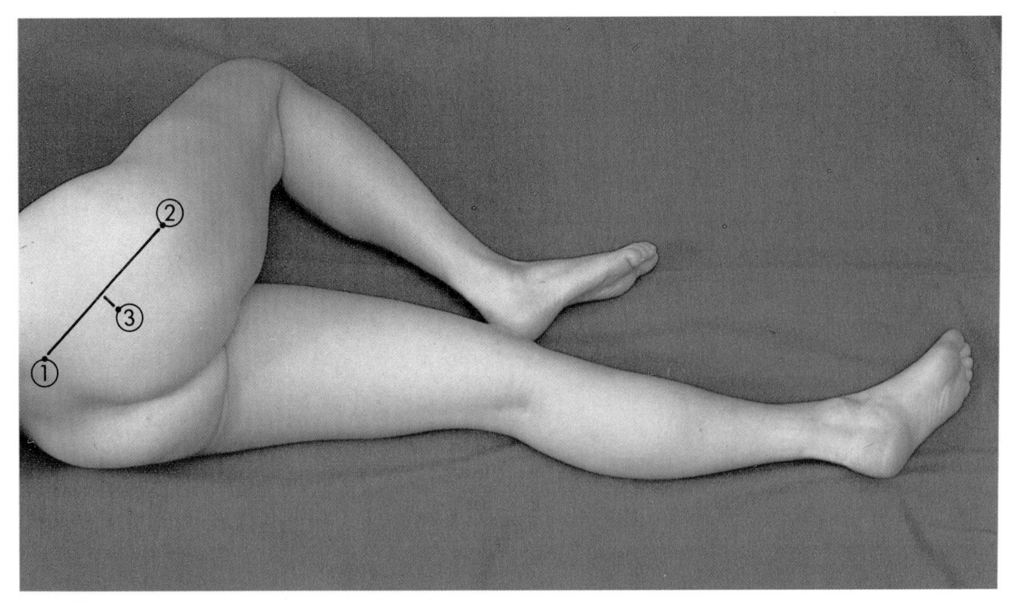

FIG 60.
1. Posterior superior iliac spine
2. Greater trochanter
3. Point of entry.

A. The posterior sciatic block

3.4 Positioning

Lateral position, resting on side that is not to be anesthetized: flexion of the extremity to be blocked 20–30° at the hip and 90° at the knee.

3.5. Landmarks

Posterior, superior iliac spine
Greater trochanter
(Fig 61)

3.6. Technical Procedure

Preparing the skin with a suitable antiseptic solution. The patient is on his/her side, the side to be blocked is "up" with a 20°–30° flexion at the hip and a 90° flexion at the knee.
The entry point is 3–4 cm at right angles and caudad from the midpoint of a line drawn between the greater trochanter and the posterior, superior iliac spine (Fig 60). After raising a skin wheal, a 10–12 cm long thin needle is introduced at right angles to the skin surface. After paresthesias have been elicited at a depth of 6–8 cm, and after a negative aspiration, the local anesthetic solution is injected.

3.7. Dosage

20–30 ml local anesthetic solution, e.g., prilocaine 1%, bupivacaine 0.5%.

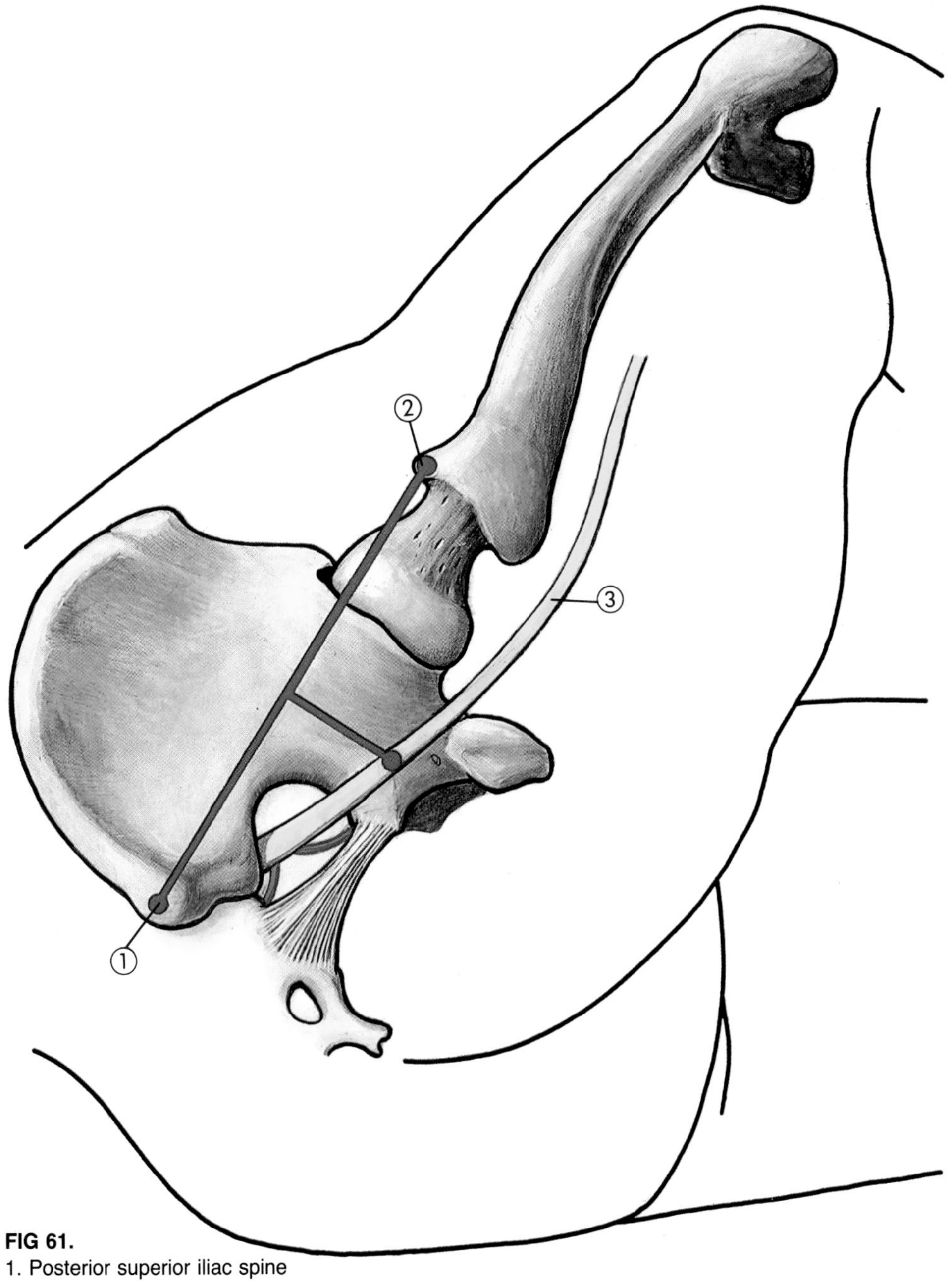

FIG 61.
1. Posterior superior iliac spine
2. Greater trochanter
3. Sciatic n.

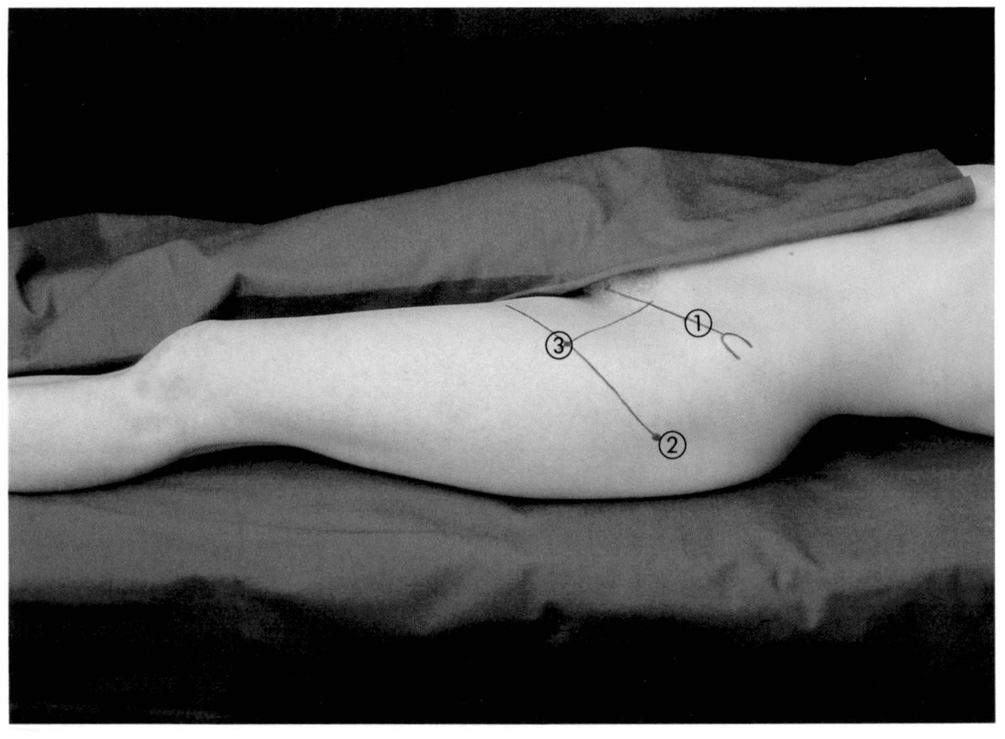

FIG 62. 1. Inguinal ligament 2. Greater trochanter 3. Point of entry

B. The anterior sciatic block

3.4. Positioning

Supine with the legs extended

3.5. Landmarks

Anterior superior iliac spine
Pubic tubercle
Greater trochanter
(Fig 63)

3.6. Technical Procedure

Preparing the skin with suitable antiseptic solution. The anterior superior iliac crest and the pubic tubercle are connected by a line (inguinal ligament) and the distance is divided into thirds. A parallel line is drawn through the greater trochanter. At the point between the medial third and the middle third, a line is drawn at a right angle to the greater trochanter line (Fig 62). The site of injection is at the point where these two lines cross. After a skin wheal is made, a 10–12 cm long needle is introduced at this point and advanced slightly laterally until bony contact is made on the anterior surface of the femur.

The needle is withdrawn into the subcutaneous area and its direction is adjusted until it glides off the femur. After advancing it another 5 cm and eliciting paresthesias, an aspiration test is performed and,

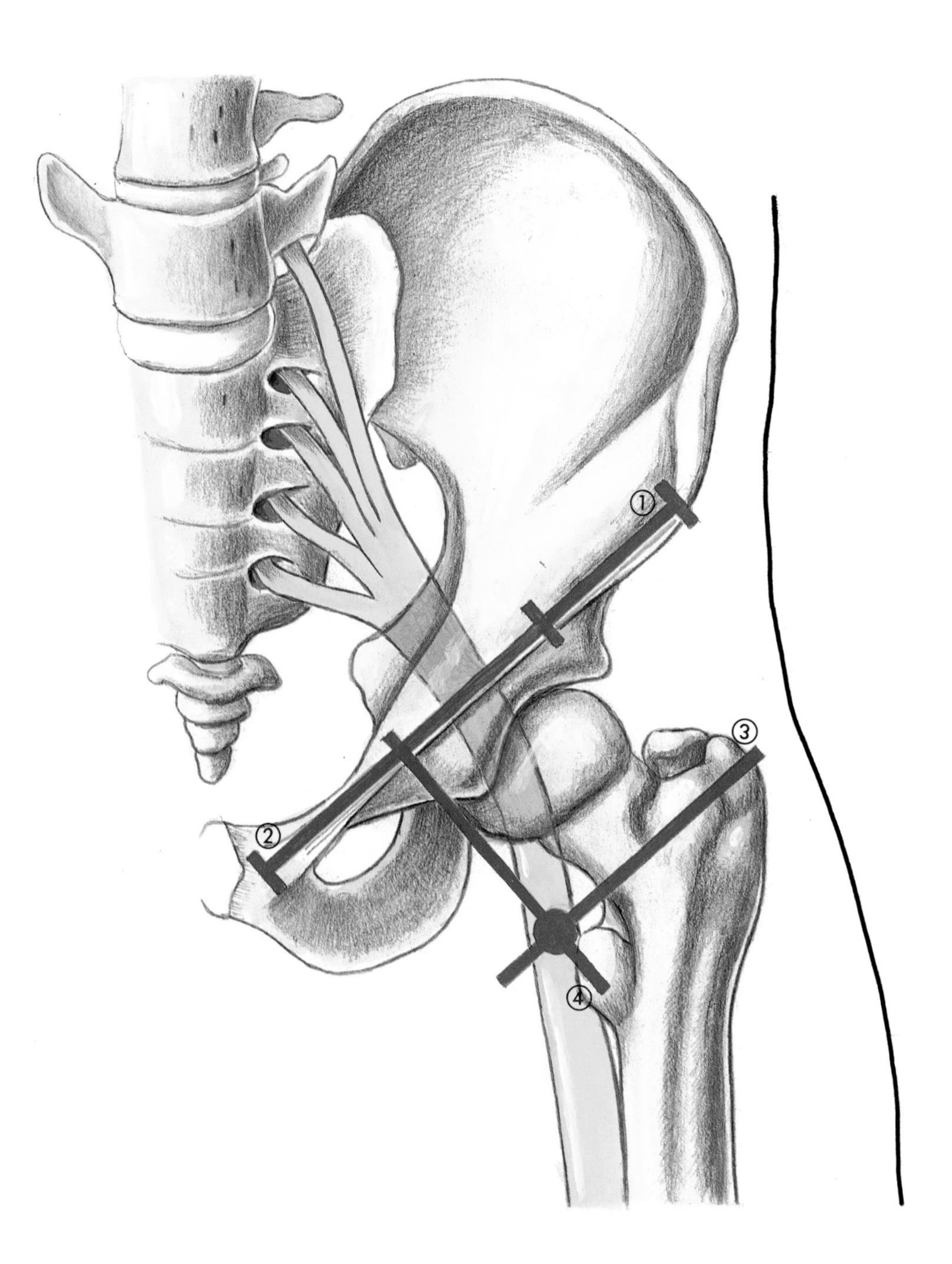

FIG 63.
1. Anterior superior iliac spine
2. Pubic tubercle
3. Greater trochanter
4. Sciatic n.

if the test is negative, the local anesthetic solution is injected. If there is resistance to the injection, the needle should be marginally adjusted since the tip of the needle is probably within the gluteus maximus m.

3.7. Dosage

10–20 ml local anesthetic solution, e.g., prilocaine 1%, bupivacaine 0.5%.

4. Special Complications

None

5. Indications

In combination with the 3-in-1 block all surgical procedures can be performed on the lower extremity, even those which require a tourniquet.

6. Special Contraindications

None

7. Advantages–Disadvantages

Advantages

(In combining of the 3-in-1 block and the sciatic n. block)

a. Suitable for outpatients
b. If the anterior approach is used, both blocks can be performed with the patient in the supine position (e.g., fracture patients)

Disadvantages

A combination of the 3-in-1 block and the sciatic n. block results in an elevated local anesthetic level in the serum.

References

1. Beck GP: Anterior approach to sciatic nerve block. *Anaesthesia* 1963; 18:222–224.
2. Chayen D, Nathan H, Chayen M: The psoas compartment block. *Anesthesiology* 1976; 15:95–99.
3. Gjessing J, Harly N: Sciatic and femoral nerve block with mepivacaine for surgery on the lower limb. *Anaesthesia* 1969; 24:213–218.
4. Winnie AP, Ramamurthy S, Durrani Z: The inguinal paravascular technic of lumbar plexus anesthesia. The "3-in-1 block." *Anesth Analg* 1973; 52:989–996.

Block of the Peripheral Nerves in the Area of the Knee Joint

W. Hoerster

I. The common peroneal nerve

1. Definition

Block of the common peroneal n. (L_4–S_2) at the head of the fibula.

2. Topographic Anatomy

The common peroneal n. is a mixed nerve which originates from the distal components of the lumbosacral plexus, and runs jointly with the tibial n. and the sciatic n. from the pelvis through the infrapiriform sinus on the dorsal aspect of the shaft of the femur.

In the proximal angle of the popliteal fossa, the peroneal n. separates from this joint course and proceeds laterally under the biceps femoris m. on the lateral edge of the gastrocnemius m. in a distal direction. It appears under the tendon of the biceps femoris, gives off a sensory branch to the skin, and the lateral cutaneous sural n., and makes a half turn around the neck of the fibula, ventrally over the tendon insertion of the fibularis longus m. It disappears through the muscular insertion in the fibular space deep in the muscles of the leg, having divided into its two terminal branches, the superficial peroneal n. and the deep peroneal n.

3. Technique

3.1. Anesthesiologic Assessment

Careful anesthesiologic assessment including the identification of any contraindication.

3.2. Preparation

Intravenous cannula, intubation setup, ventilation equipment with O_2 connection, atropine, sedative, succinylcholine, vasopressor, catecholamine.

3.3. Equipment

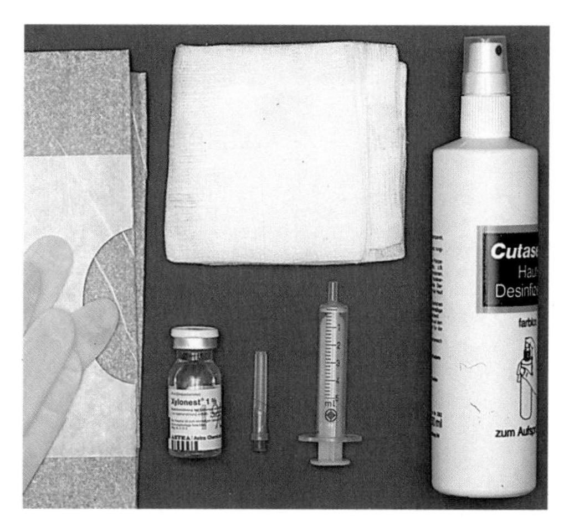

FIG 64.

Drape with hole
Sterile gloves
Skin prep equipment
5 ml syringe
2–3 cm (16–18 g) needle

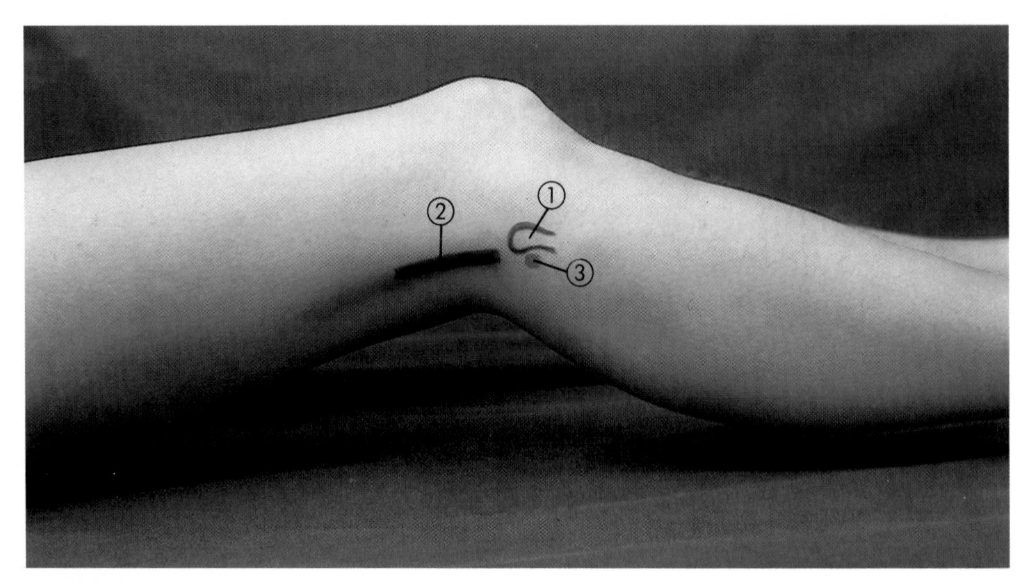

Fig 65.
1. Head of the fibula
2. Tendon of the biceps femoris m.
3. Point of entry (peroneal block)

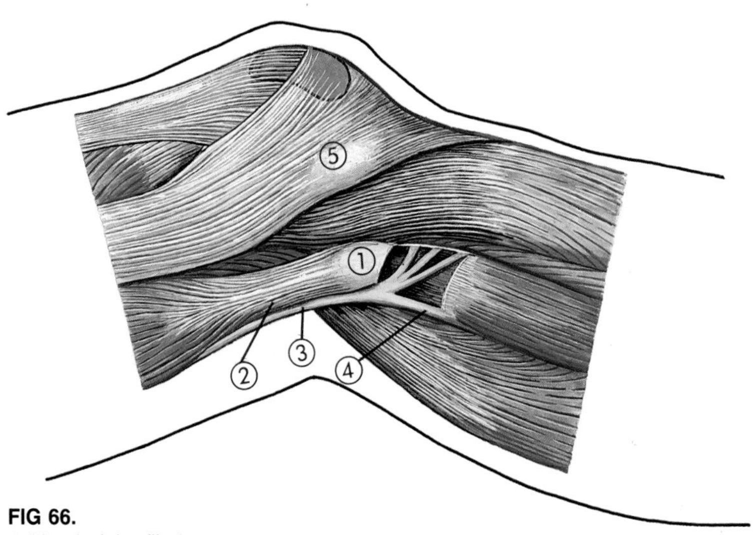

FIG 66.
1. Head of the fibula
2. Tendon of the biceps femoris m.
3. Common peroneal n.
4. Lateral sural cutaneous n.
5. Tibial tubercle

3.4. Positioning

Patient in the supine position with legs extended.

3.5. Landmarks

Head of the fibula
Tendon of the biceps femoris m.
Tubercle of the iliotibial tract

3.6. Technical procedure

Topographic orientation, palpation and marking of the landmarks.
Preparing the skin with a suitable antiseptic solution. After making a skin wheal 2 cm below the head of the fibula, the needle is introduced vertically and advanced about 1 cm at the dorsal edge.
After paresthesias have been elicited and the aspiration test is negative in two planes, 5 ml of local anesthetic solution are injected into the space directly behind the head of the fibula.

3.7. Dosage

5 ml local anesthetic solution e.g., prilocaine 1%, bupivacaine 0.5%.

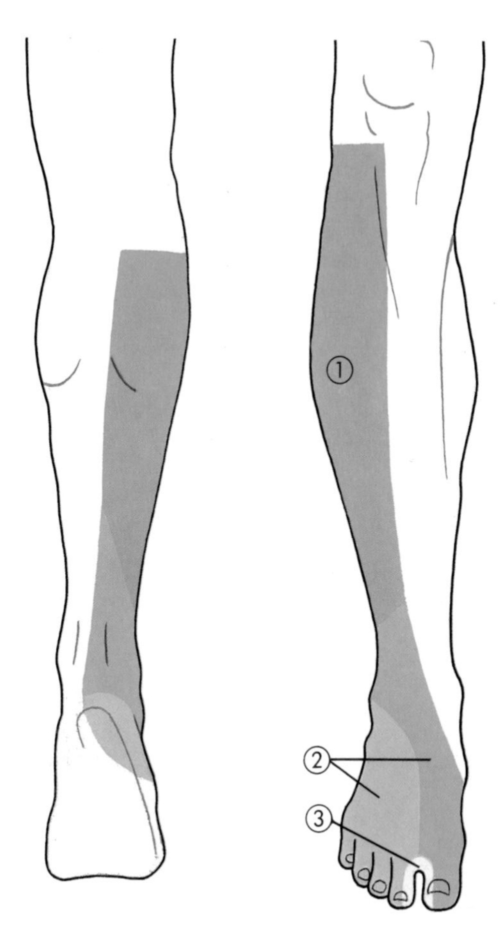

FIG 67.
Area of cutaneous sensory innervation, common fibular n.
1. Lateral sural cutaneous n.
2. Superficial peroneal n.
3. Deep peroneal n.

4. Special Complications

Peroneal neuritis
Peroneal paresis (difficult to distinguish from damage caused by the pressure of a cast or malposition)

5. Indications

Supplementation of an incomplete sciatic n. block.
Supplementation of an incomplete epidural anesthetic.
Diagnostic, therapeutic, and surgical procedures in the sensory area of innervation, particularly for external malleolar fracture and external ligament rupture.

6. Special Contraindications

Peroneal paresis
Peroneal neuritis

7. Advantages–Disadvantages

Advantages

Very simple technique with guaranteed success, particularly suitable for outpatient surgery.

Disadvantages

Peroneal neuritis and paresis are possible.

II. The tibial nerve

1. Definition

Block of the tibial n. (L_4–S_3) in the distal angle of the popliteal fossa.

2. Topographic Anatomy

The tibial n. is a mixed nerve which originates from the distal components of the lumbosacral plexus and which emerges jointly with the common peroneal n. and the sciatic n. from the pelvis through the infrapiriform foramen onto the dorsal aspect of the shaft of the femur.
In the area of the knee joint, the tibial n. appears at the proximal corner of the popliteal fossa and transverses it superficially in the middle, surrounded by fat and connective tissue in the company of the popliteal a. and v. It disappears between the two heads of the gastrocnemius m., passes below the arcus tendineus of the soleus m., and proceeds between the superficial and deep plantar-flexors in the direction of the ankle.

3. Technique

3.1. Anesthesiologic Assessment

Careful anesthesiologic assessment including the identification of any contraindication.

3.2. Preparation

Intravenous cannula, intubation set-up, ventilation equipment with O_2 connection, atropine, sedative, succinylcholine, vasopressor, catecholamine.

3.3. Equipment

Drape with hole
Sterile gloves
Skin prep equipment
2 ml, 5 ml, and 10 ml syringes
Needle 2–3 cm long (25 g) for skin wheal
Needle 3–5 cm long (20 g)
"Immobile needle" (Winnie)

3.4. Positioning

Patient in prone position.
The extremity to be blocked is extended.

3.5. Landmarks

Medial epicondyle of the humerus
Lateral epicondyle of the humerus
Medial and lateral head of the gastrocnemius

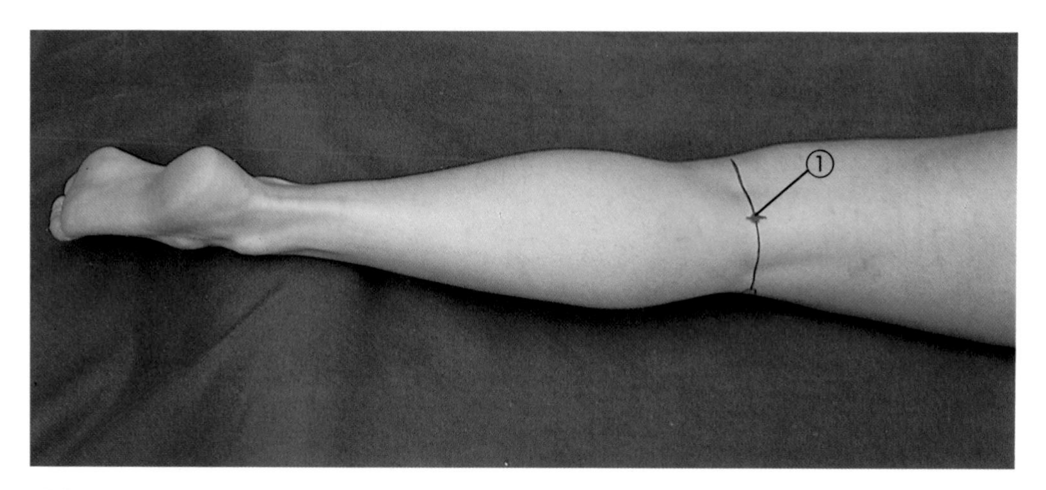

FIG 68.
1. Popliteal a.

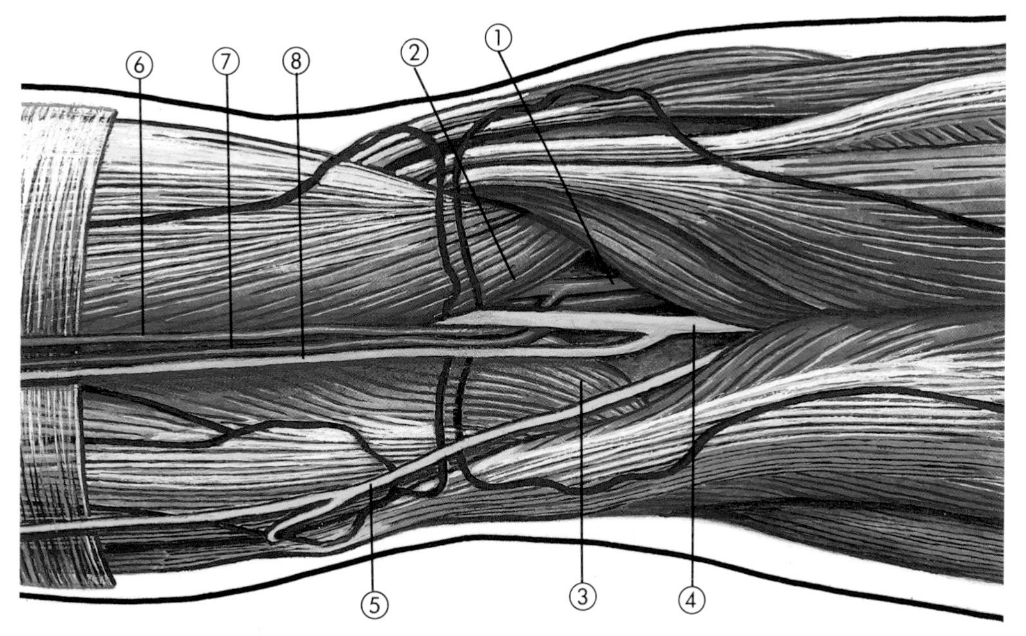

FIG 69.
1. Popliteal a.
2. Medial head of the gastrocnemius m.
3. Lateral head of the gastrocnemius m.
4. Tibial n.
5. Common peroneal n.
6. Sural a.
7. Lesser saphenous v.
8. Sural n.

3.6. Technical Procedure

Topographic orientation, palpation and marking of the landmarks; drawing a line between the medial and lateral epicondyle of the femur, marking the midpoint of this line.

Preparing the skin with a suitable antiseptic solution. Placing a skin wheal at the midpoint of the line across the popliteal fossa. The needle is introduced vertically at this point and advanced approximately 1.5–3 cm. After eliciting paresthesias and following a negative aspiration test in two planes, 10 ml of local anesthetic solution are injected. If the needle is in the body of the popliteus m. or in one of the heads of the gastrocnemius m., a springy resistance is felt on injection. If the tip of the needle is in the fat/connective tissue area, resistance to injection should be minimal.

3.7. Dosage

5–10 ml local anesthetic solution, e.g. prilocaine 1%, bupivacaine 0.5%.

4. Special Complications

None

5. Indications

Supplementation of an incomplete sciatic n. block. Supplementation of an incomplete epidural block. Diagnostic, therapeutic, and surgical procedures in the area of sensory innervation. In combination with a common peroneal n. and saphenous n. block, any procedure in the region of the leg and foot.

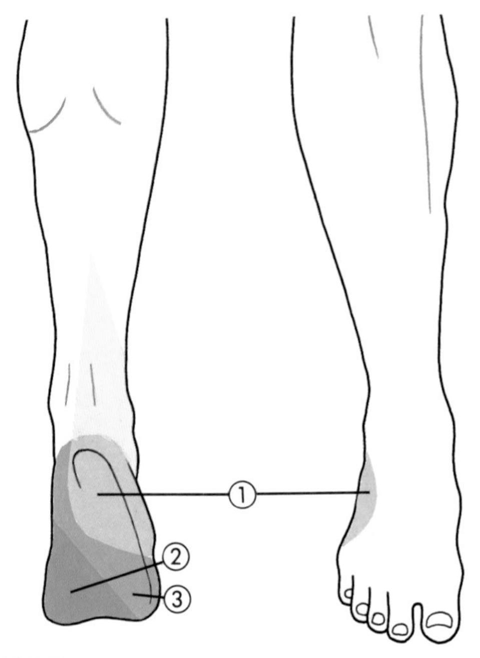

FIG 70.
Area of sensory cutaneous innervation, tibial n.
1. Sural n.
2. Medial plantar n.
3. Lateral plantar n.

6. Special Contraindications

None

7. Advantages–Disadvantages

Advantages

Particularly suitable for outpatient surgery.

Disadvantages

Technically demanding block.

III. The saphenous nerve

1. Definition

Block of the saphenous n. (L_1–L_4) at the pes anserinus, over the medial condyle of the tibia, proximal to the greater saphenous vein.

2. Topographic Anatomy

The saphenous n. is the sensory terminal branch of the femoral n. From the common course with the femoral artery and vein it proceeds medially, passes under the sartorius m., and pierces the fascia of the knee between the tendons of the sartorius m. and gracilis m., slightly below the popliteal fossa. It passes over the pes anserinus (tendon insertion of the gracilis, semitendinosus and semimembranosus mm.) and follows the greater saphenous v. subcutaneously, on the surface of the tibia medially to the gastrocnemius m., in the direction of the medial aspect of the ankle. The infrapatellar and medial cutaneous branches provide sensory innervation to the medial and anterior portions of the leg.

3. Technique

3.1. Anesthesiologic Assessment

Careful anesthesiologic assessment including the identification of any contraindication.

3.2. Preparation

Intravenous cannula, intubation setup, ventilation equipment with O_2 connection, atropine, sedative, succinylcholine, vasopressor, catecholamine.

3.3. Equipment

Drape with hole
Sterile gloves
Skin prep equipment
10 ml syringe
Needle 3–5 cm long (20 g)

3.4. Positioning

Patient in prone position with legs extended.

3.5. Landmarks

Medial condyle of the tibia
Pes anserinus
Tibial tuberosity
Gastrocnemius m.
(Figs 71, 72)

3.6. Technical Procedure

Topographic orientation, palpation and marking of the landmarks. Preparing the skin with a suitable antiseptic solution. Subcutaneous infiltration of the area from the medial aspect of the tibial tuberosity, over the medial condyle of the tibia, in the direction of the gastrocnemius m.

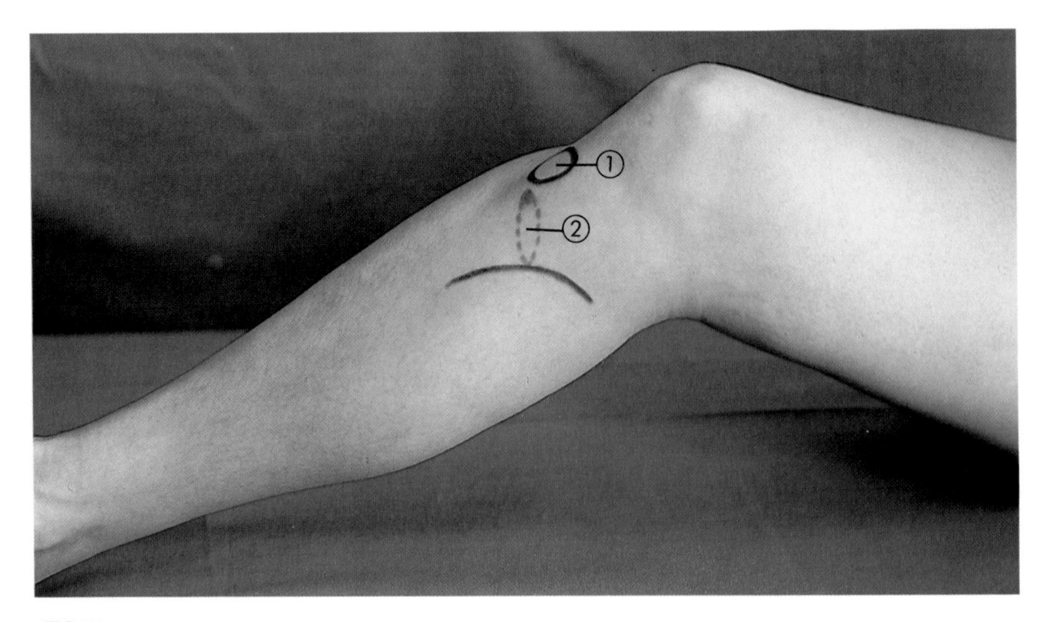

FIG 71.
1. Tibial tuberosity
2. Subcutaneous infiltration

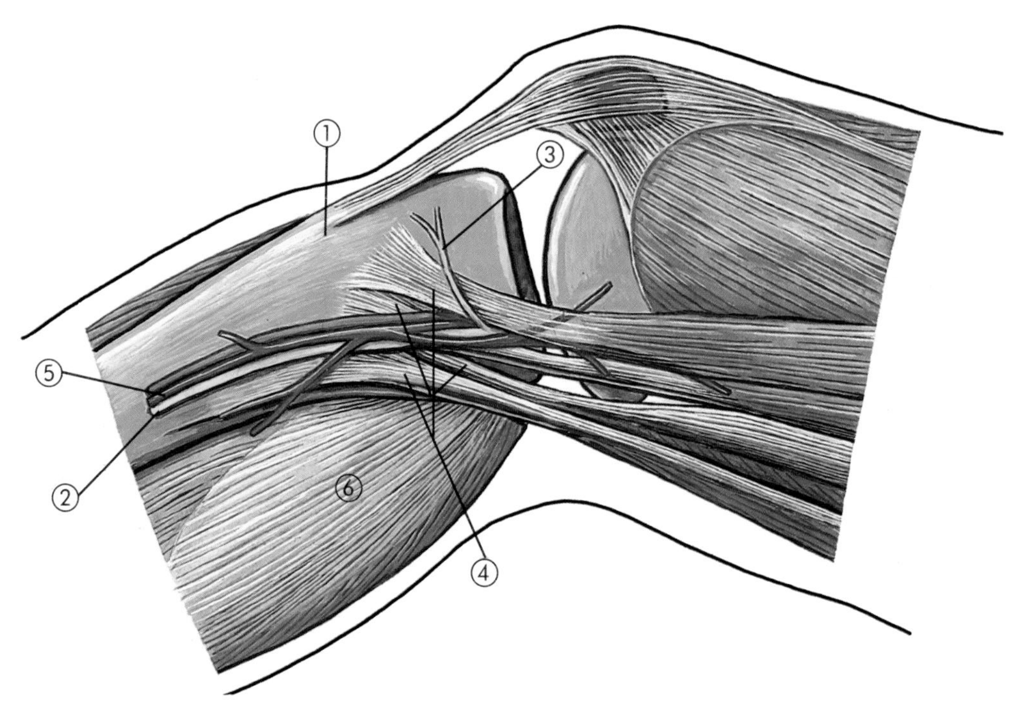

FIG 72.
1. Tibial tuberosity
2. Saphenous n.
3. Infrapatellar branch
4. Pes anserinus
5. Greater saphenous v.
6. Gastrocnemius m.

3.7. Dosage

5–10 ml local anesthetic solution, e.g., prilocaine 1%, bupivacaine 0.5%.

4. Special Complications

None

5. Indications

Supplementation of an incomplete femoral n. block. Diagnostic, therapeutic, and surgical procedures in the area of sensory innervation on the medial surface of the leg and the medial area of the ankle. Particularly suitable for varicose vein procedures.
In combination with blocks of the tibial and peroneal nn., any surgical procedure on the entire leg and foot.

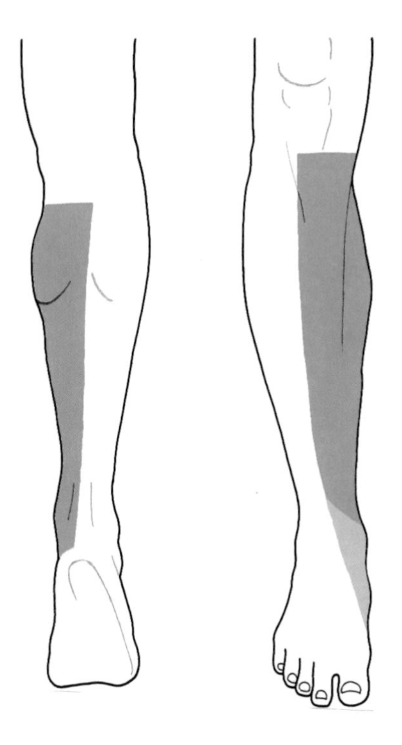

FIG 73.
Area of cutaneous sensory innervation, saphenous n.

6. Special Contraindications

None

7. Advantages–Disadvantages

Advantage

Technically simple procedure, particularly suitable for outpatient surgery.

Disadvantage

Increased danger of intravascular injection in patients with varicose vessels.

Blocks in the Area of the Ankle (Foot Block)

W. Hoerster

The foot is innervated by the five terminal branches of the primary nerves of the lumbosacral plexus.

In view of the wide anatomic variations in the location of these nerves, and in view of the possible anastomoses between them, it is advisable to perform a complete foot block for all diagnostic, therapeutic, or surgical procedures on the foot and not to limit the block to just a single nerve.

The "Technical Procedure" section will therefore be handled as a unit, following the discussion of the topography.

1. Definition

Blockade of all the nerves serving the foot at the level of the proximal ankle joint.

It includes the following nerves:

Tibial n.
Deep peroneal n.
Superficial peroneal n.
Sural n.
Saphenous n.

2. Topographic Anatomy

Tibial nerve

The tibial n. crosses the leg between the superficial and deep plantar–flexors and reaches the medial aspect of the ankle between the Achilles tendon and the tendons of the flexor digitorum longus and tibialis posterior mm, immediately adjoining the tibial a. and v. It proceeds distally around the internal malleolus, gives off the medial calcaneus branches to the heel, and then divides into two main branches, the median and lateral plantar nn. which supply the sensory innervation to the sole of the foot (Fig 74).

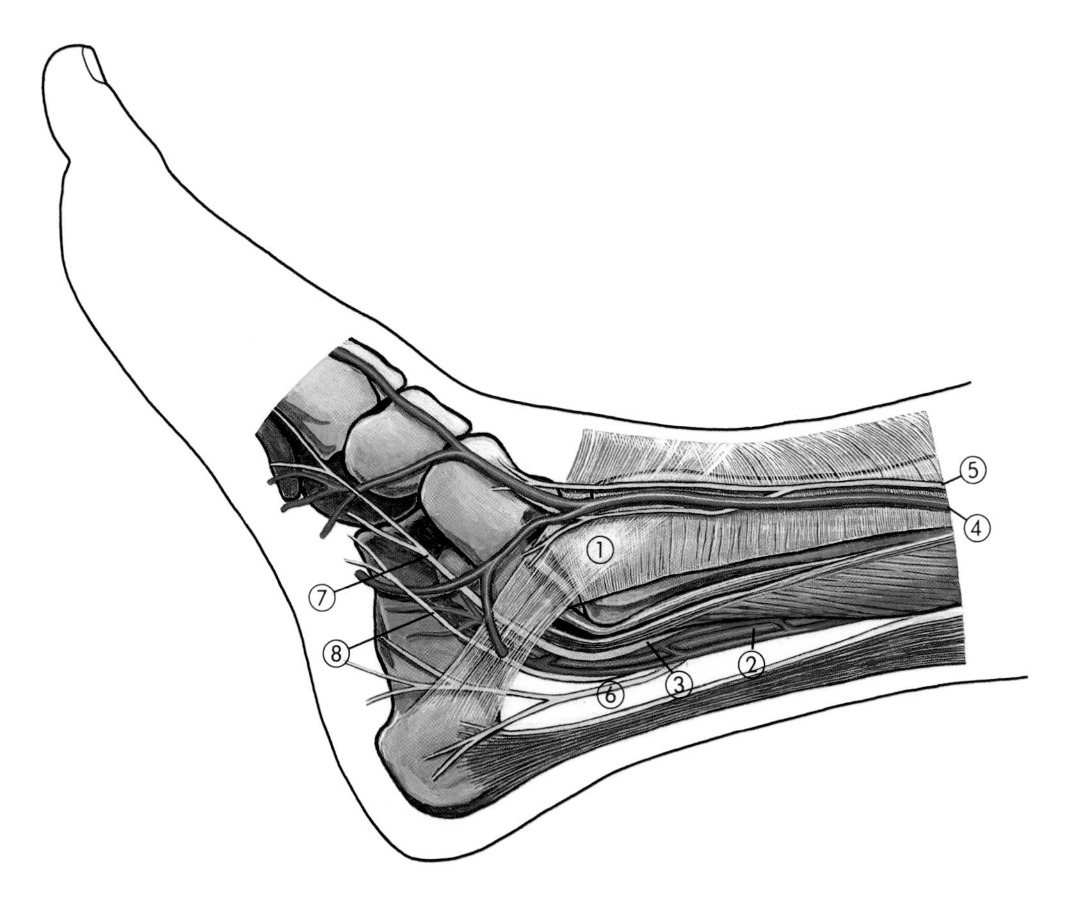

FIG 74.
1. Internal malleolus
2. Tibial a.
3. Tibial n.
4. Greater saphenous v.
5. Saphenous n.
6. Medial calcaneous branches
7. Medial plantar n.
8. Lateral plantar n.

The deep peroneal nerve

The deep peroneal n. runs in the leg in the dorsiflexor space and reaches the surface between the tendons of the extensors of the toes above the ankle.
It passes under the cruciform ligament together with the dorsalis pedis a. and proceeds along the dorsum of the foot, directly below the fascia, between the tendon of the extensor hallucis longus m. and the tendon of the extensor digitorum communis m. It follows the dorsalis pedis a., lying either laterally or inferiorly to it, to the area between the great toe and the second toe, for both of which it provides sensory innervation.

Superficial peroneal nerve

The superficial peroneal n. reaches the lateral area of the distal portion of the leg under the fibularis longus and brevis mm. After perforating the fascia cruris it spreads out in a fan-shaped fashion, runs subcutaneously, and provides sensory innervation to the dorsum of the foot and of the toes through its terminal branches, the medial and intermedial dorsal cutaneous nerves (Fig 75).

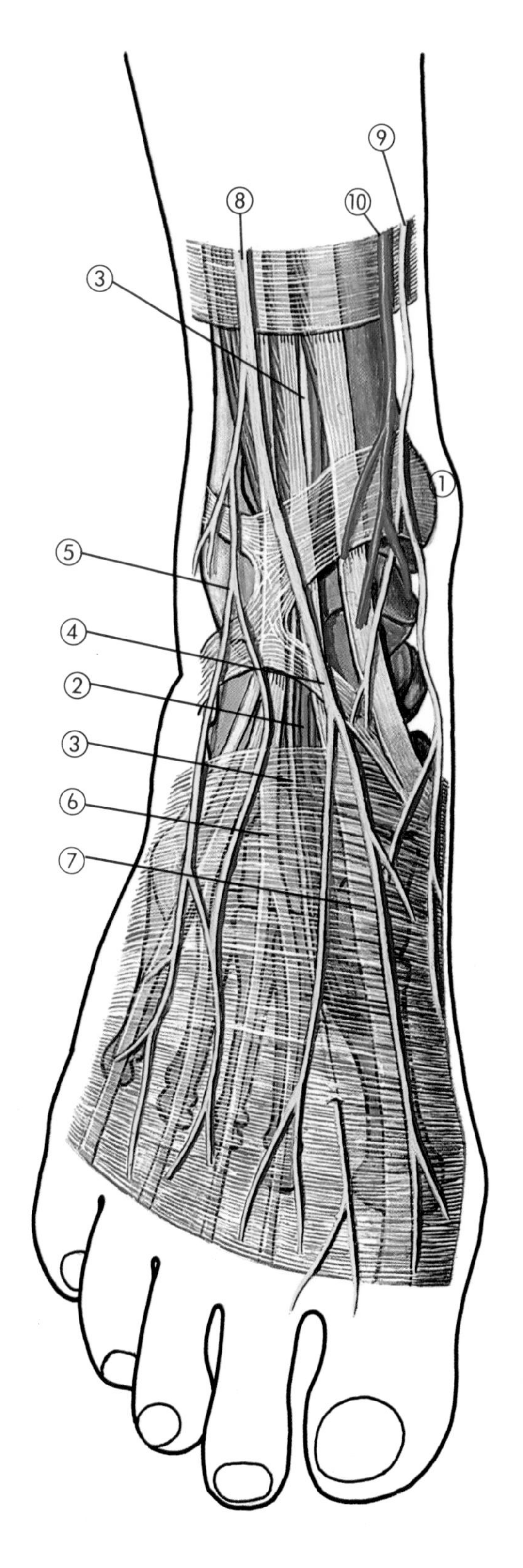

FIG 75.
1. Internal malleolus
2. Dorsalis pedis a.
3. Deep peroneal n.
4. Medial dorsal cutaneous n.
5. Intermediate dorsal cutaneous n.
6. Tendon of the extensor digitorum communis m.
7. Tendon of the extensor hallucis longus m.
8. Superficial peroneal n.
9. Saphenous n.
10. Greater saphenous v.

The sural nerve

The sural is the joint terminal branch of the tibial nerve and the superficial peroneal nerve. The anastomosis usually takes place in the middle third of the leg, at the level of the extensor muscles of the toes. The sensory terminal branch perforates the fascia cruris below the gastrocnemius m. and runs between the Achilles tendon and the external malleolus distally. At this point it divides into its sensory terminal branches, the lateral calcaneus branches which provide the heel with sensory innervation, and the lateral dorsal cutaneous n. which innervates the lateral edge of the foot to the fifth toe (Fig 76).

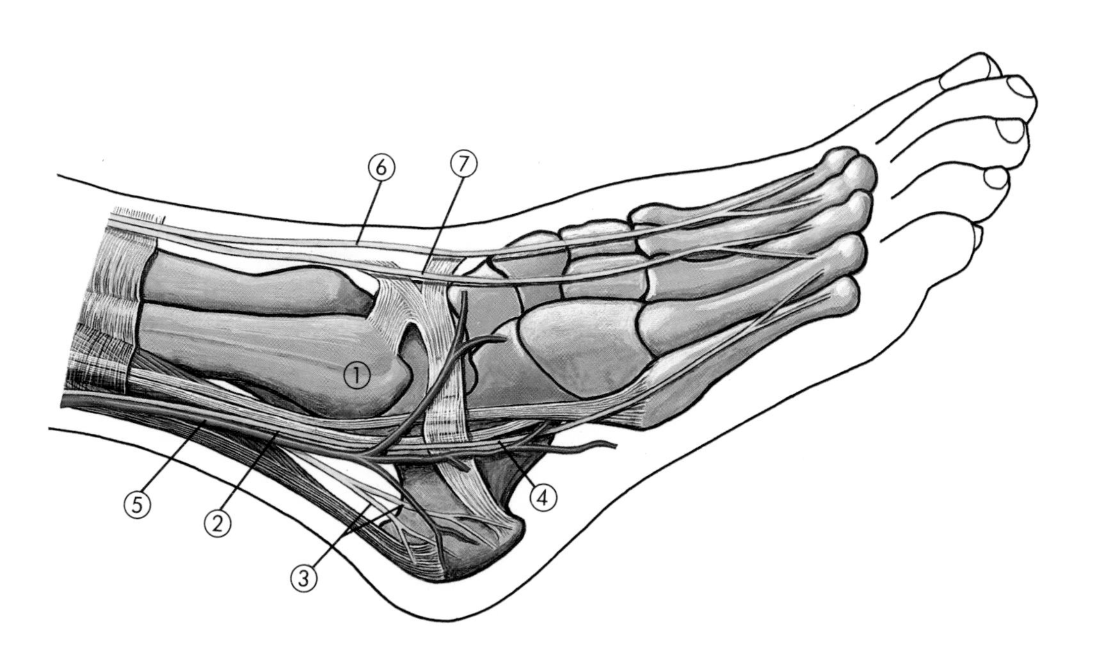

FIG 76.
1. External malleolus
2. Sural n.
3. Lateral calcaneous branches
4. Lateral dorsal cutaneous n.
5. Lesser saphenous v.
6. Medial dorsal cutaneous n.
7. Intermediate dorsal cutaneous n.

The saphenous nerve

The saphenous n. accompanies the greater saphenous vein and reaches the medial surface of the ankle between the edge of the tibia and the internal malleolus. It divides into its terminal branches in the subcutaneous tissues above the fascia cruris and provides the area of the internal malleolus and the medial aspect of the dorsum of the foot, including the medial edge with sensory innervation.

3. Technique

3.1. Anesthesiologic Assessment

> Careful anesthesiologic assessment including the identification of any contraindication.

3.2. Preparation

> Intravenous cannula, intubation setup, ventilation equipment with O_2 connection, atropine, sedative, succinylcholine, vasopressor, catecholamine.

3.3. Equipment

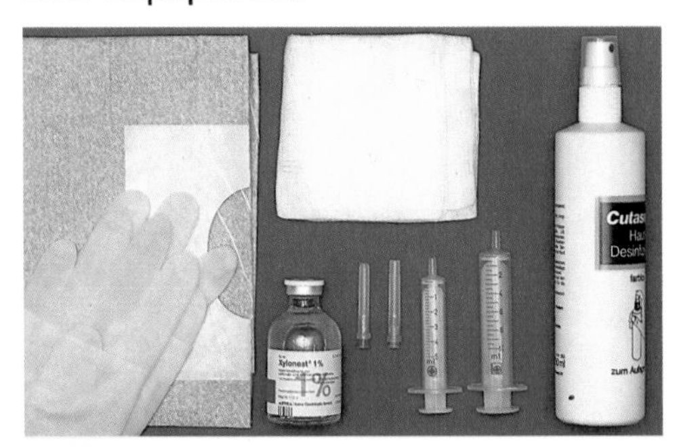

FIG 77.

Drape with hole
Sterile gloves
Skin prep equipment
5 ml syringe
25 g needle
10 ml syringe with 21 g needle
Sponges

3.4. Positioning

Patient in prone position with legs extended.

3.5. Landmarks

Internal malleolus
External malleolus
Edge of the tibia
Achilles tendon
Tibial a.
Dorsalis pedis a.

3.6. Technical Procedure

Topographic orientation. Palpation and marking of the landmarks, particularly the pulsations of the tibial and dorsalis pedis arteries. Preparing the skin with a suitable antiseptic solution.

Tibial nerve

Immediately medial to the tibial artery, a 2–3 cm long, fine needle is introduced at right angles to the skin and advanced 0.5–2 cm. The tip of the needle should be directly next to or below the artery. After negative aspiration in two planes, 2–3 ml local anesthetic solution are injected.
Because of anatomic variations, repeat on the opposite side (Fig 78).

Deep peroneal nerve

Immediately medial to the dorsalis pedis a., on the dorsum of the foot, a thin, 2–3 cm long needle is introduced at right angles to the skin, and the tip of the needle is advanced to lie directly next to or just under the artery.
After negative aspiration, 2–3 ml local anesthetic solution are injected. Because of anatomic variation, the injection should be repeated on the other side of the artery (Fig 79).

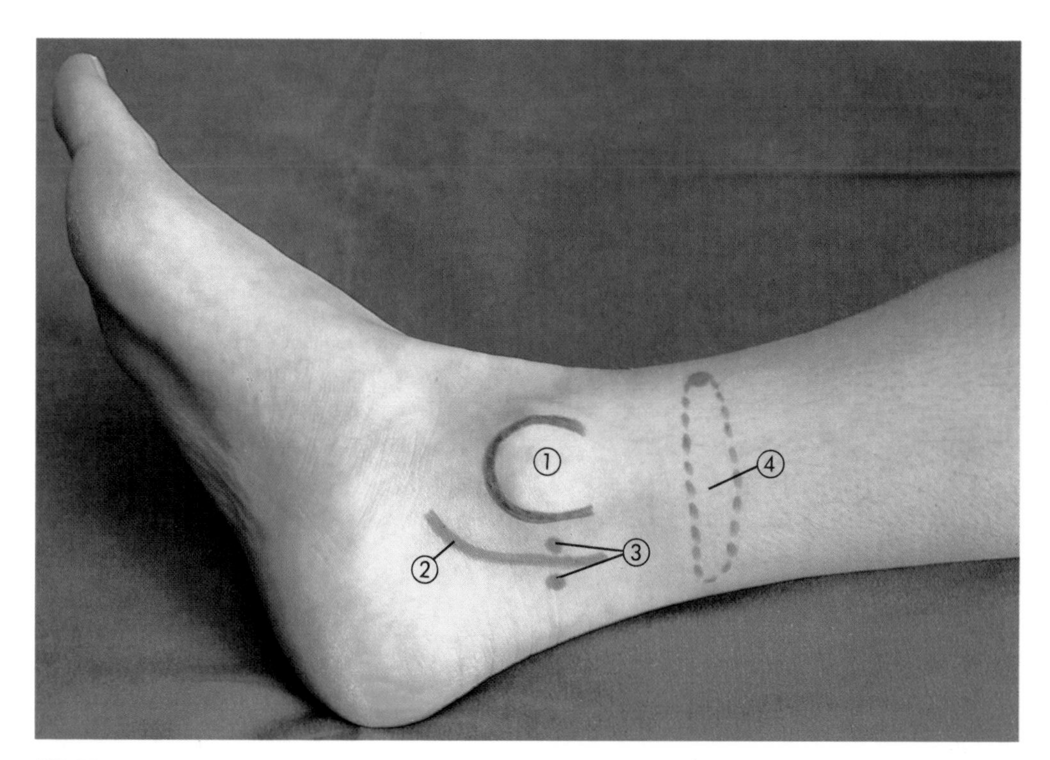

FIG 78.
1. Internal malleolus
2. Tibial a.
3. Point of entry (tibial block)
4. Subcutaneous infiltration (saphenous block)

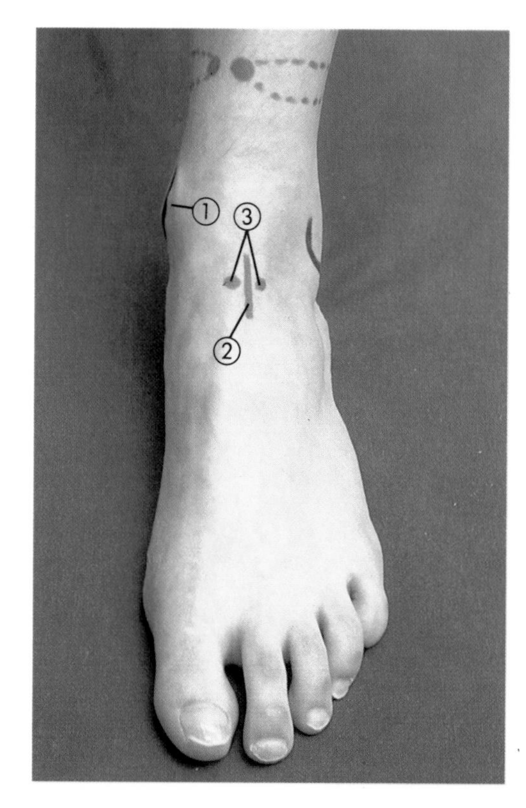

FIG 79.
1. Internal malleolus
2. Dorsalis pedis a.
3. Point of entry (deep peroneal block)

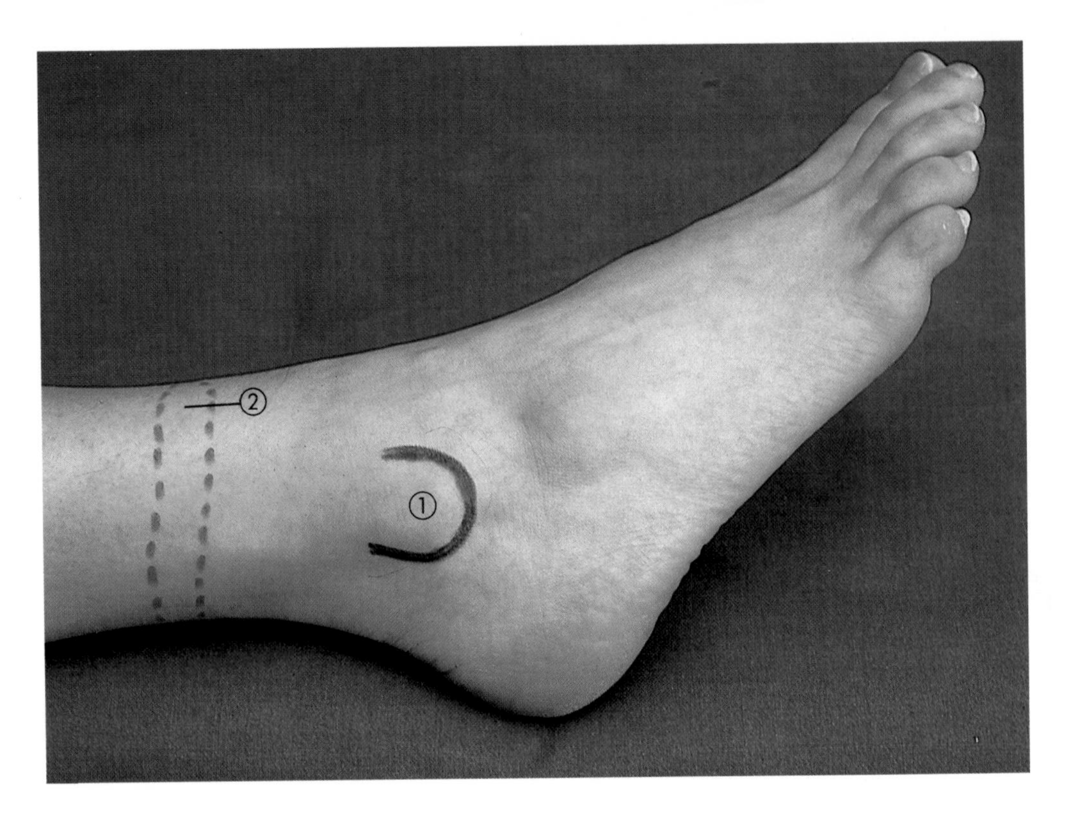

FIG 80.
1. External malleolus
2. Point of entry

Superficial peroneal and sural nerves

From the edge of the tibia to the Achilles tendon, a subcutaneous ring block is performed approximately one hand's breadth from the external malleolus and parallel to the upper ankle joint (Fig 80).

Saphenous nerve

From the edge of the tibia to the Achilles tendon, a subcutaneous ring block is performed approximately one hand's breadth above the inner malleolus (Fig 78).

3.7. Dosage

For the tibial n. and the deep peroneal n., 5 ml local anesthetic solution each. For the subcutaneous ring block, 10–20 ml local anesthetic solution, e.g., prilocaine 1%, bupivacaine 0.25–0.5%.

4. Special Complications

None

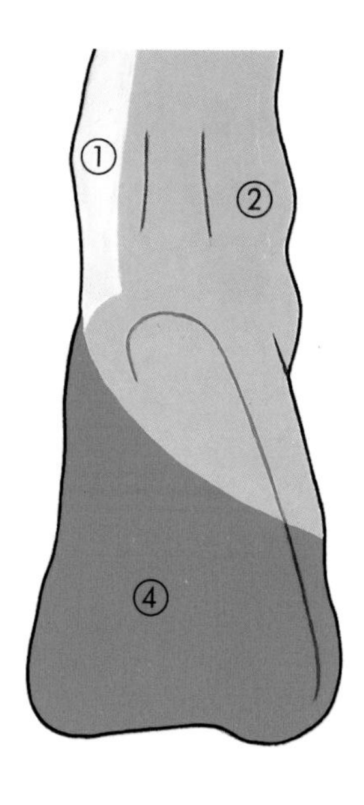

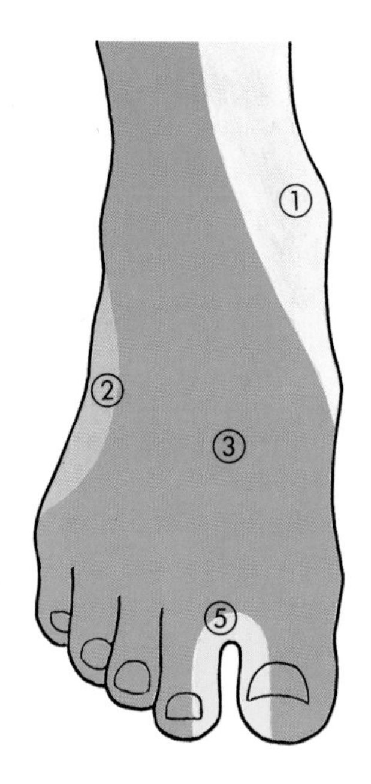

FIG 81.
Area of analgesia, foot block:
1. Saphenous n.
2. Sural n.
3. Superficial peroneal n.
4. Tibial n.
5. Deep peroneal n.

5. Indications

Supplementation of an incomplete lumbosacral plexus block.
Supplementation of an incomplete epidural block.
Diagnostic, therapeutic or surgical procedure on the foot, particularly orthopedic surgical procedures.

6. Special Contraindications

None

7. Advantages–Disadvantages

Advantage

Ideal procedure for outpatient surgery, very suitable for high risk anesthesia patients.

Disadvantage

Procedures requiring a tourniquet are limited to 60 min operating time.

References

1. Auberger HG, Niesel HC: *Praktische Lokalanästhesie.* Thieme, Stuttgart, 1982, pp 125–127.
2. Cousins M, Bridenbaugh PO: *Neural Blockade.* JB Lippincott Co, Philadelphia, 1980, pp 334–339.
3. Eriksson E (Hrsg): *Atlas der Lokalanästhesie.* Berlin–Heidelberg–New York, Springer, 1980, pp 111–115.
4. Nolte H, Meyer J, Würster J: *Die peripheren Leitungsanästhesien.* Stuttgart, Thieme, 1974, pp 77–81.

Spinal Anesthesia

D. Theiss, E. Lanz

1. Definition

Regional anesthesia in the proximity of the spinal cord. The local anesthetic solution is injected into the subarachnoid space in the lumbar area and blocks neural conduction in the nerve roots in the area of its spread in the cerebrospinal fluid.

Synonyms:

Lumbar anesthesia
Subarachnoid anesthesia

2. Topographic Anatomy

See Figures 82, 83, and 84.

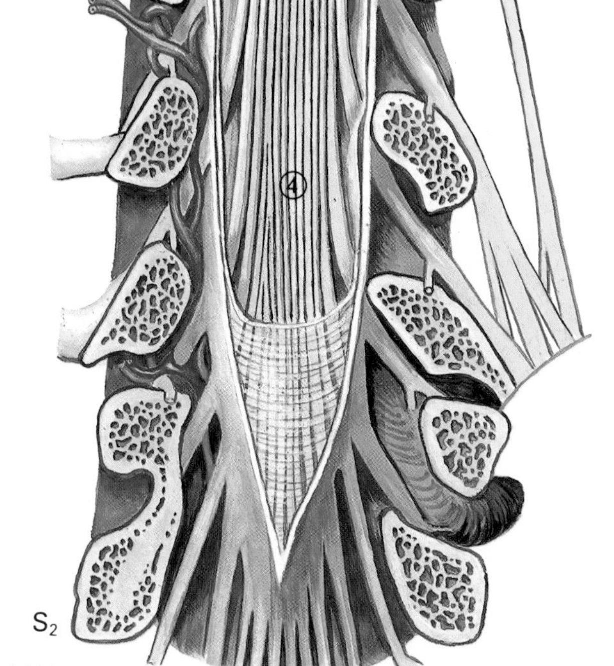

FIG 82.
(after Hafferl)
1. Epidural venous plexus
2. Conus medullaris (caudal extension is variable)
3. Open dura mater and arachnoid membrane
4. Cauda equina

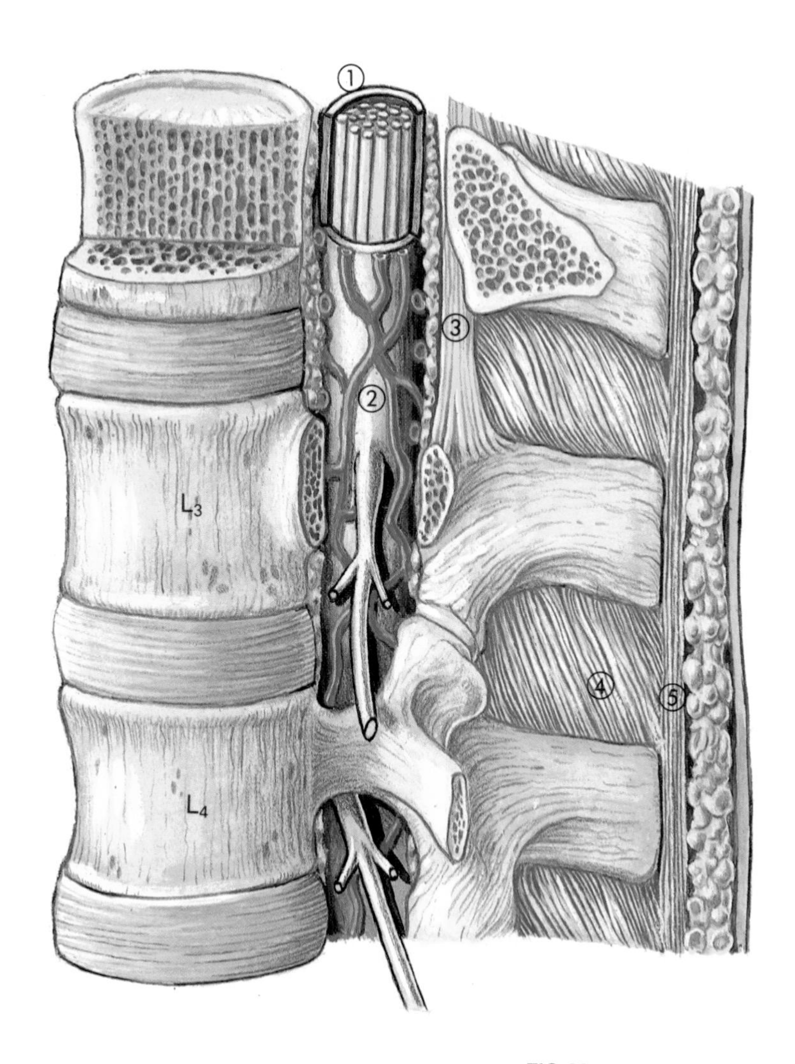

FIG 83.
(after Lee and Atkinson)
1. Dura mater and arachnoid membrane
2. Epidural space
3. Ligamentum flavum
4. Interspinal ligament
5. Supraspinal ligament

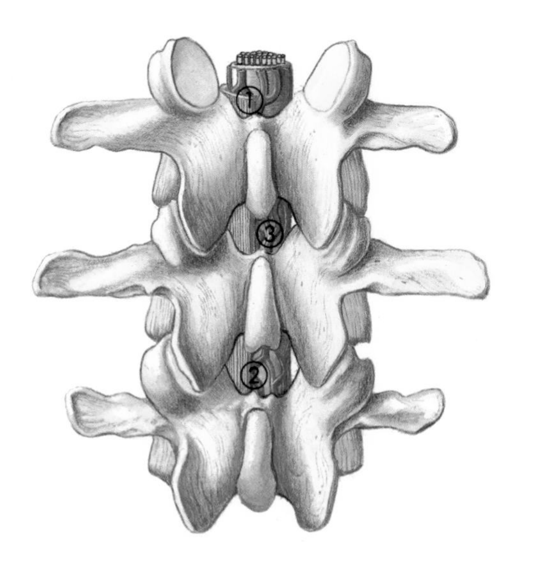

FIG 84.
1. Ligamentum flavum
2. Interlaminar foramen
3. Epidural space

3. Technique

3.1. Anesthesiologic Assessment

Careful anesthesiologic assessment including the identification of any contraindication.

3.2. Preparation

Intravenous cannula, infusion of a balanced electrolyte solution, intubation equipment, ventilation equipment with O_2 connection, atropine, sedative, succinylcholine, vasopressor, catecholamine.

3.3 Equipment

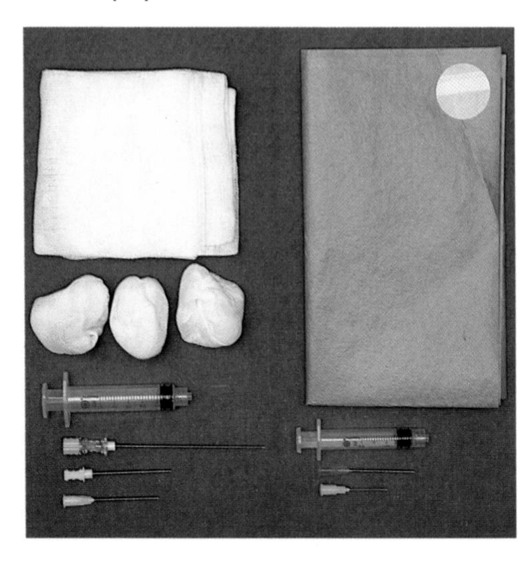

FIG 85.

Spinal set

If the antiseptic solution is not to be sprayed, a container for antiseptic solution, sponges, and spongeholder for application and for wiping must be provided
Sponges
Drapes
Syringes
Needles for drawing up drugs and for skin infiltration
Introducer needle
Spinal needle 25 g, i.e., 0.5 mm E.D.
In rare instances a 22 g spinal needle (= 0.8 mm) should be available
Spinal needles with a conical tip penetrate the fibers of the dura without cutting them
Gloves
Antiseptic solution

Medication set (sterile, if at all possible)

Local anesthetic solution for infiltration
Local anesthetic solution for spinal anesthesia
Optional Glucose 5%
Vasoconstrictor

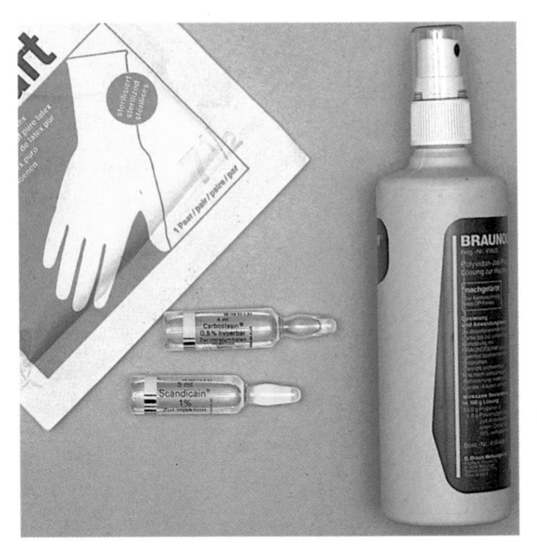

FIG 86.

Local anesthetic solution and spinal needle should be selected on the basis of individual requirements

3.4. Positioning

"Cat's back" and "chin on the chest." This position eliminates the lumbar lordosis; the interlaminal foramina and the interspace are enlarged.

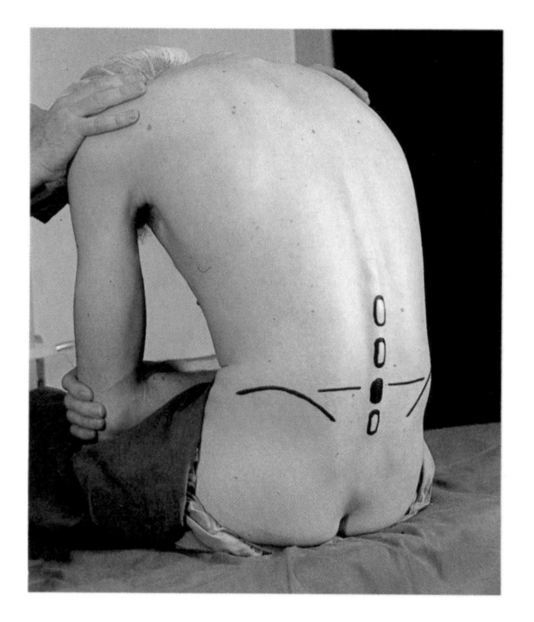

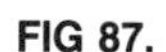
FIG 87.

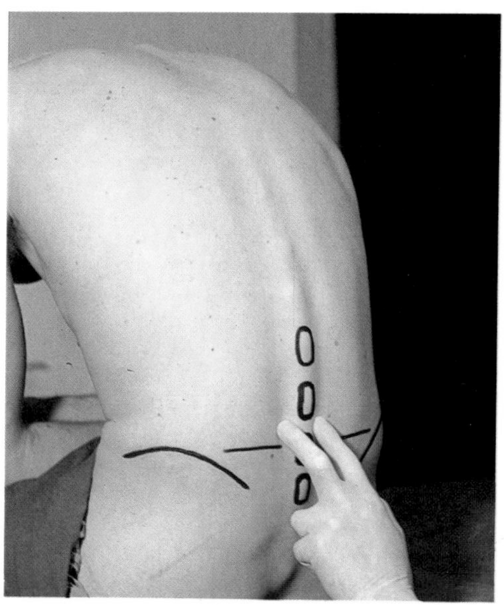

FIG 88.

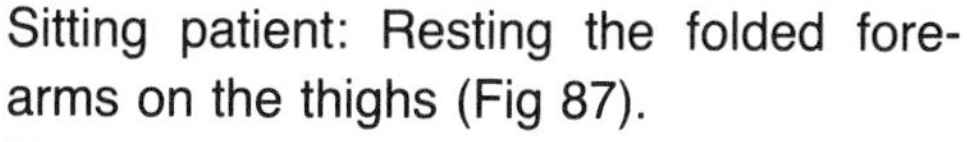
Sitting patient: Resting the folded forearms on the thighs (Fig 87).
Horizontal patient: Head and knees as close to each other as possible (Fig 97).

Advantages of spinal puncture in a sitting patient

The lines of the spinal processes and the midline are more readily identified.
Less painful for patients with lower limb trauma.
More rapid "descent" of a hyperbaric solution.
Anesthesia can be limited to the sacral segments.

Advantages of the spinal puncture in the horizontal patient

Less likelihood of syncope.
With hyperbaric solution, unilateral anesthesia is possible.

Spinal puncture with the patient in the prone position is useful only for the rare hypobaric spinal.

3.5. Landmarks

The line between the iliac spines is usually at the level of the spinous process of L_4 (Fig 88). The spinous processes and the spaces between them are visible and palpable in the slender patient. In the obese patient the sitting position facilitates the identification of the midline and the localization of the spinous process with the tip of the introducer or the needle used for the infiltration (Fig 87).

3.6. Technical Procedure

Skin preparation through threefold scrub or spray. Avoid antiseptic solution on the spinal tray or on the gloves. The antiseptic solution should be wiped away from the area of the puncture.
Localization of the puncture site (Fig 88).
Skin wheal and infiltration, between the spinous processes.

Puncture

The puncture should not be performed above L_2 (conus medullaris). It is generally performed between L_{2-3} or L_{3-4}, depending on the level of anesthesia which is to be achieved.

An introducer needle should be used with the finer spinal needles since it eliminates skin contact with the spinal needle and since its use makes the maintenance or correction of the direction of the puncture easier. The spinal needle should be advanced carefully with the hand braced against the back (Fig 89).

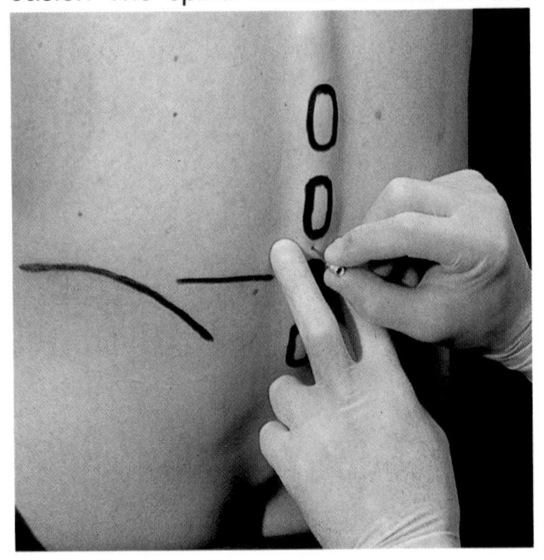

FIG 89.

Beyond 3 cm, entry into the ligamentum flavum should be noted. It feels like the entry of a needle into a soft rubber eraser.

At some time prior to the perforation of the dura (usually at a depth of 4–6 cm), the bevel of the needle should be directed laterally. A "hanging drop" is placed into the hub of the needle and the needle is advanced. As soon as the dura is pierced, the "hanging drop" will become larger (Figs 90 and 92). As soon as a "drip" is observed, the needle is advanced an additional mm to assure that the entire bevel is within the subarachnoid space.

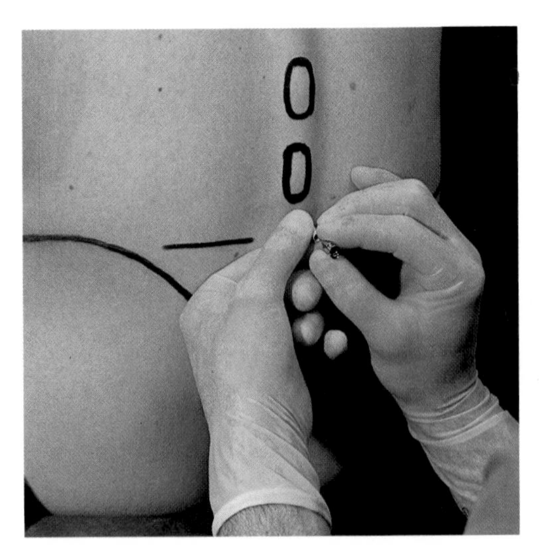

FIG 90.

If the supraspinal ligament is ossified, the *lateral (= paramedial) approach* is selected:

Puncture is made approximately 1.5 cm from the midline and the needle is directed medially to the extent that the tip of the needle perforates the dura approximately in the midline (Figs 91 and 93).

FIG 91.

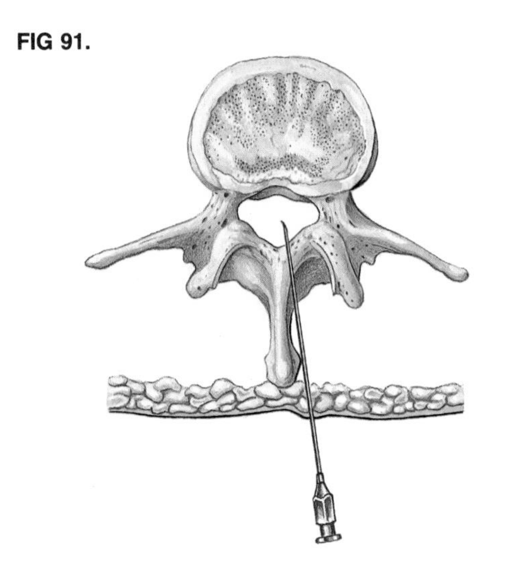

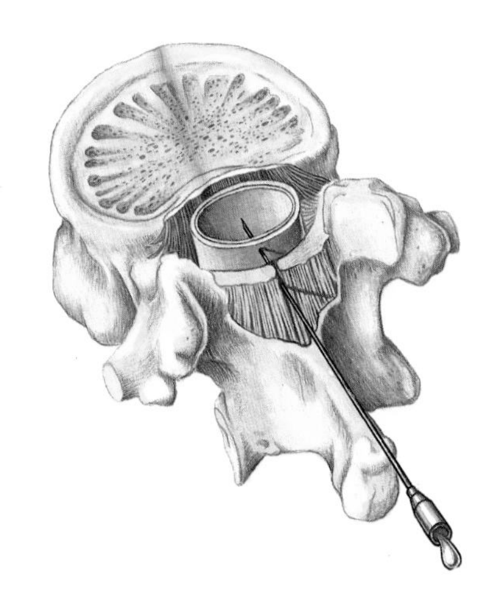

FIG 92.

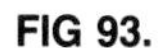

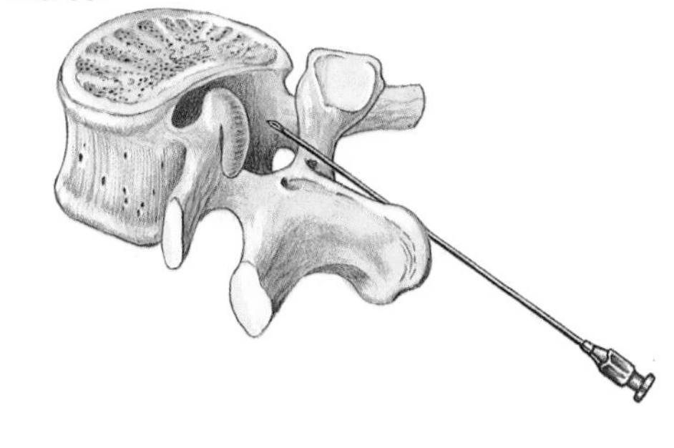

FIG 93.

Difficulties in accomplishing the dural puncture

If no introducer is used, the spinal needle must be withdrawn into the subcutaneous tissue every time its direction is to be changed. If an introducer is used, the tip of the spinal needle must be withdrawn only so that it lies within the introducer sheath. The direction can now be changed without pulling back the introducer. If bony contact is made several times, a new spinal needle should be used since the bony contacts may have caused a hook to be formed at the tip of the original needle.

Paresthesia without CSF return suggests a peridural contact with a nerve root.

If the paresthesia is elicited in the subarachnoid space, the needle should be withdrawn 1 mm.

If the first drop of blood, followed by blood mixed with CSF, followed by clear CSF, the local anesthetic solution may be injected.

Bloody CSF that does not clear after a few drops suggests injury to a blood vessel in the subarachnoid space. Spinal anesthesia may mask the development of neurologic symptoms and is contraindicated.

Injection

The syringe should be free of air bubbles and should be attached firmly to the needle with a rotary motion.
Aspiration of approximately 0.2 ml of CSF to ascertain the subarachnoid position of the tip of the needle.
During injection the needle should be stabilized by bracing one hand against the back of the patient (Fig 94).
If hyper- or hypobaric solution is used, the injection should be performed very slowly to allow the appropriate layering of the local anesthetic solution and the CSF.
If isobaric solution is used, the injection should be as rapid as possible to produce a mixing of the local anesthetic solution with the CSF. Intrathecal or extrathecal barbotage is used only when an isobaric technique is used.

Controlling the spread of the block

In hyper- and hypobaric techniques by:
Extent and duration of tilting the spinal column from the horizontal during and after injection.
Level of the puncture.
Concentration and volume of the local anesthetic solution.
Lateral positioning may achieve unilateral or mostly unilateral anesthesia.

In isobaric technique by:
Volume of the solution and the level of the puncture. Consideration must be given to the length of the spinal column and to the presence of increased intraabdominal pressure (e.g., obesity, pregnancy). In the average patient, 4-5 ml of approximately isobaric local anesthetic solution injected at $L_{2/3}$ or $L_{3/4}$ produce level of anesthesia to about T_{10}. In obese patients, the volume should be reduced by 25%.

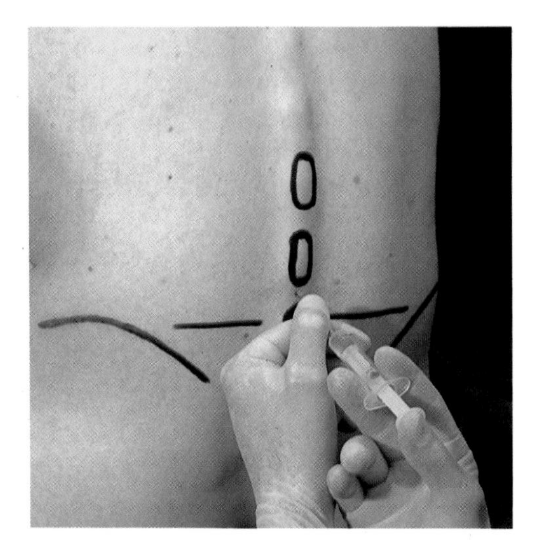

FIG 94.

3.7. Dosage

Hyperbaric solution (dextrose added):	*Isobaric solution:*
Bupivacaine 0.5%	Bupivacaine 0.5%
Lidocaine 5%	Lidocaine 2%
Mepivacaine 4%	Prilocaine 2%
Tetracaine 0.5%	Tetracaine 0.5%

OPERATIVE AREA	LEVEL OF ANESTHESIA	DOSE HYPERBARIC*	DOSE ISOBARIC**
Anal region	S_3 (saddle block)	0.5–1 ml	—
Lower extremity without tourniquet	T_{12} (low spinal)	1–1.5 ml	3 ml
Lower extremity with tourniquet, groin, genitalia	T_{10} (middle spinal)	1.5–2 ml	4 ml
Lower abdomen	T_6 (high spinal)	2 ml	5 ml

*When injecting in sitting position use upper dose range. When injecting in lateral position use lower dose range, particularly when unilateral anesthesia is sought.

**When using L_{2-3} interspace in smaller patients or increased abdominal pressure (obesity, pregnancy, abdominal neoplasm), the volumes must be reduced.

Duration of surgical anesthesia

Lidocaine, mepivacaine and prilocaine 1.5 to 2.5 hr. Vasoconstrictor, e.g., epinephrine 0.2 mg, extends the effective range by 30 to 50%.

Signs of onset, of latency and of fixation

Signs of onset, in the form of a sensation of warmth, frequently already during the injection.
Maximal spread of the block after 15 to 20 min. After 20 min further spread is unlikely but cannot be excluded.

Insufficient level and failure

If the required level of anesthesia is not achieved in spite of appropriate dose, level of injection and positioning, a second administration using half of the original dose may be performed.
If in 10 min there is no evidence of any block, the spinal anesthesia may be repeated using the entire initial volume.

Atraumatic technique:

Needle should be introduced into the subarachnoid space only for a distance of 2–3 mm. If paresthesias have been elicited, the greatest care must be exercised, and intramural injection must be avoided by assured free flow of CSF. Consideration must be given to the variable length of the conus medullaris. Correct choice of drug and dosage.

4. Special Side Effects and Complications

	COMPLICATION	THERAPY	PREVENTION
During induction	Vasovagal reaction	Vasoconstrictor Atropine	Puncture in lateral position Infusion Vasoconstrictor Atropine
After induction	Hypotension	Vasoconstrictor IV fluids	IV fluids Keep level as low as possible
	Bradycardia	Atropine Metaproterenol	Atropine
	Nausea and vomiting	Atropine Droperidole	Antiemetic premedication Sedatives Atropine
	Dyspnea in high spinal	O_2 by nasal cannula PRN mask ventilation and sedation	Keep level as low as possible
	Apnea in total spinal	Intubation Ventilation Sedation	Keep level as low as possible
Late complications	Urinary retention	Timely catheterization	Appropriate IV Infusion—commensurate to length of block
	Spinal headache	Horizontal position Hydration Epidural Blood patch	Fine needle Conical tip, e.g., Whitacre needle Single dural puncture
	Cranial nerve palsy	By neurologist	As in spinal headache
	Other neurologic complications	By neurologist	Aseptic technique Atraumatic technique

5. Indications

Procedures involving the lower half of the body (see 3.7)

Particularly in:

Inebriated patients
Patients with preexisting cardiac or pulmonary disease
Metabolic diseases
Liver or kidney insufficiency
In anticipated intubation difficulties
Patients whose jaws are wired shut (wire cutters must be immediately available)

6. Special Contraindications

Absolute

Uncorrected hypovolemia
Significant coagulopathy

Relative

Sepsis
Chronic and recurrent spinal cord and peripheral nerve disease
Neurologic deficit
Lumbar spine—complaints and lumbar spine anomalies
Previous lumbar spine surgery
History of headaches
Young patients (spinal headache is more common)

7. Advantages-Disadvantages

Advantages over epidural anesthesia

Simpler technique
Fewer failures
Shorter latent period
Better muscular relaxation
Reliable surgical anesthesia
Smaller total local anesthetic dose

Disadvantages in comparison to epidural anesthesia

Post spinal headache
Catheter technique is not recommended
More profound circulatory effects
Segmental block is not possible

References

1. Bergmann H: Die Komplikationen, Fehler und Gefahren der Spinalanästhesie, in Nolte H, Meyer J (Hrsg): *Die rükkenmarksnahen Anašthesien.* Stuttgart, Thieme, 1972, p. 45.
2. Bridenbauch PO, Kennedy WF: Spinal, subarachnoid neural blockade, in Cousins MJ, Bridenbaugh PO (eds): *Neural blockade in Clinical Anesthesia and Management of Pain.* Philadelphia–Toronto, Lippincott, 1980, p. 146.
3. Greene NM: *Physiology of Spinal Anesthesia,* ed 3. Baltimore, Williams and Wilkins, 1981.
4. Macintosh Sir R, Lee JA, Atkinson RS: *Lumbalpunktion, intradurale und extradurale Spinalanalgesie.* Stuttgart, Fischer, 1982.
5. Lund, PC: *Principles and practice of spinal anesthesia.* Springfield, Charles C Thomas, 1971.

Lumbar Epidural Anesthesia

H. Chr. Niesel

1. Definition

Epidural anesthesia represents the administration of a local anesthetic solution into the so-called epidural space.

The local anesthetic solution spreads in a caudal and cranial direction (in the lumbar and thoracic space). In caudal injection (caudal anesthesia) the spread is only craniad (Fig 95).

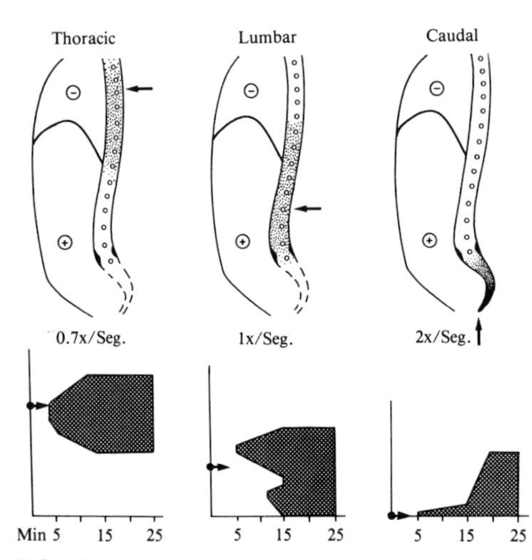

FIG 95.
Typical pattern of spread of epidural anesthesia (after Bromage).

The injected local anesthetic agent acts:

1. by diffusion through the dura mater just as in a spinal (subarachnoid) block.
2. by spread through the intervertebral foramina as a paravertebral block.
3. by diffusion in the area of the dural sleeves directly on the spinal nerves.

2. Topographic Anatomy

The epidural space is located along the entire extent of the spinal column, between the dura mater and the external dural (periosteal) layer. It contains fat, connective tissue, and numerous vessels, primarily veins (Fig 83).

It is limited dorsally by the ligamentum flavum, which connects the upper and lower lips of the lamina and which is most strongly developed in the lumbar area and least developed in the cervical area.

The spread of the local anesthetic solution depends essentially on the anatomy of the space and on the volume of the injected solution. The injected solution can spread over the intervertebral foramina, more easily in the young patient, but much less so in the old patient in whom sclerosing of the foramina forces a spread of the injected volume caudad and, more particularly, craniad. Anatomic variations of the spinal cord (conus medullaris) must be kept in mind.

3. Technique

3.1. Anesthesiologic Assessment

Careful anesthesiologic assessment including the identification of any contraindication.

3.2. Preparation

Intravenous cannula, infusion of a balanced electrolyte solution, ventilation equipment with O_2 connection, intubation equipment, atropine, sedative, succinylcholine, vasopressor, catecholamine.

3.3 Equipment

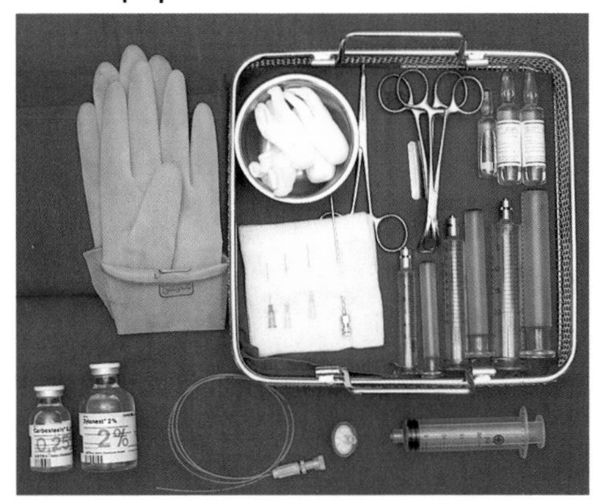

FIG 96.

Disposable sets or individually assembled sets (Fig 96).

Contents (example):

Syringes: 5 ml syringe for infiltration
- 10 ml syringe—loose glass or plastic
- 20 ml syringe for injection of the local anesthetic solution

Needles: Thin needles
- Epidural needle with dull bevel ("single shot" needle)
- Tuohy needle (with bent tip for catheter technique)
- The epidural needles must have a stylette to avoid the cutting and introducing of a skin plug into the deeper spaces
- Needles to draw up the solutions
- (It is useful to teach and to get used to a single technique)

Other: Drapes with clips or with adhesive stripe, cup for antiseptic solution
- Sponges and dressing for skin preparation and for dressing; forceps
- Two 10 ml ampules of 0.9% NaCl
- Local anesthetics; the ampules can be sterilized with the set

In catheter technique, additionally in the set:
Scissors (for the optimal preparation of the dressing; to cut the plastic envelopes containing the connectors and syringes).
Since the epidural catheter and the filter cannot be autoclaved, they must be added after the set is open.

Catheter-epidural anesthesia (continuous epidural)

Equipment as in single shot epidural set, plus:
Catheter—Vinyl, nylon or Teflon (stylette is usually not needed and should be avoided since it can cause a dural perforation, particularly if it is pushed too close to the tip of the catheter)

3.4. Positioning

Lateral position

The lateral position is preferable, even though the technical aspects of the puncture are somewhat more demanding. More comfortable for the patient; no danger of syncope.

FIG 97.

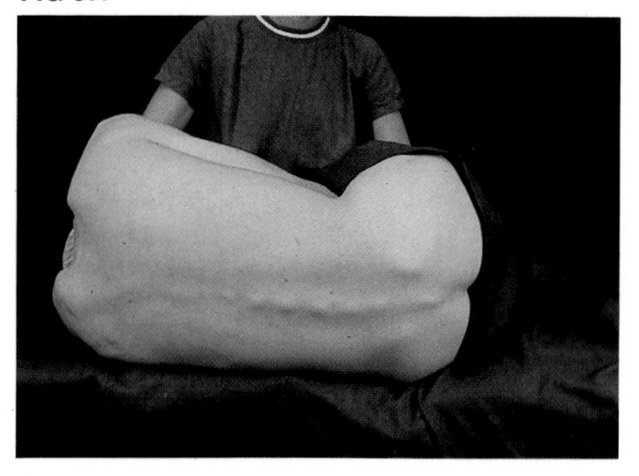

Sitting position

Recommended only in exceptional cases and when technical difficulties are encountered (relatively ineffective premedication). Relaxed, ideal positioning is very important. Assistant must support the patient. In the sitting position, the forearms should rest on the thighs. Support for the feet is essential (see Fig 87, p. 99).

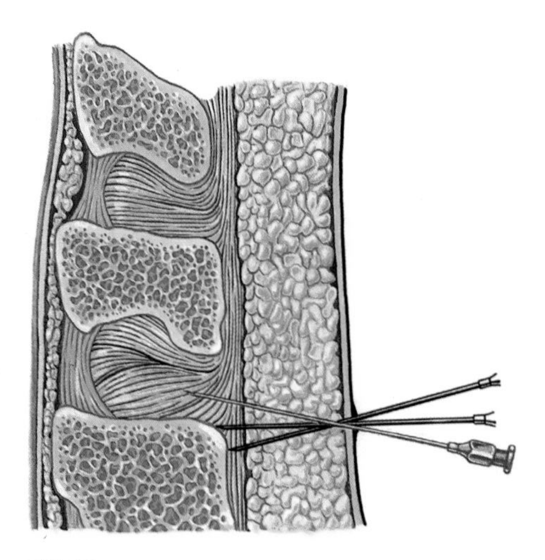

FIG 99.

3.5. Landmarks

(See also "Spinal anesthesia," p. 99.) Localization of the spinous processes through lateral definition as well as cranial-caudal (midline) identification (Fig 98). In the obese patient, the spinous process should be identified by the insertion of a long infiltration needle making bony contact. The epidural needle can then usually be advanced craniad from the identified spinous process in the direction of the interspinal ligament (Fig 99).

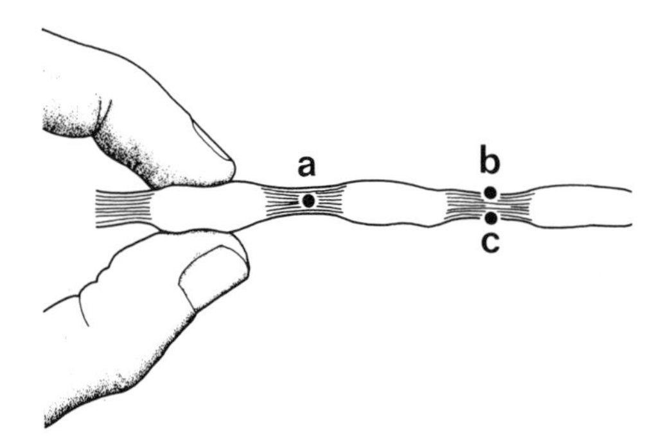

FIG 98.
Palpation of the spinous processes to locate the midline (a).
(after Bromage)
b, c: incorrect placement of the needle.

3.6. Technical Procedure

Single shot epidural anesthesia

Absolutely aseptic technique is mandatory for epidural anesthesia. Sterile gloves are required; surgical scrub of the hands, sterile gown, and mask is recommended. Careful preparation of a large skin surface on the back. Intracutaneous infiltration. Locating the midline by identifying the interspinal ligament with the infiltration needle. Advancing the epidural or Tuohy needle until it enters the interspinal ligament. Perforating the skin by a rotary motion or through an opening made with a larger needle. This is followed by the attachment of a NaCl solution-filled 5 or 10 ml syringe to the epidural needle. The needle should be rotated sideways so that the fibers of the ligament can be separated rather than transsected. The position of the needle tip can be determined by the gap in the hub. Under continuous pressure on the plunger (Fig 100), the needle is advanced until the epidural space is reached. The resistance will be marked in the interspinal ligament and almost solid in the ligamentum flavum. As soon as the epidural space is reached, there is an unmistakably obvious loss of resistance and the salt solution will be emptied into the epidural space (Fig 101). If the needle is advanced very slowly, the stepwise approach to the epidural space can be observed very plainly. During the advancement of the needle, the hand (usually the left) securing the needle is braced against the back. If the tissues are tough and the hand is weak, advancements in 1 mm steps can be made and pressure is exerted on the plunger after every advance (Tremolo advance). If there is any pain during the advancement of the needle, it is likely that the tip of the needle is in the vicinity of the sensitive periosteum. The direction of the needle should be adjusted. If bone is encountered at a shallow depth in the midline, it is probably the lower spinous process. If the bony contact is at a deeper depth it is probably the upper spinous process. If the bony contact is even deeper, it is probably the vertebral arch or the lamina, and it means that the needle has deviated laterally. If the epidural space is reached, 2–3 ml salt solution are injected, and injection and aspiration are performed in two planes to make certain that the resistance is negligible and that no blood can be aspirated.

The lateral approach can also be used in the lumbar area. It may become necessary if the interspinal ligament is impenetrable or if there is a developmental anomaly.

Concerning the technique, see "Thoracic epidural anesthesia" (p. 120).

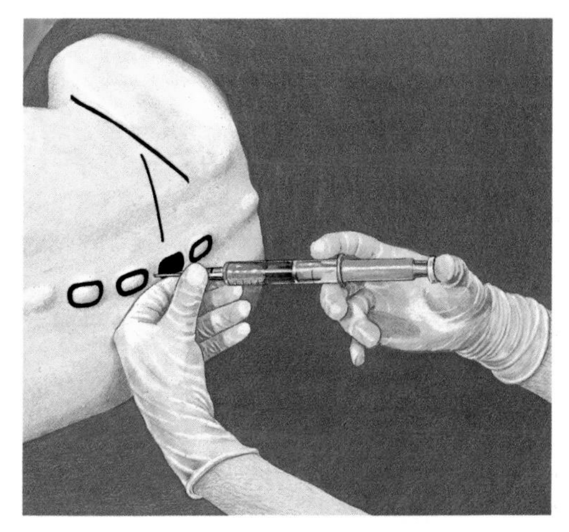

FIG 100.

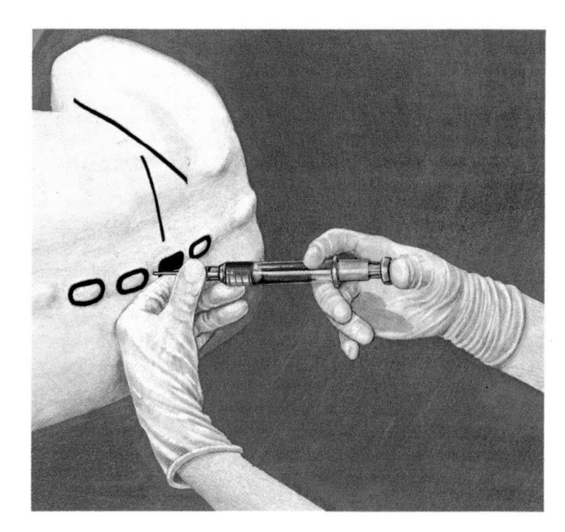

FIG 101.

After aspiration, a test dose is administered.

If the test dose contains epinephrine, accidental IV injection will become rapidly manifest by the appearance of tachycardia.

Wait 5 min. Inject the remainder of the local anesthetic solution.

Factors which can simulate a loss of resistance:

1. Reaching a loose part of the interspinal ligament (Fig 102).
2. Lateral deviation of the tip of the needle beyond the interspinal ligament (Fig 103).
3. The distance between the skin and the epidural space can vary from 2–9 cm (and even more)
4. The width of the peridural space in the lumbar area is 1–6 mm, with a mean of 3–5 mm.

Other methods to identify the epidural space

1. Loss of resistance, using air-filled or air and salt-water filled syringe.
2. Loss of resistance being indicated by a mechanical device (balloon indicator).
3. Negative pressure in epidural space: e.g., use of hanging drop technique or mechanical indicator.

For point 1: Air being compressible does not transmit the feeling of change in resistance well. Air spreads in the epidural space in irregular pockets. The dura is not displaced by the tip of the needle. Advantages: There is no drip of fluid if the epidural pressure is elevated, and thus escape of CSF is easier to recognize.

For point 2: There is no stepwise change in the pressure relationships.

For point 3: Negative intrathoracic pressure can be assumed in the sitting patient.

Monitoring the Patient

Verbal contact with the patient to recognize speech disturbances which may be an early indication of a developing total spinal.

Blood pressure measurements at frequent intervals.

Checking the level of anesthesia.

Watching the motor activity of the patient.

Precise recording of the level of anesthesia and motor function.

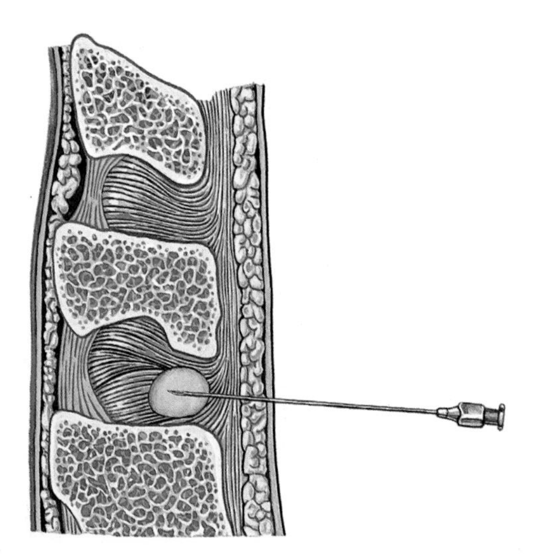

FIG 102.
Perceived loss of resistance in the area of the interspinal ligament

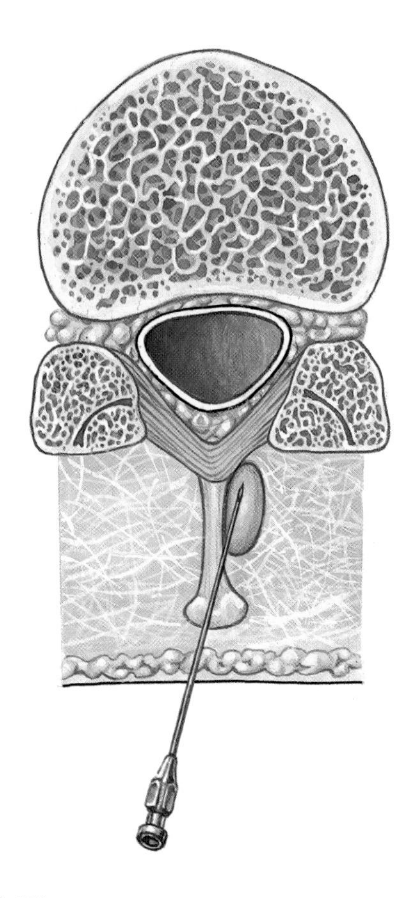

FIG 103.
Lateral deviation of the needle from the interspinal ligament

Catheter epidural anesthesia

(So-called continuous epidural anesthesia)
Test catheter and needle for fit and patency. The epidural space is reached and identified in exactly the same way as in "single shot" epidural anesthesia. Loss of resistance is checked in two planes, in order to be able to introduce the catheter easily (approx. 3–4 cm). Further advance of the catheter may lead to lateral deviation (i.e., paresthesias through contact with nerve roots). The catheter should only be advanced cranially; caudal advancement frequently leads to lateral deviation (Fig 104).

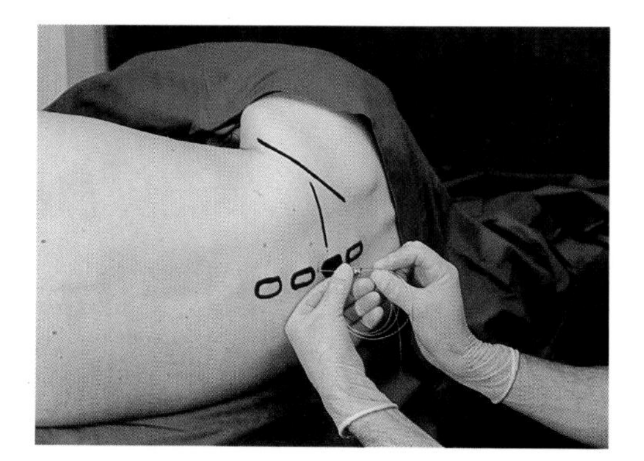

FIG 104.

If there are difficulties in inserting the catheter, simultaneous injection of saline should be performed. Next the needle is withdrawn while the catheter is fixed in place. (Never withdraw the catheter while the needle is in place, because of the danger of shearing the catheter.) Use sterile dressing, making sure that all connections are also covered by a sterile plastic cover (Fig 105).
To assess the advantages and disadvantages of the different types of catheters, see "Thoracic epidural anesthesia" (p. 122).

Disadvantages

Technically more demanding, since the needle must be in a perfect position. Possibility of vascular injury and perforation. Lateral deviation of the catheter, catheter breakage.

Advantages

Variable dose which can be adjusted for the individual patient (particularly important in old patients or in pregnant patients). The anesthesia can be prolonged, and incomplete blockade of some segments can be eliminated. Postoperative or therapeutic analgesia can be provided.

3.7. Dosage

Test dose

Not a guaranteed safety factor to eliminate the possibility of a subdural injection. Necessary with the catheter technique in view of the danger of dural perforation. Negative aspiration is also no guarantee against accidental subarachnoid puncture.

Anesthetic dose

The intensity of the block depends on the concentration of the local anesthetic solution.
With prilocaine, mepivacaine, and lidocaine: 0.5% provides primarily a sympathetic block; 1% provides a sympathetic and sensory block; 2% provides a sympathetic, sensory, and motor block.

FIG 105.

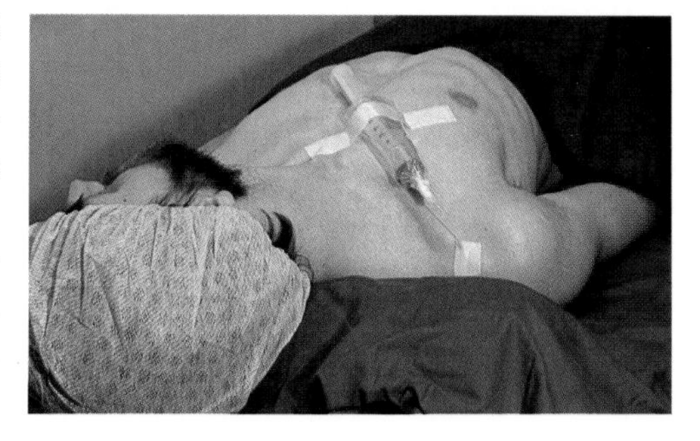

With bupivacaine: 0.125% provides a sympathetic block; 0.25% provides a sympathetic and sensory block; 0.5% (to 0.75%) provides a sympathetic, sensory, and motor block.

Dose requirements

The required dose depends on the concentration of the local anesthetic solution. The following suggestions refer to 2% lidocaine with epinephrine or bupivacaine 0.5%:

Example:

20 year old: 1.5 ml/segment
40 year old: 1.3 ml/segment
60 year old: 1.0 ml/segment
80 year old: 0.7 ml/segment

The spread is divided between the cranial and caudal components of the epidural space. If there is a long time lapse between the test dose and the main dose, the test dose should not be included in the main dose calculation (individual variations are possible, Fig 106).

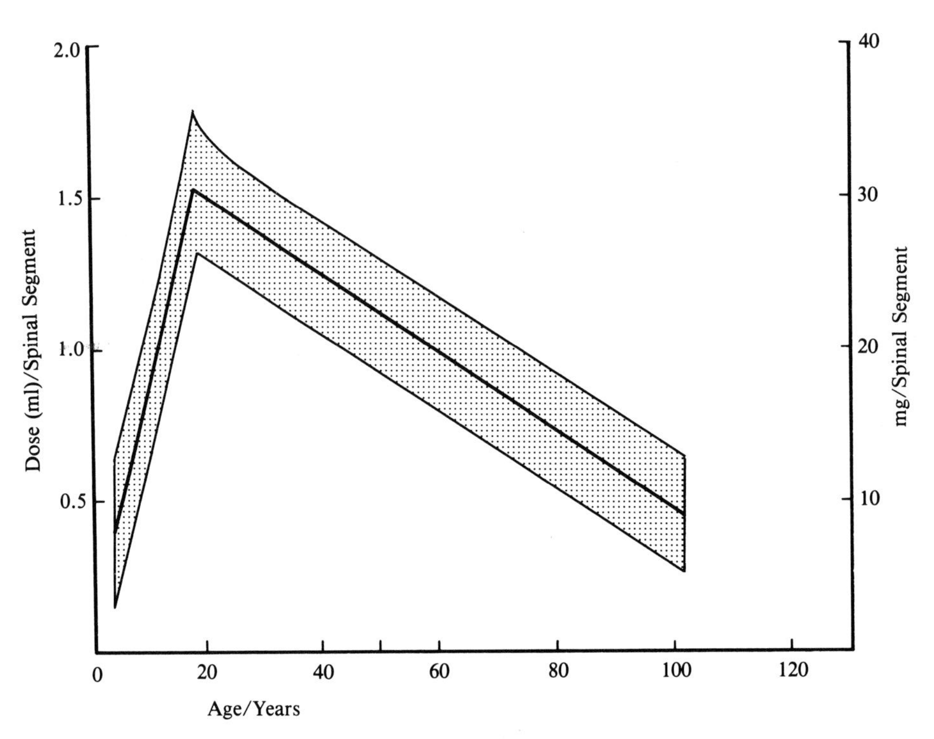

FIG 106.
The relationship of the dosage requirements to the age of the patient (lumbar injection, 2% solution) (after Bromage).

Duration of effect

In intermediate-acting local anesthetics 45 min to 2 hr. In long-acting local anesthetics 1.5 to 7 hr.

Latent period

In intermediate-acting local anesthetic 12-20 min; in long-acting local anesthetics 15–25 min.

Conditions affecting the dose

a. Arteriosclerosis
   A reduction in dose is required and the reduction may be as much as one third. The latency period may be prolonged.
b. Pregnancy
   A reduction in dose by 25% is desirable. For cesarean section, an increase in block from S_5 to T_{6-7} is necessary.
   The accidental IV injection of large amounts of highly concentrated, long-acting local anesthetic solution can produce severe cardiac toxicity. Injection should, therefore, be in stages. Use a test dose.
c. Concentration
   Reduction of the concentration to 1% requires an increase in the volume administered, as compared with a 2% solution. The increase may be as much as 30%.
d. The addition of epinephrine
   Strengthens the motor blockade, extends the duration of the blockade. Tachycardia after the test dose is an early warning signal.
e. Rate of injection
   Has little effect on the level of the blockade.
f. Position
   Sitting position requires an increase of the dose of up to 20%
g. Size and weight of the patient
   Questionable effect on the dose-effectiveness relationship. In individual cases the patient's body build must be taken into consideration. Obesity definitely requires a reduction of the dose.
h. Incompletely blocked segments
   L_5–S_1 are particularly favored.

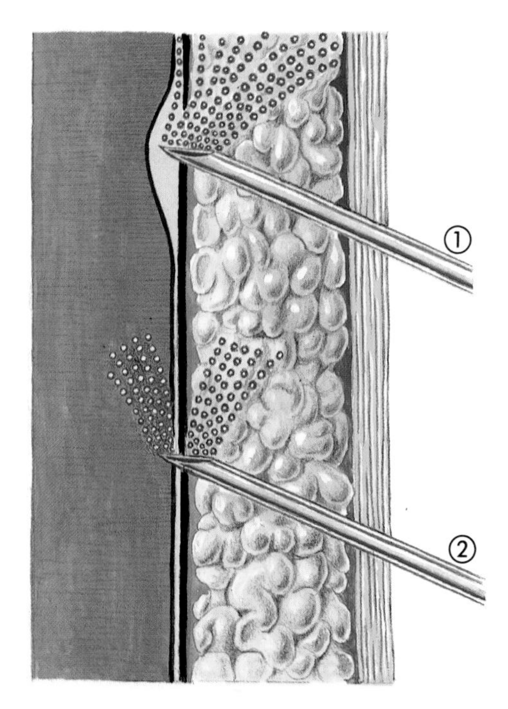

FIG 107.
Varieties of dural perforation:
1. Partial subdural injection
2. Partial subarachnoid injection

4. Special Complications

4.1. Serious early complications

	SYMPTOMS	THERAPY
Total spinal anesthesia (Subarachnoid injection) (Fig 107)	Early signs: Speech disturbances Hypotension Bradycardia Unconsciousness Apnea Mydriasis Asystole	O_2 administration Mask-intubation Vasoconstrictor Atropine Fluids Metaproterenol CPR[1]
Massive epidural anesthesia (Overdose or subdural injection) (Fig 107)	Extensive anesthesia level Hypotension Bradycardia Miosis Dyspnea-hypoventilation As above under "total spinal anesthesia"	O_2 by nasal cannula O_2 mask-ventilation PRN Vasoconstrictor Atropine Elevate the legs[2] Fluid
IV Injection	See "Complications of regional anesthesia" (p. 13)	
Vasovagal reactions	Hypotension Bradycardia Nausea and vomiting	Vasoconstrictor (ephedrine) Elevate legs Trendelenburg position[2] Fluids Atropine Sedation (diazepam) Droperidol

[1]Aspiration of local anesthetic solution through the catheter is possible, but unreliable (due to loss of time).
[2]In obstetrics: lateral position—right side "up."

4.2. Late Complications

Headaches

If the injection is done properly, the incidence is no greater than after general anesthesia. In headaches due to dural perforation, the patient should be kept in a horizontal position and should be given plenty of fluids and analgetics. An incidence of dural perforations in excess of 1% suggests faulty technique. If neurologic symptoms are present because of loss of CSF, epidural blood patch should be placed (5–10 ml, drawn under sterile conditions).

Urinary bladder dysfunction

Frequently triggered by overdistention of the bladder during anesthesia. For this reason overhydration must be avoided. Prevention of hypotension should be accomplished by a combination of fluid administration, positioning, and vasoconstrictors, particularly in normovolemic and young patients. Patients with hypertrophy of the prostate are particularly vulnerable and great care must be taken so that overhydration does not occur and result in bladder distention. If necessary, catheterization must be performed. Indwelling catheters should not be used.

Catheter breakage

Never withdraw the catheter with the needle in place!
The catheter should not be introduced further than 4 cm, particularly not in the lumbar area. If introduced further than 4 cm, loop formation, knotting, and lateral deviation may occur. This may lead to unilateral or isolated segmental anesthesia. When removing the catheter at the termination of anesthesia, the back should be bent; otherwise breakage is possible. When a small portion breaks off and remains in the epidural space, the patient must be informed. Surgical removal is usually not necessary. Neurologic monitoring must be provided.

Spinal cord injury

Caused by faulty technique and excessively deep injection. The spinal cord can extend well below L_2 and can be injured through accidental subarachnoid puncture. Complete loss of resistance can be experienced at levels deeper than the epidural space as well.

Epidural hematoma

Possible in patients with coagulopathies. It should be noted that in obstetrical anesthesia, spontaneous epidural hematoma formation is possible. If normal sensory functions do not return as expected, neurologic monitoring and possibly neurosurgical intervention may become necessary.

Complications due to decreased perfusion

(Anterior spinal artery syndrome)
The possibility of decreased perfusion of the spinal cord due to vasoconstriction in the event of systemic hypotension is much debated. The combination of vasopressor-containing local anesthetic solution and systemic hypotension is dangerous, since the anterior spinal artery is functionally an end artery.

Infections

Absolute asepsis is mandatory. In septic patients, spinal or epidural anesthesia should not be performed. In continuous epidural anesthesia the use of a bacterial filter is recommended. The entire system (connectors and tubing) must remain aseptically covered (Fig 105).

Arachnoiditis

Impurities can lead secondarily to arachnoiditis.

5. Indications

Procedures on the lower extremities
Abdominal procedures—preferentially in the lower abdomen. Upper abdominal procedures, in combination with light general anesthesia, (see "Thoracic epidural anesthesia," p. 124)
Pulmonary (and cardiac) diseases
Metabolic diseases
Obstetric analgesia
Postoperative and posttraumatic analgesia
Therapeutic blocks

6. Special Contraindications

Absolute

Shock
Coagulopathies
Sepsis
Bowel perforation
Decompensated ileus

Relative

(Must be weighed against the disadvantages of general anesthesia)

Neurologic diseases
Severe myocardial insufficiency
Anatomic difficulties
Patient reluctance—regional anesthesia should never be forced upon a patient.

7. Advantages–Disadvantages

See "Spinal anesthesia" (p. 105).

Thoracic Epidural Anesthesia

F. Wagner

1. Definition

Injection of local anesthetic solution into the epidural space of the thoracic spine. Relatively equal craniad and caudad spread of the anesthetic solution. In the sitting position and in high thoracic puncture the spread is largely caudad. See also "Lumbar epidural anesthesia" (p. 106).

2. Topographic Anatomy

See "Lumbar epidural anesthesia" (p. 106).

Peculiarities in the thoracic region: primarily the direction of the spinous processes and the angle of the lamina (Figs 108 and 109).

Craniad—increasingly thinner ligamentum flavum and narrower epidural space.

FIGS 108 AND 109.
6th thoracic vertebra:
1. Spinous process
2. Lamina
3. Arch
4. Transverse process

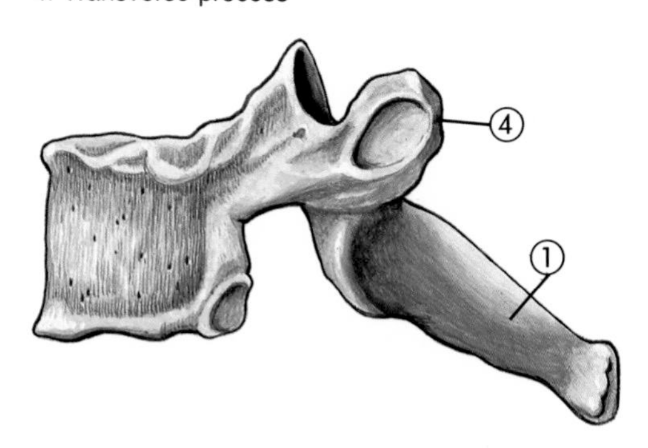

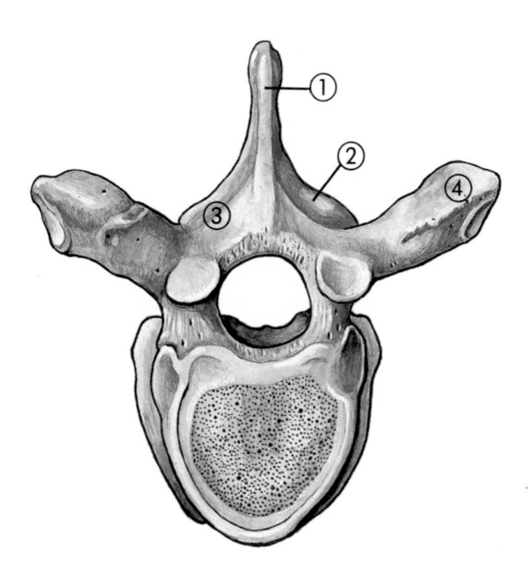

STRUCTURE	CERVICAL/UPPER THORACIC	MIDDLE THORACIC	LOWER LUMBAR/ THORACIC
Spinal cord	Sagittal diameter 9 mm	Sagittal diameter 6.5–8 mm	Sagittal diameter 7–9mm
Epidural space	Sagittal diameter 3–4 mm	Sagittal diameter 3–5 mm	Sagittal diameter 4–6 mm
Ligamentum flavum	Thin	Medium	Thick
Dura	1.5–1 mm	Approx. 1 mm	0.7–0.3 mm
Spinous process (Direction of puncture)	C_7–T_1 horizontal, then increasingly caudad	Strongly caudad Angle 40–70°	Increasingly less caudal direction

The direction and depth at which the ligamentum flavum is punctured vary considerably (2–3 to over 8 cm).

3. Technique

See: "Lumbar epidural anesthesia" (p. 106).

Peculiarities of thoracic epidural anesthesia

Positioning

Lateral position is hemodynamically advantageous, but for the novice technically more difficult (spatial visualization is lacking).
Sitting position possible only with cooperative patient. Rapid (but sure) technique desirable (danger of syncope). The patient is supported by an assistant. Back is flexed and head is slightly flexed. Arms are crossed, forearms rest on the thighs. In catheter technique, only test dose is given in the sitting position. The full dose is given after the patient is placed into a horizontal position.

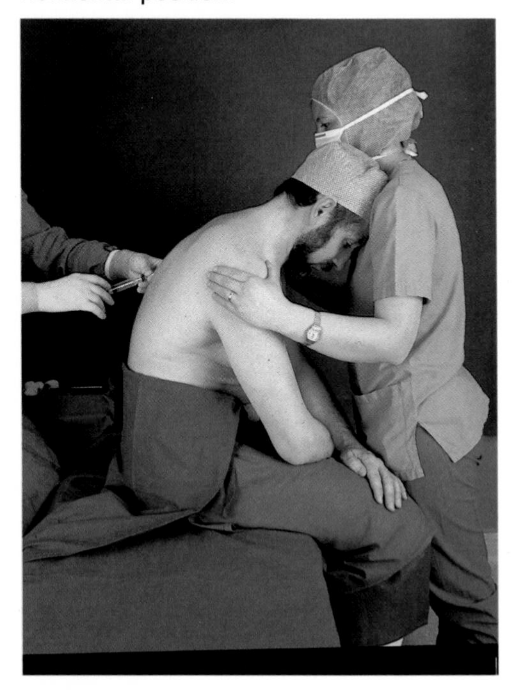

FIG 110.

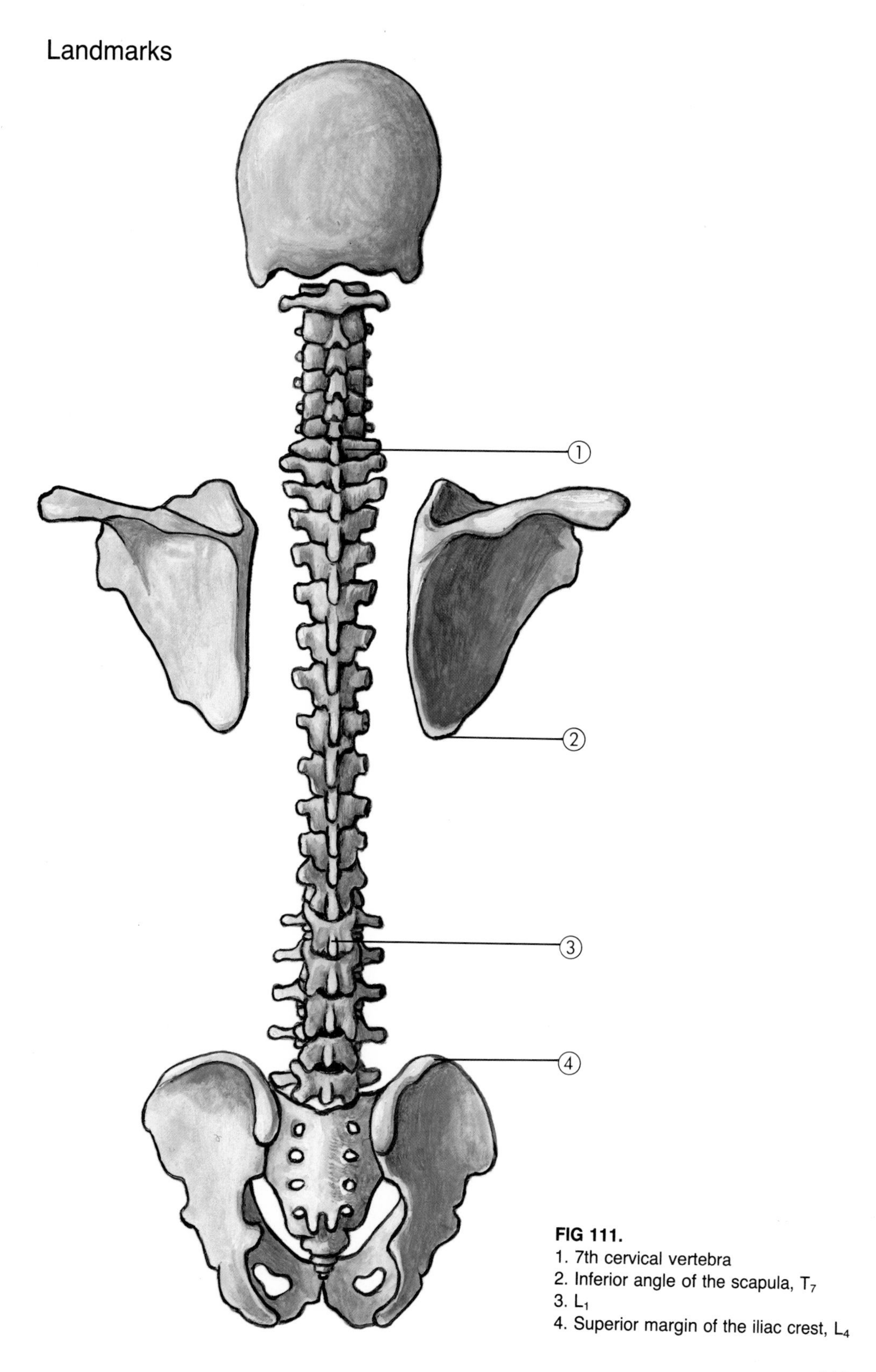

FIG 111.
1. 7th cervical vertebra
2. Inferior angle of the scapula, T_7
3. L_1
4. Superior margin of the iliac crest, L_4

Technical Procedure

See also: "Lumbar epidural anesthesia" (p. 108).

Selection of the site of puncture

The site of puncture depends on the proposed operative site. It should be as close as possible to the middle of the area of analgesia.

SURGICAL SITE	"IDEAL" PUNCTURE SITE
Arm/shoulder/neck	C_7–T_1
Thorax	T_2–T_6
Upper abdomen	T_6–T_8
Lower abdomen	T_{11}–T_{12}

A. *Median (medial) approach*

Relatively difficult in the mid-thoracic area where a paramedian technique is frequently easier.

After the appropriate interspace has been identified, the skin and the "interspinal" space are infiltrated with local anesthetic solution. The direction of the proposed approach is made by palpation and by the exploratory introduction of a thin (23–27 g) needle. Next, the epidural needle (Tuohy or Crawford) is introduced into the interspinal space (max. 2 cm). The stylette is removed and a 10 ml glass syringe filled with 0.9% saline, but also containing an air bubble, is attached to the needle. There should be a light springy resistance when gentle pressure is exerted on the plunger. Under constant pressure on the plunger by the right thumb, the needle is advanced millimeter by millimeter with the left hand until there is a sudden loss of resistance (Fig 112). (Left-handed anesthesiologists reverse the hands.)

Because of the steep orientation of the spinous processes and the lamina, the Tuohy needle is introduced with opening craniad and the Crawford needle with the opening caudad (Fig 114). This will decrease the likelihood of a dural puncture. Since in the sitting position there is almost always a negative pressure in the epidural space, the "hanging drop" technique can also be used. Deep inspirations can make several drops "disappear." (Watch out for asthmatic or emphysematic patients.) After the epidural space has been reached, a maximum of 2–3 ml of saline is injected. The syringe is then removed and the needle is advanced

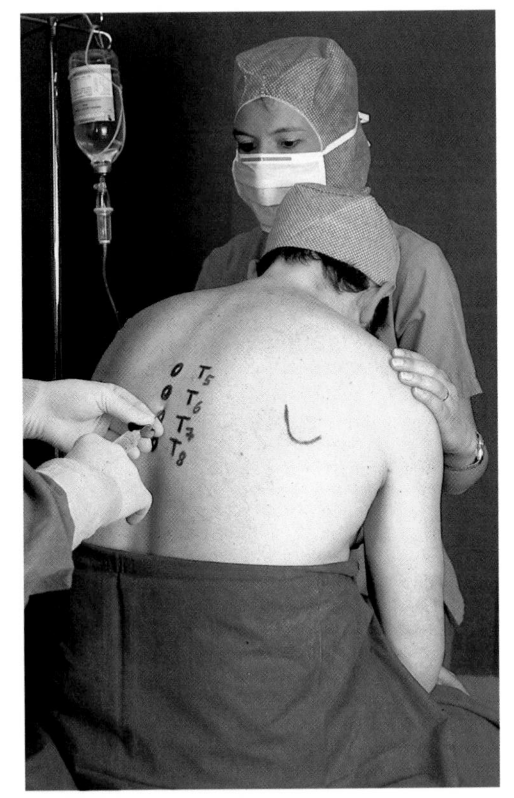

FIG 112.

0.5–1 mm to make sure that the entire bevel of the Tuohy needle is "past" the ligamentum flavum. (Crawford needle should be rotated so that the bevel points craniad.) An air-filled, loose glass syringe is attached to the needle. Injection, accomplished with the little finger of the right hand, must be easy (no springy resistance) (Fig 113). Next aspiration—cold solution = saline; warm solution = suspicion of CSF: Dextrostix!

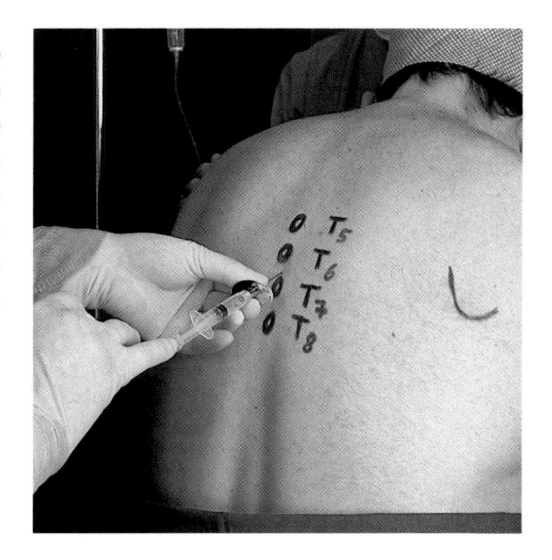

FIG 113.

FIG 114.
(after Dawkins and Steel)
1. Epidural space
2. Tuohy needle
3. Crawford needle

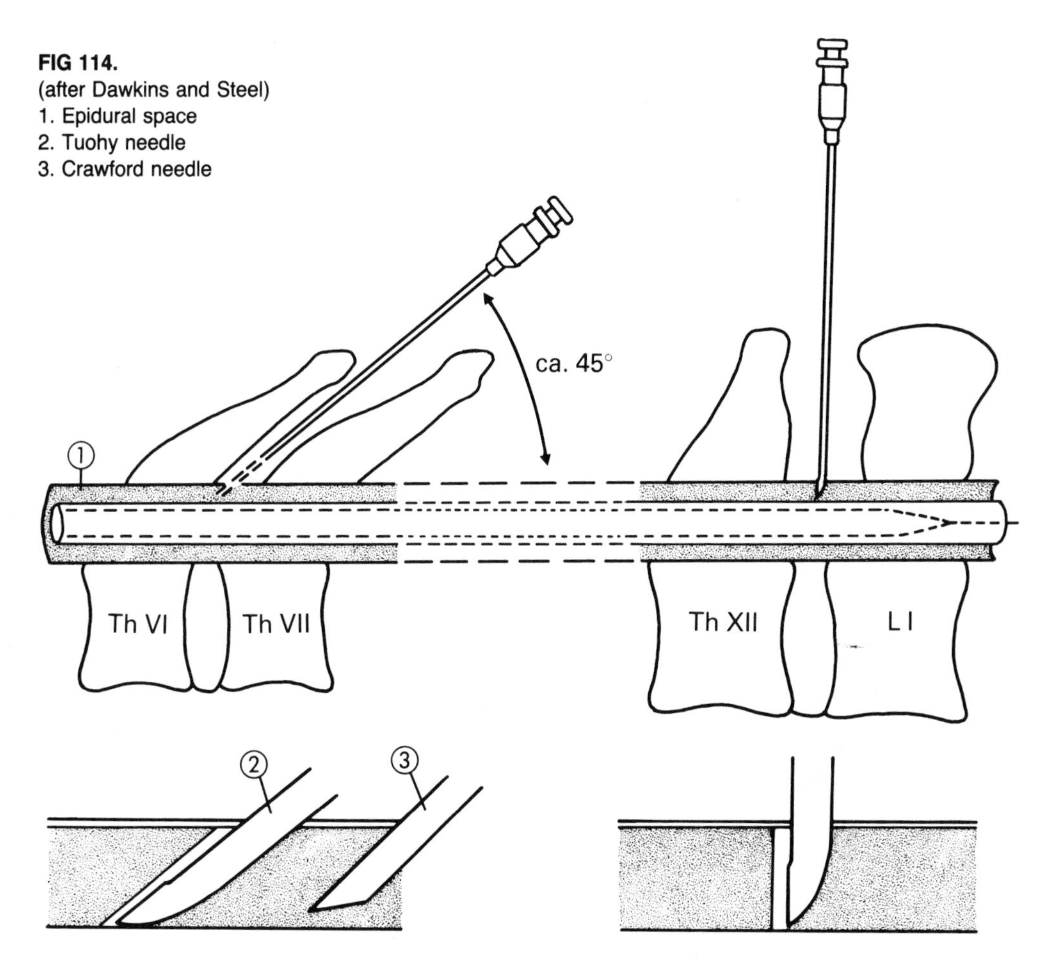

The danger of dural puncture is less in the midthoracic area, provided the needle is held correctly and the direction of entry is correct, since the steeper "path" from the ligamentum flavum to the dura is one and one half times as wide (Fig 114).

Single shot technique

Inject 2–3 ml of the local anesthetic solution as a test dose. After negative test and check of blood pressure and pulse as well as verbal contact, half the anticipated dose is injected slowly (0.3 ml/sec). The above checks are all repeated and, if satisfactory, the remainder of the dose is injected.

Catheter technique

Catheter with terminal opening: more frequent perforations are possible, particularly venous wall perforations.
Catheter with lateral openings: negative aspiration is frequent, even though placed intravenously.
After the catheter has been advanced (max. 3–5 cm = Mark III) the needle is withdrawn, while the catheter is "fed" in. A test dose is administered after aspiration (for blood or CSF). The catheter is taped, the patient is placed into surgical position (supine; in thoracic procedures with the contralateral side down). After another negative aspiration test, blood pressure and pulse monitoring, and verbal contact, half the dose is injected slowly (0.3 ml/sec). Repeat all checks, and if satisfactory, inject the remaining dose.

B. Paramedian and lateral approach

The skin wheal is placed paramedially (1 cm) or laterally (2.5 cm) from the caudal end of the spinous process. The subcutaneous tissues are infiltrated with a thin needle and the depth to the lamina is identified.
An epidural needle is slowly advanced to the ligamentum flavum at an angle of 10° (paramedian) or 20° (lateral) and up to 40° in a vertical plain (spinal column) (Fig 115). Up to this point there should be practically no resistance. When contact is made with the lamina, the depth is marked. The cannula is redirected and advanced slightly craniad.
The spinous process in the middle thoracic spine reaches to the height of the lamina of the subjacent arch. After loss of resistance, the same steps are followed as described above for the median technique. The needle should reach the epidural space in the midline.

Dosage

Test dose

It is never absolutely certain that there may not be a misdirected injection. An intrathecal position of the needle should be generally excluded by a negative aspiration test. Intravascular position (more frequent than intrathecal) can be excluded with a 2–3 ml test dose containing epinephrine. If the needle is in a vessel: tachycardia, tachyarrhythmia, hypertension within seconds (no waiting for minutes) may occur; hence: ECG monitor and measurement of pulse and blood pressure are in order.

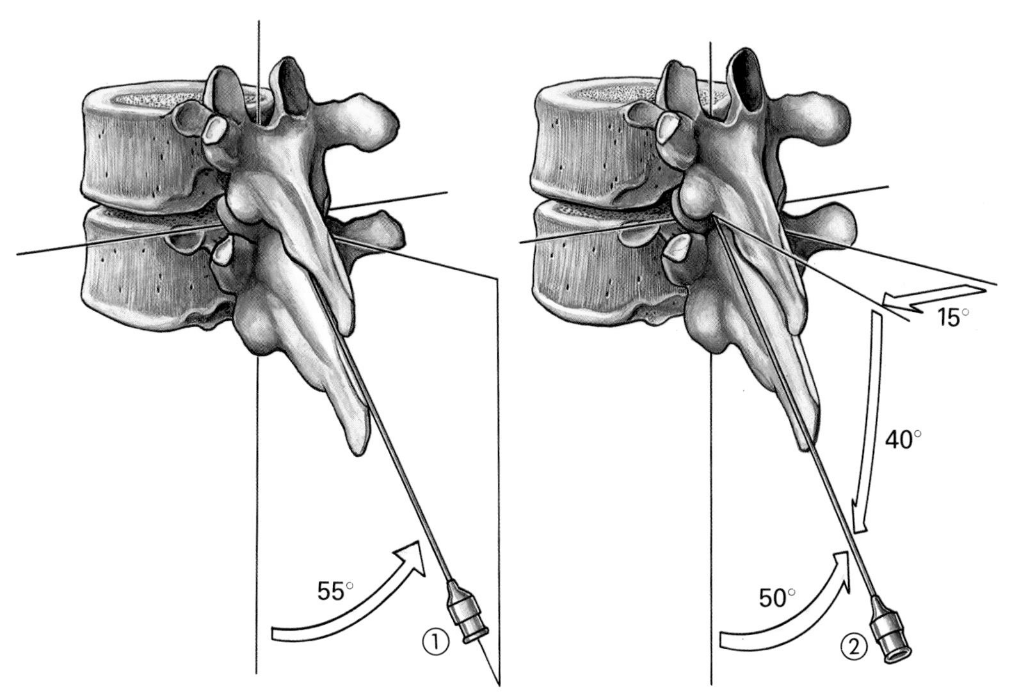

FIG 115.
(after Cousins)
Direction of the needle in:
1. Midline approach
2. Lateral approach

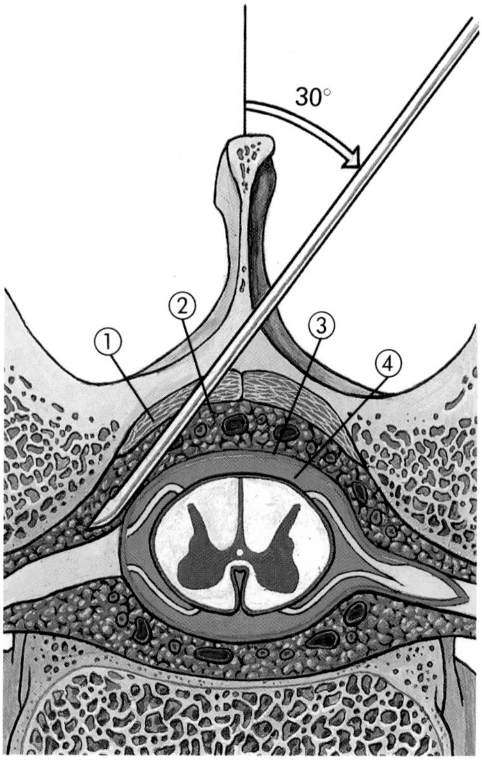

FIG 116.
(after Cousins)
Incorrect position of the needle: The bevel of the Tuohy needle points laterally
Incorrect direction: Lateral approach directed too far medially
1. Ligamentum flavum
2. Epidural space
3. Dura mater
4. Subarachnoid space

Dose

On a mg/segment basis the dose is about 30% less. Age dependence is the same as in the lumbar technique. The segmental distribution is clearly more even cranially and caudally, although the cervical segments are more resistant to a block since there is a greater density of fibers.
The time of onset for the long-acting local anesthetics, e.g., bupivacaine and etidocaine, is apparently somewhat shorter (smaller epidural space?).
The selection of the local anesthetic is largely dependent upon the desired effect and the pharmacologic properties of the local anesthetic.

4. Special Complications

See also: "Lumbar epidural anesthesia" (p. 114)
Injury to the spinal cord (extremely rare)
Dura perforation (less frequent than in lumbar epidural)
Vascular and nerve injury (most frequent with paramedian and lateral approach)
"High thoracic" above T_4 blocks the cardiac sympathetic fibers as well
Complete block to or over T_1 eliminates the cardiovascular regulatory mechanism and means additional duties for the anesthesiologist: volume loading (including plasma expander), atropine, vasoconstrictor (ephedrine), catecholamines

5. Indications

See also "Lumbar epidural anesthesia" (p. 116)
Abdominal procedures—particularly upper abdominal ones
Thoracic procedures and thoracic trauma (multiple rib fractures, unstable thorax)
Patients with pulmonary and cardiac pathology
Patients with metabolic disease (morbid obesity)
Postoperative analgesia and mobility (gut mobilization)
Therapeutic blocks (cancer pain, herpes zoster)

6. Special Contraindications

See "Lumbar epidural anesthesia" (p. 116).

7. Advantages–Disadvantages

Advantages over general anesthesia

See also "Advantages of regional anesthesia over general anesthesia" (p. 5) and "Spinal anesthesia" (p. 105).
Better ventilation intra- and postoperatively.
Less intraoperative blood loss.
Less metabolic load—less stress reaction.
Renal function is not depressed.
Lower incidence of thromboembolism
No trace gas exposure for the O.R. personnel.

References

1. Cousins MJ, Bridenbaugh PO: *Neural Blockade.* Philadelphia–Toronto, JB Lippincott Co, 1980.

2. Cheng PA: The anatomical and clinical aspects of epidural anesthesia. *Anesth Analg* 1963; 42:398.
3. Dawkins CJM, Steel GC: Thoracic extradural (epidural) block for upper abdominal surgery. *Anaesthesia* 1971; 26:41.
4. Sobotta-Becher: *Atlas der deskriptiven Anatomie des Menschen,* 1. Teil, München-Berlin, Urban & Schwarzenberg, 1957.

Caudal Anesthesia

H. Chr. Niesel, O. Schulte-Steinberg

1. Definition

See "Lumbar epidural anesthesia" (p. 106) and "Caudal anesthesia in obstetrics" (p. 143).

2. Topographic Anatomy

See "Lumbar epidural anesthesia" (p. 106) and "Caudal anesthesia in obstetrics" (p. 143).

3. Technique

3.1. Anesthesiologic Assessment

Careful anesthesiologic assessment including the identification of any contraindication.

3.2. Preparation

Intravenous cannula, infusion of a balanced electrolyte solution, ventilation equipment with O_2 connection, intubation equipment, atropine, sedative, succinylcholine, vasopressor, catecholamine.

3.3. Equipment

Disposable sets or individually assembled sets

Contents (example):

Syringes: 2 ml syringe (for infiltration)
5 ml loose glass or plastic syringe
20 ml syringe, to inject the local anesthetic solution

Needles: Thin needle for infiltration
Median length needles (20 or 22 g) or 16 g or 17 g needles or Tuohy needle (for catheter technique)
Needles to draw up solutions

Other: Drapes with clip or adhesive drape
Cup for antiseptic solution
Sponges for prep and for dressing
Ampules with 0.9% NaCl
Local anesthetic solutions

3.4. Positioning

Prone is best. Ideally on a flexed operating table, or with a pillow under the pelvic area. The legs are spread and externally rotated as far as possible. For special considerations of positioning in obstetrics, see "Caudal anesthesia in obstetrics" (p. 144).

3.5. Landmarks

The dorsal superior iliac spines are marked and are connected with a line. This line serves as the base of an equilateral triangle pointing caudad. The tip of the triangle will lie in the area of the sacral hiatus. Laterally to this point the sacral cornua should be palpable.

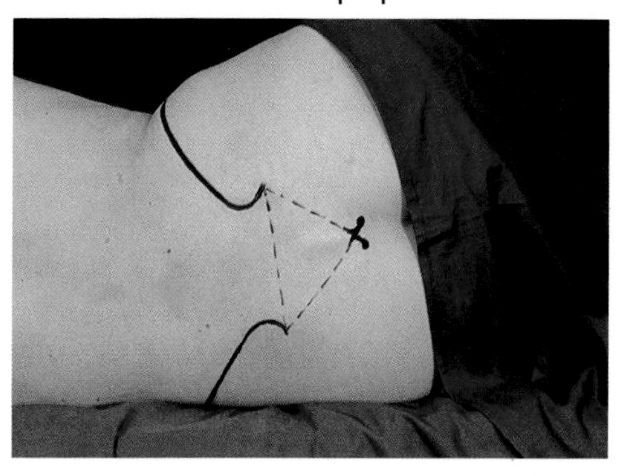

FIG 117.

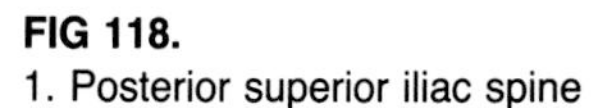

FIG 118.
1. Posterior superior iliac spine

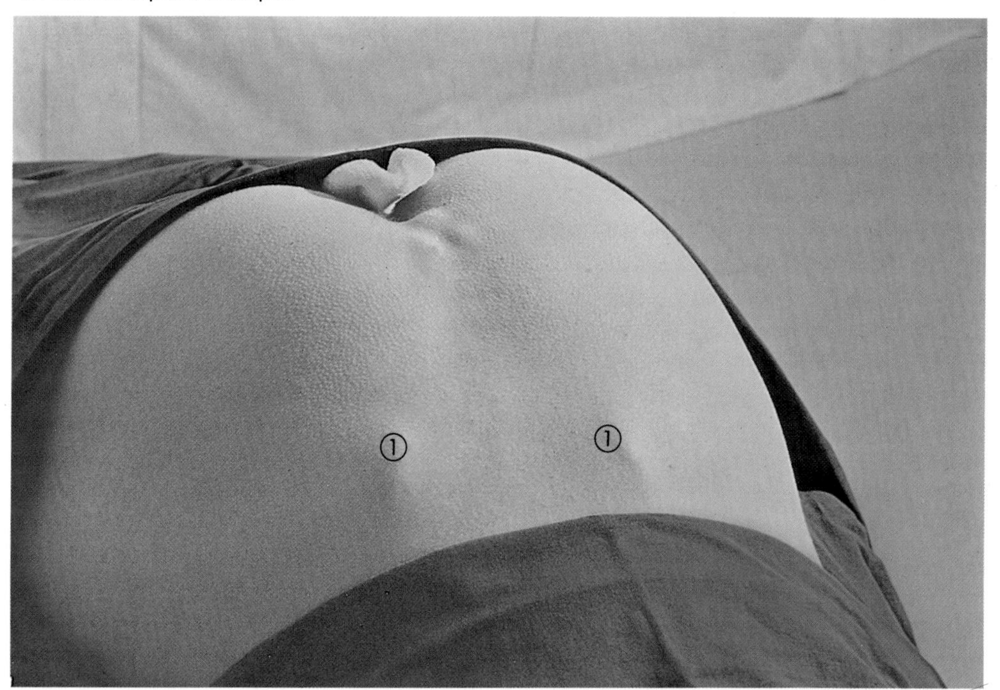

3.6. Technical procedure

Preparation as in epidural anesthesia. Intracutaneous infiltration of the skin. Introduction of the sacral needle into the sacral hiatus. If bone is encountered, the needle is slightly withdrawn, the hub is depressed, and the needle is again advanced so that it may enter the sacral canal (approx. 2 cm). See also "Caudal anesthesia in obstetrics" (p. 144).

Catheter-caudal anesthesia (continuous)

Puncture and introduction of the needle as above. Followed by introduction of the catheter to a maximum of 2 cm beyond the tip of the needle. Withdraw the needle without any tension on the catheter. Connect the catheter to a filter and to a syringe under sterile cover (see the section on catheter epidural anesthesia, p. 111).
Aspiration test. Resistance should be checked by injecting a small volume of saline solution. Injection should encounter only very little resistance. Injection of test dose. After a delay of 5 min the rest of the dose is injected.
Technical difficulties: superficial dorsal deviation of the needle. This can be recognized by a subcutaneous swelling during and after injection. Superiostial injection inside the sacral canal can be recognized by increased resistance to injection. Presacral injection, perforation of the rectum. No caudal anesthesia should be administered if the leading part of the fetus is already at a presacral level. Technical difficulties are more frequent in caudal anesthesia than in spinal or epidural anesthesia.

3.7. Dosage

Test dose

3–5 ml local anesthetic solution. Wait 5 min after the test dose.

Dose

The intensity of the block is determined by the concentration of the local anesthetic solution, exactly as in lumbar or thoracic epidural anesthesia. The level of anesthesia depends on the volume injected, since the anesthesia must spread from caudal to cranial. With 15–20 ml the level will be from S_5–L_2. With a volume of 25 ml, the level will be from S_5–T_{10}. For special consideration in children, see p. 130. For special considerations in pregnant patients, see "Caudal anesthesia in obstetrics" (p. 146).

Special considerations in caudal anesthesia in children

In children, both single shot and continuous caudal anesthesia can be performed surpisingly simply and with remarkable dispatch.

First, a light general anesthetic is given with nitrous oxide, oxygen, halothane, enflurane, ketamine (4 mg/kg), i.m., or with rectal methohexital (10% solution—100 mg/ml;/25 mg/kg—0.25 ml/kg). In children, for single shot caudal anesthesia, the position of the needle is not changed after the sacral canal has been entered (Fig 119). In this respect, the technique in children differs from the one described in "Caudal anesthesia in obstetrics" (p. 144).

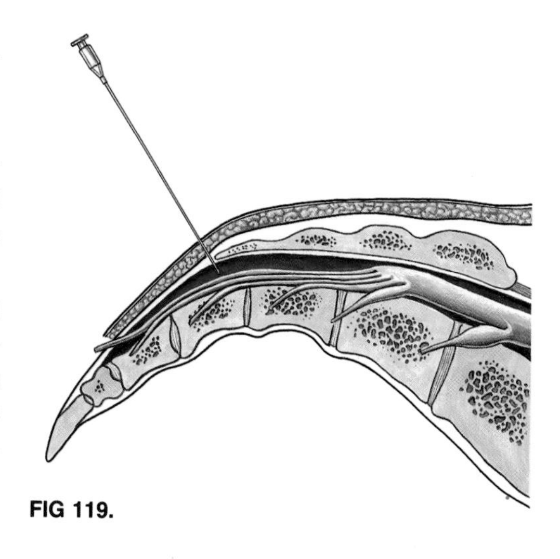

FIG 119.

For continuous anesthesia, a 1.4 mm plastic needle is introduced into the sacral canal. The stylette is partially withdrawn

FIG 120.
Plastic cannula placed into the caudal canal. Measurement of the catheter.

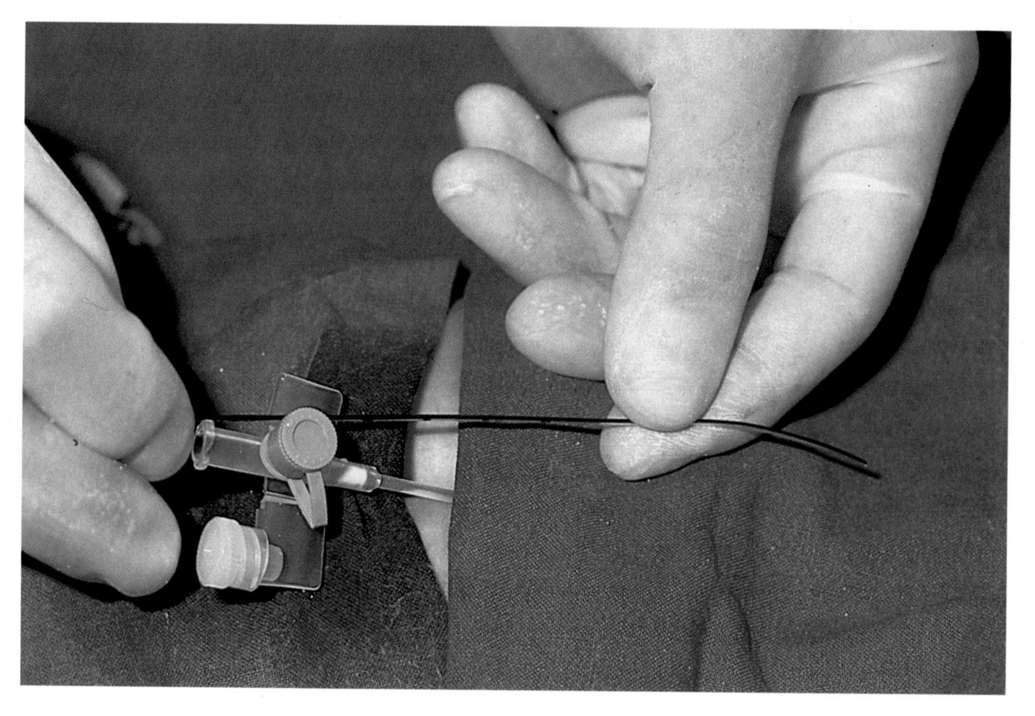

and the plastic sheath is advanced 1–2 cm. If the plastic needle is in the correct position, an 18 g epidural catheter can be introduced through this needle with ease and advanced to the level of the lumbar vertebrae. The loose structure of the epidural fatty tissues makes the introduction of the catheter easy in children.

Depending on the position of the tip of the catheter, lumbar epidural anesthesia can be administered through the caudal approach. The structure of the fatty tissue is such that it allows a further spread of the injected local anesthetic solution than that found in the adult. In fact, depending on the volume injected, high thoracic anesthesia can be achieved.

During long surgical procedures it is possible to administer a second dose—usually half of the initial dose. Because of the possibility of infection through urine and feces, the catheter should always be removed at the end of the procedure. To rule out the possibility of an intravascular position of the needle or of the catheter, a test dose of 1–2 ml of local anesthetic solution with epinephrine must be administered.

If the needle is in a vessel, monitoring with a precordial stethoscope, blood pressure cuff, and ECG will reveal arrhythmias, hypertension, and tachycardia within 1 min. Upper abdominal procedures may require endotracheal intubation and ventilation, depending on the circumstances. Muscle relaxants are usually not needed.

The dose to be used in children is given in the diagram (Fig 121) in ml per segments to be blocked. Nevetheless, in calculating the dose, the maximum permissible amount must always be determined on the basis of body weight and the volume suggested by the curve may have to be given in a more dilute solution.

4. Special Complications

The complications are similar to those discussed under lumbar and thoracic epidural anesthesia. This is particularly true for the severe early reactions.

Total spinal anesthesia

Massive epidural block (relative overdose)

Hypotension, bradycardia

Disturbances in bladder function, a particular concern in obstetrics (see also "Lumbar epidural anesthesia," p. 114)

Catheter breakage

(Never withdraw the catheter while the needle is still in place.)

Neurologic damage

(Mechanical injury after multiple punctures or in the case of an anatomic variation.)

Infection

(In view of the proximity to the anal region, which can never be kept clean, the danger of infection is relatively great. Hence the utmost care must be taken. Otherwise, similar to epidural anesthesia.)

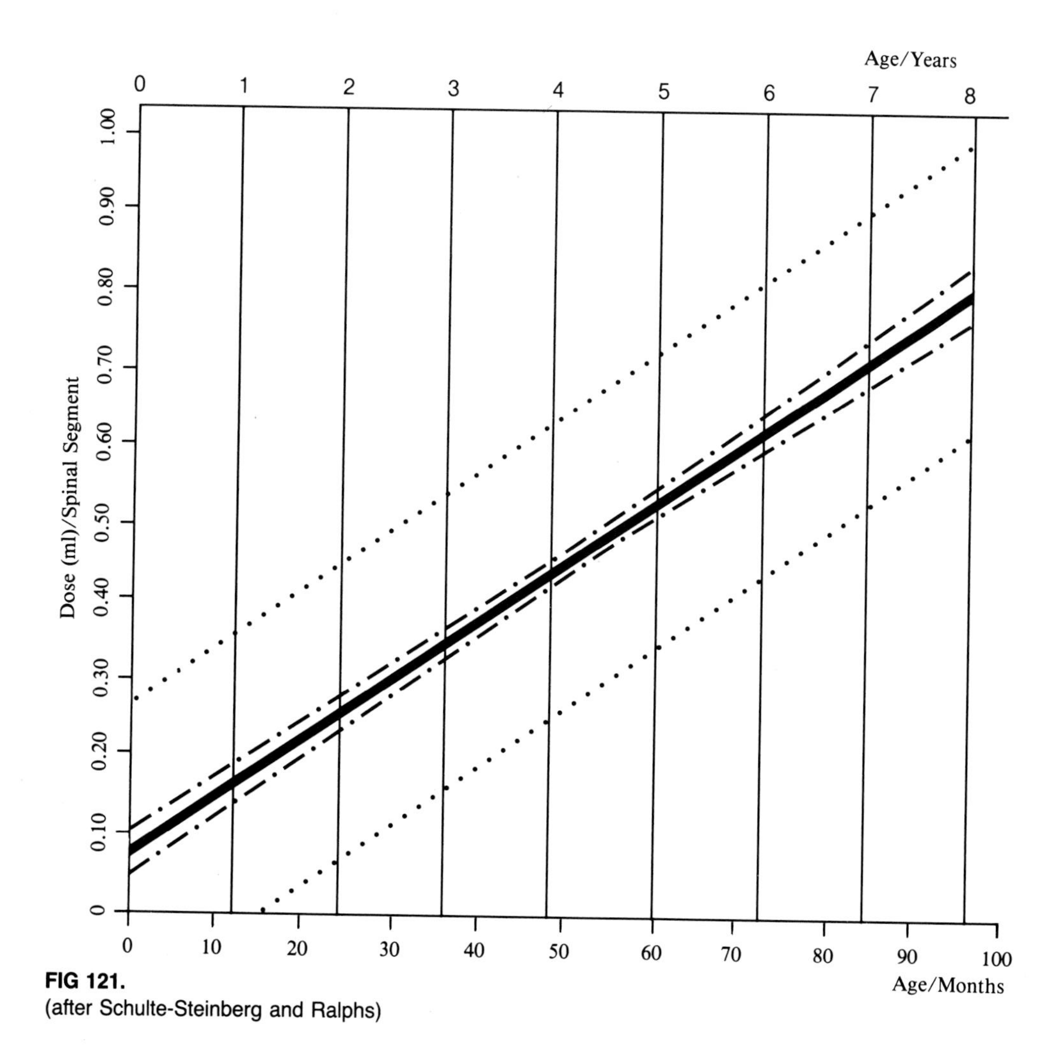

FIG 121.
(after Schulte-Steinberg and Ralphs)

5. Indications

Surgical procedures in the perineal area, on the lower extremities, and in the lower abdomen
Therapeutic blocks

6. Special Contraindications

Shock
Coagulopathies
Sepsis
Neurologic disease
Anatomic difficulties
See also "Lumbar epidural anesthesia" (p. 111)

Obstetrics

Lumbar Epidural Anesthesia in Obstetrics

W. Müller-Holve, O. Schulte-Steinberg

1. Definition

Providing relief for the pain associated with labor and delivery by the administration of a local anesthetic into the epidural space. The local anesthetic solution is placed primarily into the lumbar and lower thoracic area so that the painful sensations of the first stage (T_{11}–L_1) and of the second stage (S_2–S_4) are blocked.

2. Topographic Anatomy

See "Lumbar epidural anesthesia" (p. 106).

Special considerations for epidural anesthesia in obstetrics

a. During pregnancy, venous pressure is elevated and thus the pressure in the epidural space is also increased, since this area is very rich in veins. During uterine contractions in labor, the pressure is further increased by the retrograde pressure in the venous system.
b. During pregnancy, there is an increased fluid content in the tissues which keeps increasing until delivery. Both of these factors make it more difficult to locate the epidural space.

3. Technique

See "Lumbar epidural anesthesia" (p. 106).

Special considerations in epidural anesthesia in obstetrics

Preparation

Anesthesia machine and all equipment and supplies for general anesthesia. Defibrillator.
Drugs ready to be injected: diazepam, succinylcholine, ritodrine (because of a possible increase in the force of the contractions).
Monitoring the fetus with cardiotokography and pH determinations.

Equipment

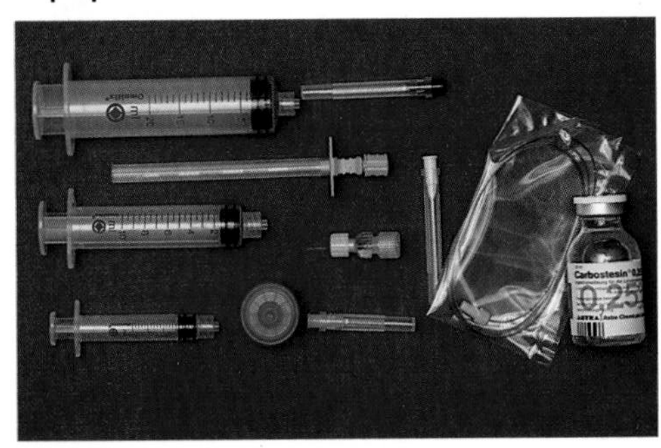

FIG 122.
Perifix^R, Fa. B. Braun Melsungen AG.

Positioning

Since women in labor are subject to circulatory problems, a lateral position is preferable. On the other hand, the sitting position makes it easier to obtain a suitable curvature of the spine in a pregnant woman at term. The administration of anesthesia in both positions must be mastered.
An assistant is always required.

Technical procedures

No premedication is given to obstetric patients.
For reasons of safety, only the continuous epidural technique should be considered.

Prerequisites

1. Continuous fetal monitoring with ECG tokography.
2. Facilities for pH monitoring.
3. No oxytocin drip during the administration of the local anesthetic. (Fetal complications are increased if oxytocins and local anesthetics are administered simultaneously.)
4. No amniotomy for 30 min before and after the administration of the local anesthetic solution.
5. Aseptic technique.
6. Monitor bladder function. (Atony of the bladder is somewhat more frequent under epidural anesthesia, since the sensitivity of the bladder is decreased during labor and delivery and in the postpartum period.)

Administration

Preloading with 500 ml of an electrolyte solution.
The test dose should be administered with the patient in the lateral position, so that only unilateral motor blockade should ensue if the catheter was inadvertently placed intrathecally.
The main anesthetic dose should be given in the period between contractions, since at the time of uterine contractions the pressure in the epidural space is increased, and the level of the anesthesia may become extremely high.

In order for the anesthetic to spread equally to both sides, the patient is placed in the supine position and the uterus is displaced to the left to avoid the vena cava compression syndrome (Fig 123).

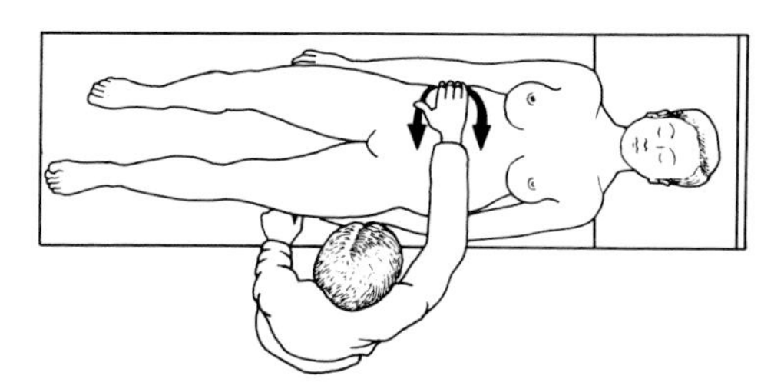

FIG 123.

If signs of the vena cava compression syndrome still appear, the patient should be turned from side to side in rapid sequence. (The patient should stay no more than 2 min on each side.)

In the early stages of dilatation, the main dose can be given with the patient in an almost supine position (Fig 124).

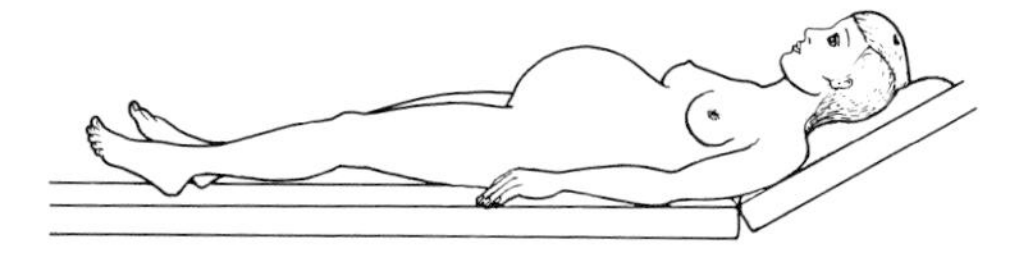

FIG 124.

In the later stages of dilatation (station 1 or more), and in the expulsive stage, the upper part of the patient's body should be elevated by approximately 30–60° so that the lower segments are affected.

If additional local anesthetic administration becomes necessary during the expulsive stage because of the need for operative vaginal delivery and/or for the repair of the episiotomy, the patient should be placed in a sitting position (Fig 125).

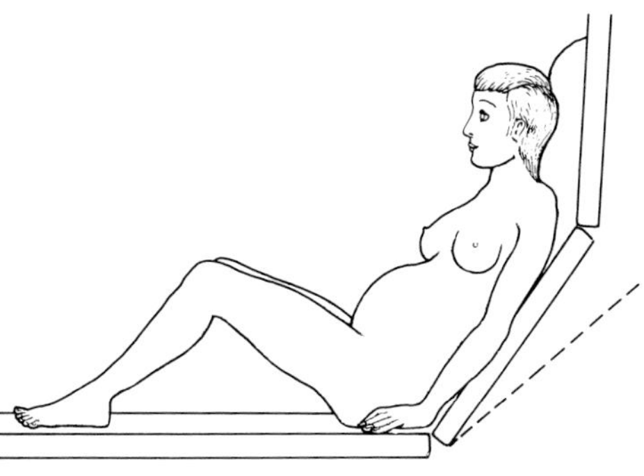

FIG 125.

The followup administrations should be in the same volume as the initial dose, i.e., 6–10 ml. Exception: after the full dose has been administered, the patient still complains of unilateral or bilateral pain at the time of contractions. In this case, 2–4 ml of additional local anesthetic solution can be given 20 min after the administration of the initial dose. This additional dose should be injected with the patient in the lateral position, i.e., lying on the less anesthetized side.

Important

1. After each dose, including the supplemental doses, verbal contact must be established with the patient and a hearing test should be performed (whispered questions) so that changes in cranial nerve function as a consequence of a total spinal can be recognized early.
2. Blood pressure must be monitored frequently (3–5 min) during the first 30 min after the administration of the full dose.

3. Crude estimation of the level of anesthesia (pinching, needle stick, cold–warm test, test of motor power), since in pregnant women the level of the analgesia in epidural anesthesia may be very variable.
   Further administrations of local anesthesia should be done on the request of the patient and in relation to the birthing process.

If the bearing down reflex is severely limited

The hands of the pregnant woman should be placed on the fundus of the uterus, so that she may feel the contractions and bear down synchronously with the contractions.
It is important to record accurately the circulatory status, the doses administered, the level of anesthesia, and the motor function.

Variations in the dose during the time of contractions

To interfere with the contractions as little as possible, and to maintain the motor function in the lower extremities, a further dilution of bupivacaine to a 0.125% solution and a volume of 10–16 ml, administered in the sitting position has proven satisfactory.

Chronic placental insufficiency

The administration of 4–6 ml of 0.125% bupivacaine per hour, with an infusion pump and with the patient in the lateral position (if possible with patient lying on the left side). This will maximize uterine perfusion.

When the contractions must be stopped

2–3 × 4 ml of 0.5% bupivacaine or etidocaine (1%, administered in the sitting position).

Dosage

A. Vaginal Delivery

In view of the recent reports of unfortunate incidents, particularly after the use of the local anesthetic bupivacaine, the primary dose and all subsequent doses should be given as fractional doses: the volume of a single injection should not exceed 4 ml.
The dose of the local anesthetic solution on a "per segment" basis is about one-third less in the pregnant woman than in the nonpregnant one.
In a patient less than 1.60 m tall, a primary dose of 6 ml (2 × 3 ml with a 10 min interval) of 0.25% bupivacaine is recommended.
Alternatively: 2 × 3 ml lidocaine 0.5%.
In larger patients, 8–10 ml may be used.

B. Cesarean Section

See "Regional anesthesia techniques for cesarean section" (p. 150).

4. Special Complications

See "Lumbar epidural anesthesia" (p. 114).
All these problems may also occur with epidural anesthesia in obstetrics. The highest consideration should be given to the possibility of producing circulatory complications.
If in doubt: rapidly infuse electrolyte solution and give vasoactive medication.

COMPLICATIONS	THERAPY
a. Excessive increase in the intensity of labor after the primary dose is given (polysystolia; rise in the CTG base line)	Left lateral position, IV administration of a tokolytic agent (e.g., ritodrine)
b. Vena cava compression syndrome (only in the supine position; practically never present when uterus is displaced to the left)	Lateral position, on the left side if possible at first, and then alternating (to assure even spread of the anesthetic solution). If the basal uterine tone increases, a tokolytic should be given; in persistent fetal bradycardia—O_2 administration
c. Pathologic CTG	Left lateral position, O_2 administration, tokolysis, preparation for cesarean section
d. Massive spread of the anesthetic level in spite of a normal dose	Ample fluid administration, circulatory support (ephedrine 1–5 mg IV). This drug does not reduce uterine perfusion

5. Indications

A. Vaginal delivery

Chronic placental insufficiency

If the fetus is poorly developed (e.g., in toxemia or nicotine abuse) the decreased uterine perfusion can be improved with epidural anesthesia.
In preeclamptic mothers with a poorly developed fetus, epidural anesthesia for several weeks (e.g., 2–4 wk) can produce good therapeutic results. The epidural anesthesia results in improved uterine perfusion, and thus in accelerated fetal growth. It also leads to a decrease in maternal blood pressure and a decreased tendency of convulsions.

Premature birth

The decreased tone of the muscular components of the pelvic floor represents an important reduction in birth trauma for the premature infant.
The premature fetus is also particularly sensitive to even transient hypoxia. Epidural anesthesia reduces the risk of hypoxia by improving uterine perfusion.

When the contractions must be stopped

In all cases of natural or operative vaginal deliveries, where for maternal or fetal reasons the uterine contractions must be stopped.

a. Maternal indications:
   Threatening retinal separation, retinal hemorrhage, cerebral hemorrhage, cardiopulmonary disease, diabetes mellitus, and other metabolic diseases.

b. Fetal indications:
   Vaginal breech presentation, twins with probable operative delivery, forceps delivery of a premature infant.

Predictable high analgetic use in patients who are very sensitive to pain

High serum level of analgetic agents leads to respiratory depression in the newborn. On the other hand, uncontrolled labor pains can lead to fetal hypoxia through increased catecholamine levels, resulting in increased uterine contractions.

Vaginal delivery in a patient with the history of a previous cesarean section

Under epidural anesthesia, it is possible to palpate the uterine scar during labor alongside the leading fetal part, without pain to the patient. This allows the recognition of a threatening rupture (Fig 126).

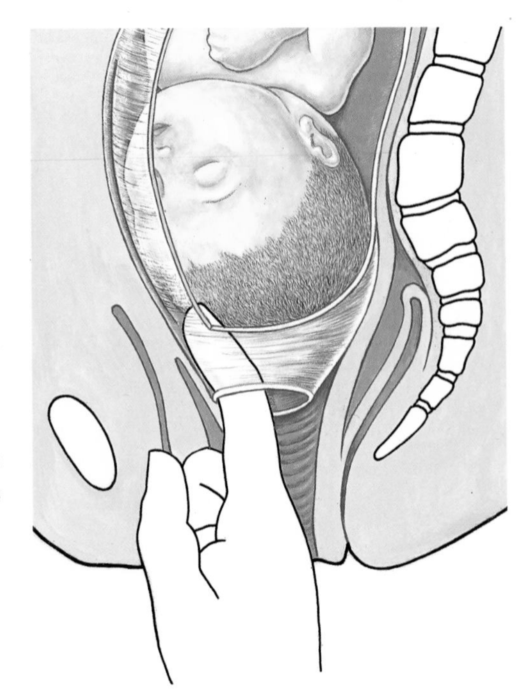

FIG 126.
Modified after Mehan (1976).

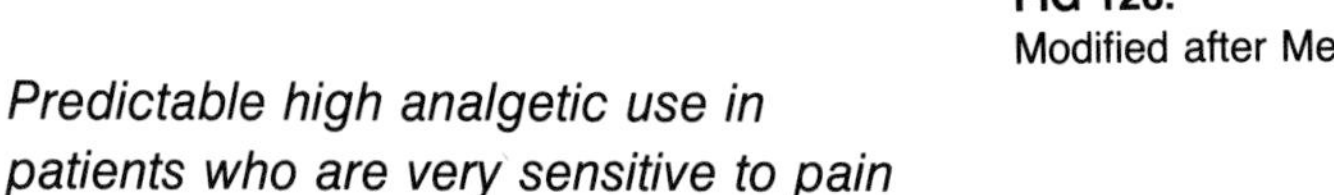

B. *Cesarean section*

See "Regional anesthesia techniques for cesarean section" (p. 151).

6. Special Contraindications

Coagulopathies, uterine bleeding due to placenta previa or premature separation of the placenta, orthopedic problems in the lumbar spine area, CNS disease, hypovolemia, acute placental insufficiency (late or variable deceleration), need for an urgent operative delivery.

References

1. Jaschevatzky OE, Shalit A, Levy Y: Epidural analgesia during labour in twin pregnancy. *Brit J Obstet Gynec* 1977; 84:327.
2. Moir DD, Victor-Rodrigues L, Willocks J: Epidural analgesia during labour in patients with pre-eclampsia. *J Obstet Gynec Brit Cmwlth* 1972; 79:465.
3. Müller-Holve W: Physiologische, biochemische und klinische Parameter zur Einwirkung der Epiduralanalgesie auf den Feten. *Habilitationsschrift,* München, 1979.
4. Strasser K, Albrecht H: Die lumbale Peridural-, die Kaudal- und Spinalanästhesie, in: Beck L, Albrecht H (Hrsg): *Analgesie und Anästhesie in der Geburtshilfe.* Stuttgart–New York, Thieme, 1982.

Caudal Anesthesia in Obstetrics

P. Berle

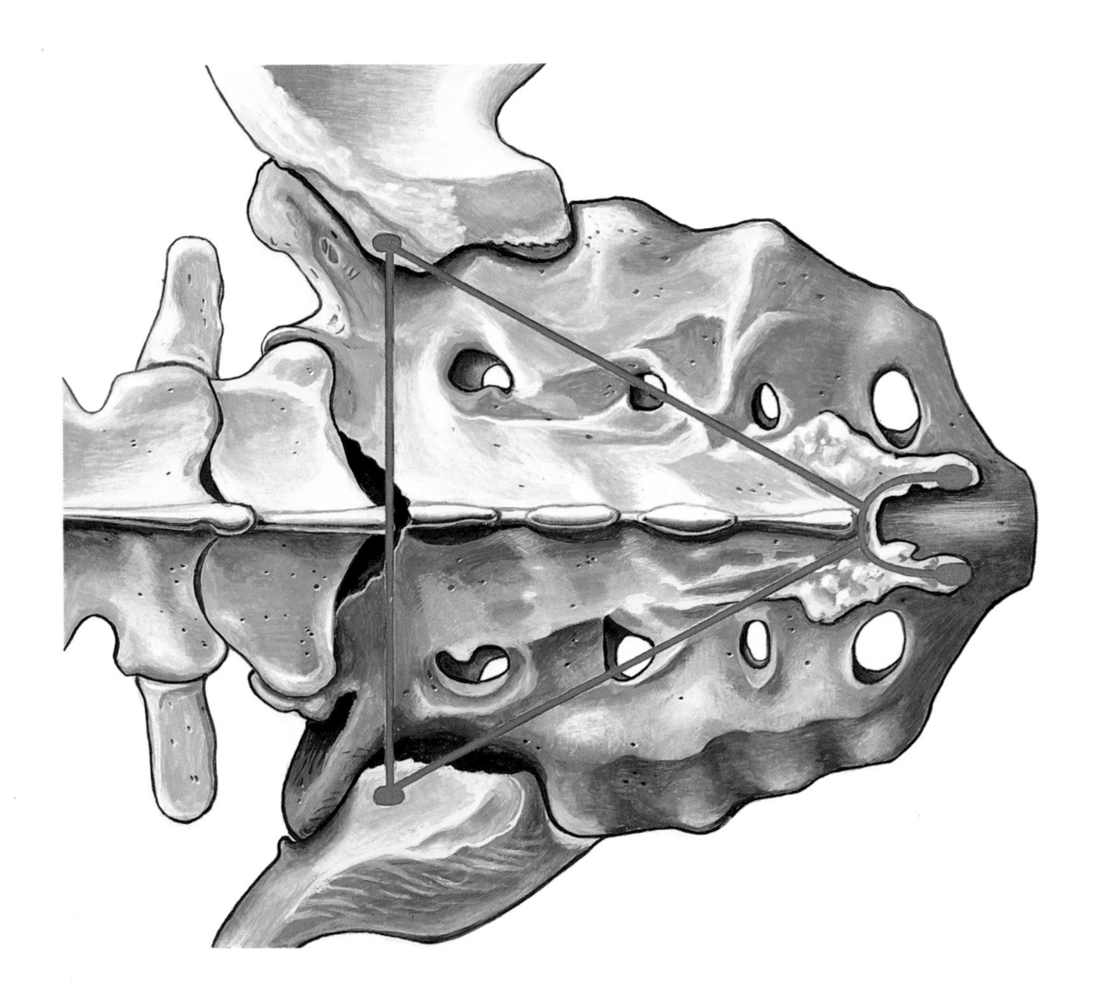

FIG 127.
The tip of an equilateral triangle, based on a line between the posterior superior iliac spines, lies in the area of the sacral hiatus.

1. Definition

Caudal anesthesia is a form of epidural anesthesia where the local anesthetic solution is administered from a caudal direction through a needle placed in the sacral canal.

2. Topographic Anatomy

At the level of the first sacral vertebra, the vertebral canal becomes the sacral canal, which ends between the sacrum and the coccyx.

Dorsal border: the fused transverse and spinous processes of the first four sacral vertebrae and their periosteum; at the level of the fifth sacral vertebra: the dorsal sacrococcygeal ligament. The articular processes of the fifth sacral vertebra form the sacral cornua between which the exit portal of the sacral canal, the sacral hiatus, is located (Fig 127). The ventral border of the sacral canal is formed by the periosteum of the bodies of the five sacral vertebrae.

Deviations from the norm occur in 10% of the cases and this may make caudal anesthesia difficult or impossible.

The sacral canal contains the filum terminale of the dura, the fifth sacral nerve, and the coccygeal nerve. The dural sack ends between S_1 and S_2, i.e., 2–3 cm below the palpable superior processes in only 43% of all cases. In 32%, the dural sack ends in the middle of S_2; in 23%, between S_2 and S_3; and in 2% between S_3 and S_4.

3. Technique

3.1 Anesthesiologic Assessment

Careful anesthesiologic assessment including the identification of any contraindication.

3.2. Preparation

Intravenous cannula and infusion of a balanced electrolyte solution.
Ventilation equipment with O_2 connection; intubation equipment, atropine, sedative, succinylcholine, vasopressor, catecholamine.

The explanation of the procedure and of the possible complications should take place, if possible, during the pregnancy so that the patient can be admitted to the labor room with the consent form already signed. Regional anesthesia in obstetrics must be preceded by a thorough discussion with the patient.

3.3. Equipment

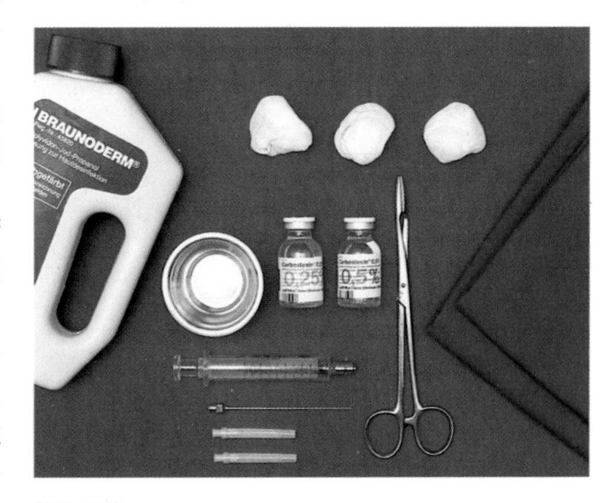

FIG 128.

One 10 ml glass syringe
Two 10 cm, flexible, 0.8 mm diameter, short bevel needles
Two disposable needles, 23 g or 25 g
One small steel cup
Sponge forceps
Several sponges
Drapes
Three ampules of 0.25% and three ampules of 0.5% bupivacaine (a 0.375% concentration can be used as a mixture of the two)

3.4. Positioning

Left lateral position facilitates the needle placement for the right-handed physician. Advancement of the needle into the sacral canal can be performed carefully by the right hand. Identification of the sacral hiatus by palpation is made easier in the left lateral position by flexion of the right hip and knee joints, since this opens up the anal fold. (The reverse position for left-handed physicians.)

3.5. Landmarks

The sacral cornua are easily palpable in the slender patient. The finger palpating the fused spinous processes can readily identify the midline hiatus between the sacral cornua.

A prominent coccyx can also serve as a guideline but the distance between the coccyx and the sacral hiatus is quite variable (2–5 cm.).

3.6. Technical Procedure

Surgical scrub, sterile gloves, wide area prep, sterile drapes.

The needle is introduced at right angles to the skin between the sacral cornua, and is advanced into the sacral hiatus. Injection of 1–2 ml local anesthetic solution provides anesthesia for the periosteum and the site of the needle entry. Subcutaneous injection should be avoided, since it may make the identification of the sacral cornua more difficult. After 2–3 min, the longer needle can be introduced painlessly, at right angles to the skin, into the sacral hiatus, and through the ligament. (Transversing the ligament can be felt by a more or less obvious decrease in resistance.) The space between the ligament and the posterior surface of the sacral vertebral body is very narrow. When bony contact is made with the tip of the needle, the needle is withdrawn a very short distance and is depressed 30–60°

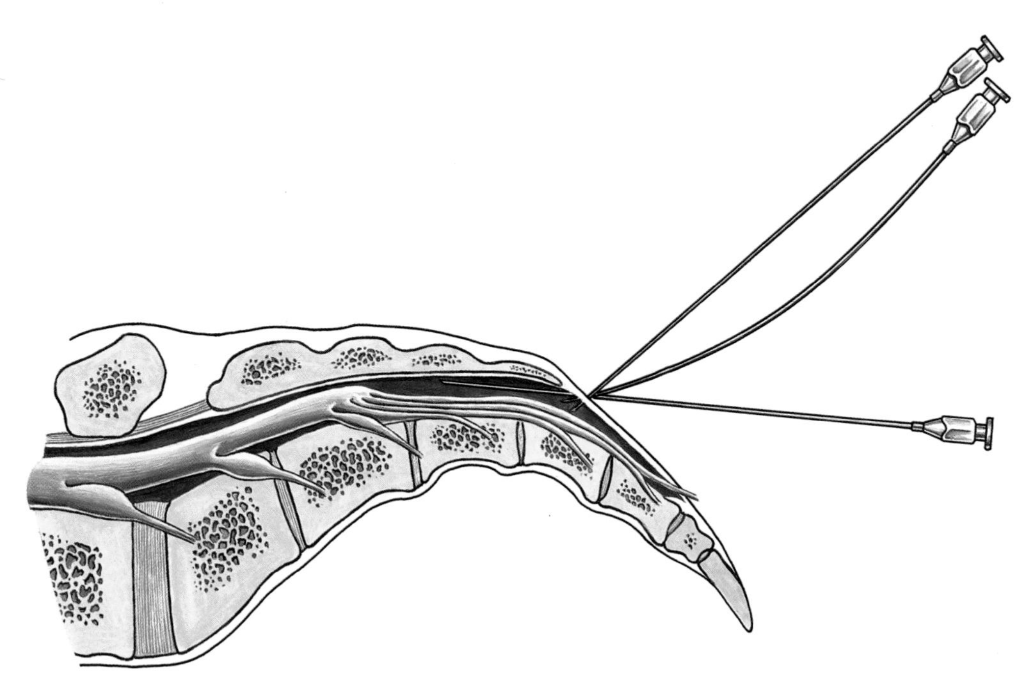

FIG 129.

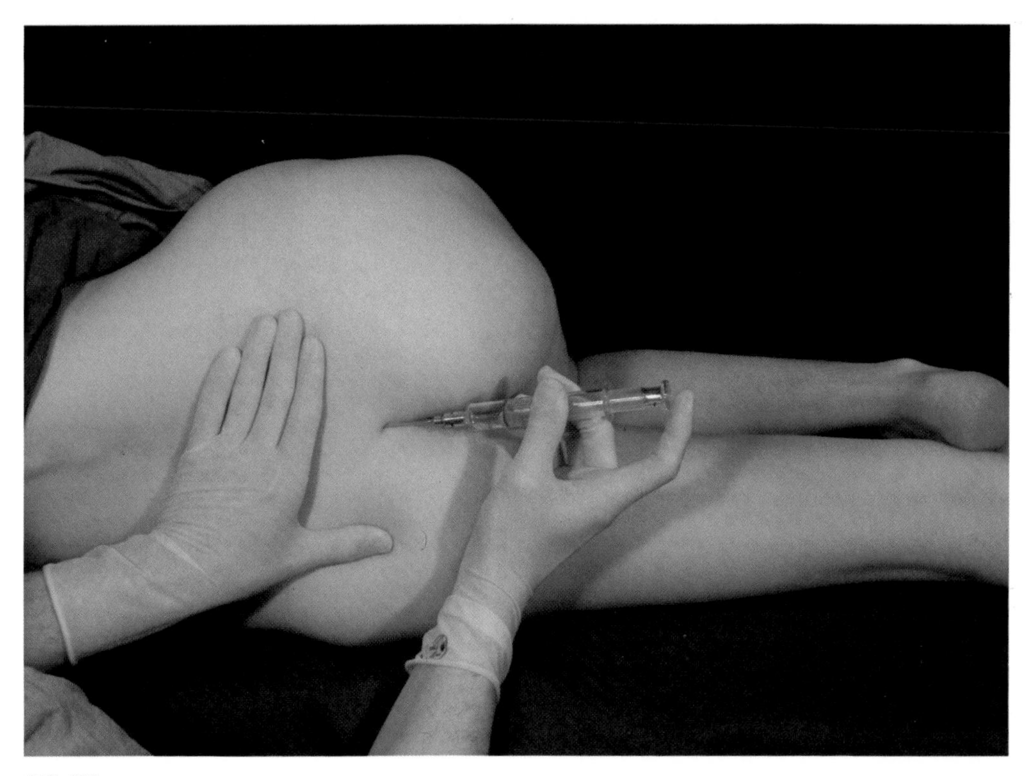

FIG 130.

in the direction of the anal fold, so that the shaft of the needle is in line with the sacrum. The needle is then advanced into the sacral canal (Fig 129). The tip of the needle should not proceed beyond S_2, and is better placed at S_3 (dural puncture). While advancing the needle, the initial resistance of the periosteum on the posterior wall of the sacral canal can be felt, so that the injection of air (5 ml) to prove the position of the needle can usually be omitted. In cases where it is desirable to perform the test, pressure with the palm of the hand (left) over the sacrum will make the entry of air into the subcutaneous tissues obvious should the needle be placed superficial to the sacrum (Fig 130). If no blood or CSF appears at the hub of the needle either spontaneously or after aspiration, a test dose of 5 ml of the anesthetic solution can be injected, to eliminate the possibility of an intravascular or intrathecal injection.

If the 5 ml test dose does not produce any undesirable reaction, the remainder of the anesthetic solution may be injected slowly. If the needle placement is correct, there is little resistance to the injection, and there may be a tingling sensation in the feet or a feeling of tightness in the thighs during the injection. If the needle is placed subperiostally, there is marked resistance to the injection and there will be some pain over the sacrum (Fig 131). If this occurs, the needle should be withdrawn slightly and advanced somewhat more ventrally.

If CSF appears at the end of the needle or in the syringe, all attempts to establish caudal anesthesia must be abandoned.

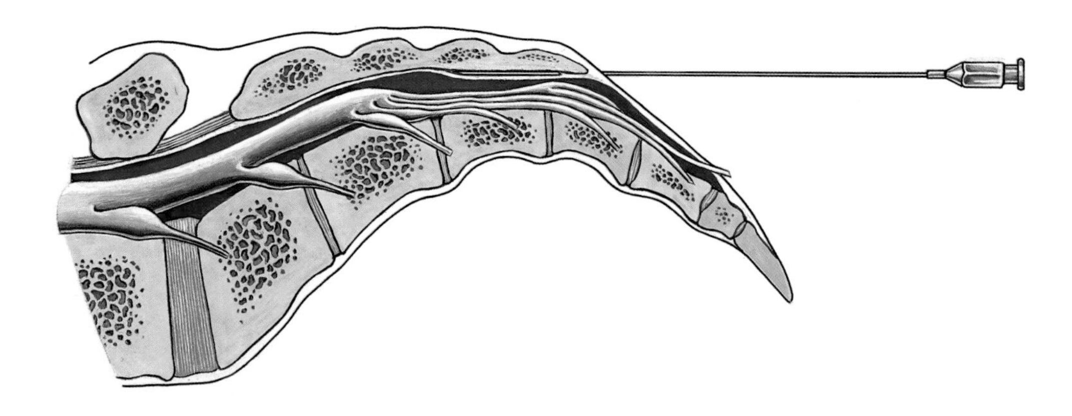

FIG 131.

The danger of a massive entry of the local anesthetic solution into the subarachnoid space is too great, even if the needle is withdrawn somewhat. If blood is withdrawn, there is no absolute contraindication to proceed after the position of the needle has been readjusted.

Since the needle lies fairly deeply in the anal fold, the use of continuous caudal anesthesia in obstetrics is questionable, due to the real danger of infection. The repeated vaginal examinations necessary during labor require that the patient be in a supine position and that the external genitalia be repeatedly cleansed with some antiseptic solution. For this reason, the possibility of infection can never be ruled out entirely for any one case. The inevitable moistness of this area makes isolation of the caudal injection site with a tight plastic seal extremely difficult, if not impossible.

3.7. Dosage

Bupivacaine 0.375%.

The volume of solution needed to achieve a level of analgesia to T_{10} (elimination of pain impulses from the urogenital area) depends on the size of the patient. For every 4 cm above 1.50 m total body height, the minimal dose must be increased by 1 ml.

HEIGHT	DOSE
1.50 m	25 ml
1.54 m	26 ml
1.58 m	27 ml
1.70 m and taller	30 ml

The injection can be repeated once or twice at intervals of 4 hours.

Onset of analgesia: 5–15 min.

Duration of analgesia: 3–4 hr.

4. Special Side Effects and Complications

Side effects

Transient decrease in uterine activity, loss of motor function in the lower extremities, and decreased ability to bear down. This leads to a prolongation of the first and second stages of labor.

Complications

In case of intravascular injection: hypertension, tachycardia arrhythmias, and headache.

Toxic reactions with convulsions (0.1%).
Dural puncture (1.2%).
Unrecognized dural puncture and total spinal block (0.1%).
Hypotension due to dehydration and/or sympathetic blockade potentiated by narcotics (2.4%).

5. Indications

Analgesia during the first and second stages of labor, particularly in eclampsia; premature or impaired fetus without pathologic cardiotokogram; ineffective, prolonged labor.
Manual removal of the placenta, curettage.

6. Special Contraindications

The contraindications are the same as in lumbar epidural anesthesia (see "Lumbar epidural anesthesia in obstetrics," p. 140).

Regional Anesthesia Techniques for Cesarean Section

W. Müller-Holve, H. Chr. Niesel,
O. Schulte-Steinberg

The obstetrical anesthesiologist is increasingly required to provide regional anesthesia for cesarean sections. There are two reasons for this:

1. In special situations (premature birth, history of previous surgical procedures with a consequent slow fetal development), regional anesthesia has the advantage of producing less stress on the fetus than general anesthesia.
2. Many mothers want regional anesthesia for cesarean section, so that they can be awake at the time the child is born and have the option of breast feeding right after delivery.

1. Definition

Epidural anesthesia, spinal anesthesia, continuous caudal anesthesia, or infiltration anesthesia, which provide sensory blockade and complete or partial motor blockade below T_8.

2. Topographic Anatomy

See "Lumbar epidural anesthesia" (p. 106), "Lumbar epidural anesthesia in obstetrics" (p. 135), "Caudal anesthesia in obstetrics" (p. 143), and "Spinal anesthesia" (p. 96).

3. Technique

3.1. Anesthesiologic Assessment

> Careful anesthesiologic assessment including the identification of any contraindication.

3.2. Preparation

> Intravenous cannula and infusion of a balanced electrolyte solution.
> Ventilation equipment with O_2 connection; intubation equipment, atropine, sedative, succinylcholine, vasopressor, catecholamine.

The explanation of the procedure and of the potential complications should take place, if possible, during the pregnancy so that the patient can be admitted to the labor room with the consent form already signed. Regional anesthesia in obstetrics must be preceded by a thorough discussion with the patient.

Special considerations in regional anesthesia techniques for cesarean section

Changes in the protein-binding capacity of the local anesthetics and changes in electrolyte and acid-base balance. Very marked reaction to the direct and indirect (sympatholytic) effects of local anesthetic agents. The accidental intravenous administration of large amounts of local anesthetic solutions, particularly those containing long-acting local anesthetics, is extremely dangerous.

3.3. Equipment

Infiltration anesthesia

Three long 19 g disposable needles (90 × 1.1 mm)
Sterile cup for the local anesthetic solution

3.4. Positioning

Epidural anesthesia and spinal anesthesia should be administered with the patient in the left lateral position, since circulatory disturbances are common during labor and the vena cava compression syndrome also occurs frequently. Furthermore, the dose of the local anesthetic solution can be smaller in this position than in the sitting position.

3.5. Technical Procedure

Premedication is not indicated for cesarean section under regional anesthesia. The premedication can have a depressant effect on the newborn. Antisialogogues are also not required, since the high level of sympathetic activity is sufficient to suppress secretions. If the maternal pulse is over 110 bpm, as is frequently the case when IV tokolytics are administered prior to the cesarean section, atropine is contraindicated.
Lumbar epidural anesthesia for cesarean section should always be performed with the catheter technique (fractional administration of large volumes of local anesthetic solution).

Prerequisites

1. Aseptic technique
2. Continuous fetal monitoring with cardiotokography
3. Facilities for pH measurements
4. No oxytocin administration while the local anesthetic is being administered

Performance of the epidural, caudal, or spinal anesthesia

Caudal anesthesia should be considered only if a continuous caudal technique has already been established at the time the decision is made to perform a cesarean section.
Left lateral position for preloading with fluids: 1000 ml of a balanced electrolyte solution; in spinal anesthesia: 1500 ml in 10–15 min before the administration of the anesthetic. In spite of these prophylactic maneuvers, hypotension is possible.
In epidural and caudal anesthesia, the patient should be kept in the lateral position and a test dose should be given.
The dose should be given in fractional increments through the catheter (e.g., 4 ml aliquots).
Injections should be done only in the interval between contractions, since otherwise, the spread of the anesthetic solution is uncontrollable and the level may become excessively high.
In order for the local anesthetic solution to spread equally to both sides, the patient may be placed into the supine position. To avoid the vena cava compression syndrome, an assistant should displace the uterus towards the left side.
In spinal anesthesia, the injection should be performed with the patient in the lateral position. The patient stays in this position until just before the start of the cesarean section.
If the injection is made in the sitting position, the patient should be placed immediately into the left lateral position.

Administration of infiltration anesthesia

This method is part and parcel of the surgical procedure. The infiltration of the tissues is performed in the area of the incision. Since the indication for this approach is frequently a need for great dispatch, the skin infiltration should take place before draping. In this way, the local anesthetic can take effect while the patient is being draped. A midline incision is preferred, since it is smaller, requires less local anesthetic, and thus is less depressant on the fetus.

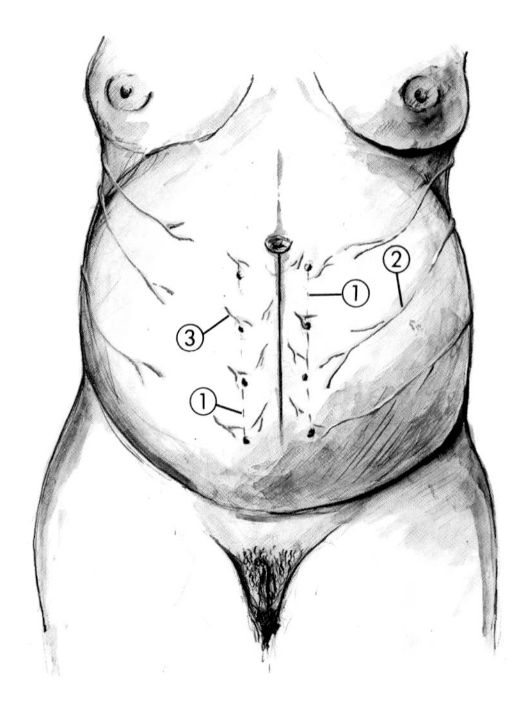

FIG 132.
1. Infiltration wall
2. Lateral cutaneous branches
3. Anterior cutaneous branches

One finger width to the left and right of the linea alba, a local anesthetic field block is performed, which reaches from the symphisis to approximately 5 cm above the umbilicus (Fig 132). Since pregnant women frequently have a diastasis recti, great care must be taken that the peritoneum not be perforated during the infiltration or that an accidental intravascular injection is not performed within the myometrium of the uterus.

After both draping and the skin incision, but before each surgical advance through the abdominal wall and the uterine peritoneum, all layers must be consecutively infiltrated.

3.6 Dosage

All local anesthetic solutions should be free of epinephrine, since this drug has a deleterious effect on uterine perfusion.

Disadvantage of the epinephrine-free solution (lidocaine, mepivacaine) is the relatively higher maternal and fetal blood level.

Epidural anesthesia

Dosage of 18–22 ml of mepivacaine 2%, lidocaine 2%, or bupivacaine 0.5%. Only 16 ml for patients weighing less than 50 kg and/or who are less than 1.50 m tall.

Never administer in a single dose; rather, always divide into individual doses at a maximum of 6–8 ml (4 ml with bupivacaine) per dose.

Caudal anesthesia

Fractional doses of mepivacaine, lidocaine or bupivacaine are given.

Additional doses and the concentration of the local anesthetic solution are the same as described above under caudal anesthesia.

Spinal anesthesia

Lidocaine 5% (heavy): 50–75 mg (1–1.5 ml)
Mepivacaine 4% (hyperbaric): 50–60 mg (1.2–15 ml)
Through barbotage with CSF, the total volume is raised to 2–2.5 ml and a level to T_7 is assured.

Infiltration anesthesia

Mepivacaine 0.25% or
Lidocaine 0.25%: 80 ml,
In large patients: up to 100 ml;
Prilocaine 0.5%: 80 ml

4. Special Complications

See "Lumbar epidural anesthesia" (p. 114), "Lumbar epidural anesthesia in obstetrics" (p. 138), "Caudal anesthesia in obstetrics" (p. 146), and "Spinal anesthesia" (p. 104).
Infiltration anesthesia may lead to toxic reactions if careful aspiration is not performed prior to every injection.
The possibility of untoward circulatory disturbances must always be kept in mind.

5. Indications

Epidural anesthesia

Long procedure can be expected (s/p prior surgery or c-section).
Poor fetal drug tolerance (section for premature birth).
The patient requests to be awake during the section and the birth of the child and to be able to breast feed soon after delivery.

Caudal anesthesia

The decision to perform a section is made after the catheter caudal is already in place.

Spinal anesthesia

Same indications as for epidural anesthesia.
Greater urgency to deliver the child (shorter preparation time).
No local anesthetic effect on the child (if hypotension develops and is not corrected, there is an indirect effect on the child).

Infiltration anesthesia

Need for immediate section when general anesthesia is not available.
Technically impossible epidural, spinal or caudal anesthesia.
Intubation difficulties.

References

1. Bonica JJ: *Obstetric Analgesia and Anesthesia.* Berlin–Heidelberg–New York, Springer Verlag, 1972.
2. Datta S, Alper MH: Anesthesia for cesarean section. *Anesthesiology* 1980; 53:142.
3. Lund PC: *Principles and Practice of Spinal Anesthesia.* Springfield, Charles C. Thomas, 1971.
4. Raney B, Stange WF: Advantages of local anesthesia for cesarean section. *Obstet Gynecol* 1975; 45:163.

Paracervical Block

H. Albrecht

1. Definition

A transvaginal form of conduction anesthesia by injection of local anesthetic solution, left and right, through the lateral vaginal vault, into the paracervical tissues. This will eliminate the pain of cervical dilatation and lower uterine contractions during the middle and later phases of the first stage of labor, but not during the second stage.

Blockade of the inferior hypogastric plexus (pelvic nerve) and its connections to the presacral nerves and to the sacral plexus.

FIG 133.
(after Bonica)
Sensory pathway during the first and second stages of labor (dilatation and expulsion).

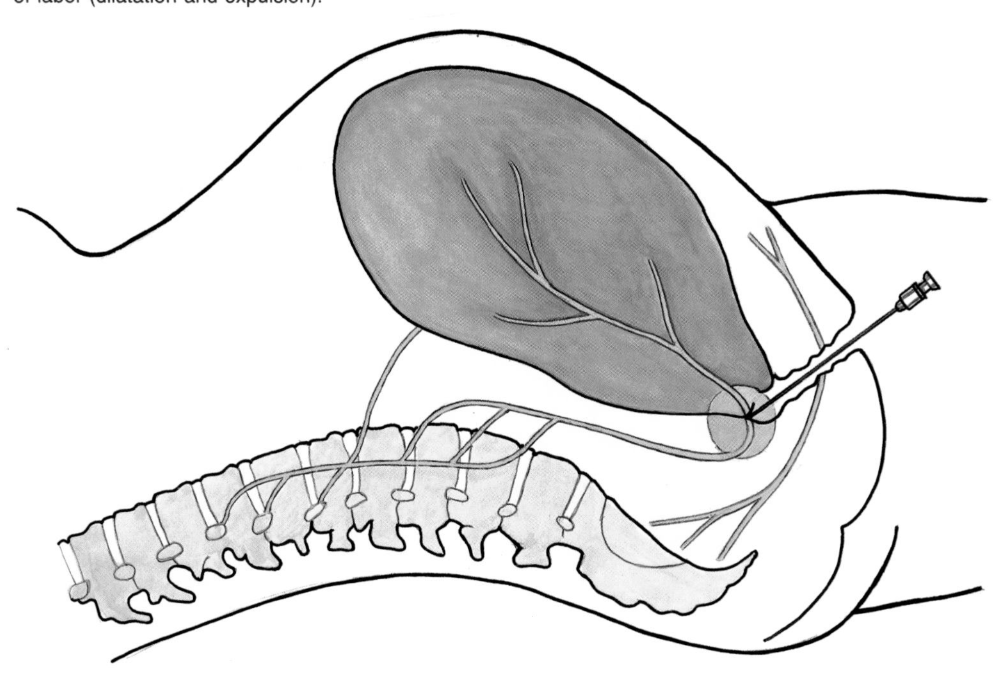

2. Topographic Anatomy

The paracervical plexus of nerves (inferior hypogastric plexus) and the superior hypogastric plexus (presacral nerves) are located in the loose connective tissue between the sacro uterine ligament, the uterine venous plexus, the ureter, the lower uterine segment, and the fetus. They are in close proximity to the uterine artery.

3. Technique

3.1. Anesthesiologic Assessment

Careful anesthesiologic assessment, including the identification of any contraindication as well as the maternal and fetal risk factors.

Findings

Cervix: 4–5 cm dilatation; regular, painful contractions; normal fetal cardiotokogram.

3.2. Preparation

Intravenous cannula and infusion of a balanced electrolyte solution. Ventilation equipment with O_2 connection; intubation equipment, atropine, sedative, succinylcholine, vasopressor, catecholamine. Infusion pumps for tokolytic solution must be immediately available.

3.3 Equipment

An assembled or a disposable set for sterilization.
The set contains a 10 ml syringe, special guide cannula, and a long, thin needle for the injection.
For example, an IOWA TRUMPET with a long needle, a KOBACK needle with a guard to prevent deep penetration. Ideally, the needle should not proceed more than 3–4 mm beyond the end of the guide cannula.

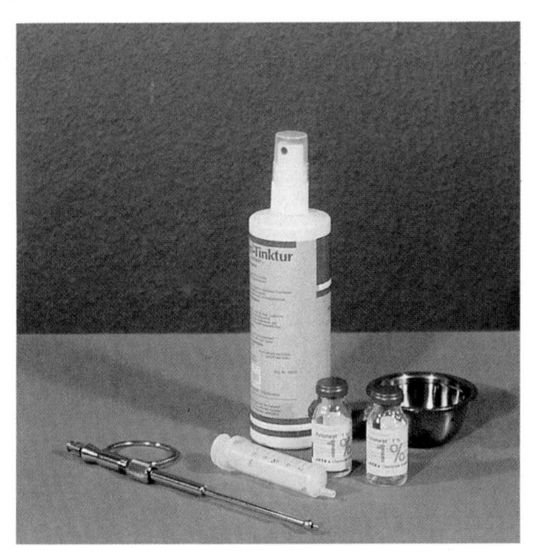

FIG 134.

3.4. Positioning

Supine position in the labor bed with the thighs flexed.

3.5. Landmarks

Lateral vaginal vault on the right between 4 and 5 o'clock or 3 and 4 o'clock; on the left between 7 or 8 o'clock or 8 and 9 o'clock.

3.6. Technical Procedure

Preparation of the perineal region. Specific preparation of the vagina is not necessary. Palpation of the effaced cervix, of the fetal head, and of the lateral vaginal vault. The needle, with the 10 ml syringe attached, is introduced into the guide cannula and advanced with gentle pressure until it enters the vaginal wall to a distance of 2–4 mm (Fig 135). Excessive pressure with the finger or with the guide cannula must be avoided since this constitutes a danger, i.e., the local anesthetic solution may be injected too deeply and into the vicinity of the paracervical vascular plexus. Bupivacaine and prilocaine are considered the safest local anesthetics from the point of view of the fetus.

Before injecting the local anesthetic, an aspiration test should be performed.

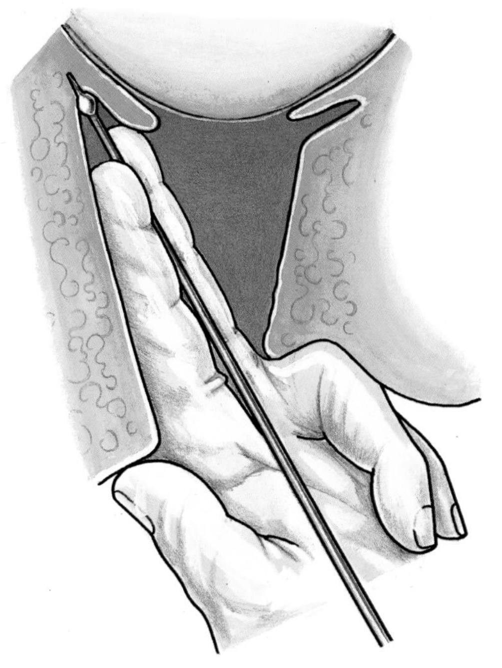

FIG 135.
The middle finger separates the cervix and the head of the fetus.

The local anesthetic solution is injected in divided doses, on the right side at 4 and 5 o'clock and on the left at 7 and 8 o'clock, or on the right at 3 and 4 o'clock and on the left at 8 and 9 o'clock. The total of 10 ml is divided according to the formula of 3-2-2-3 ml (3).

After injection the mother should be placed into the left lateral position. *Continuous monitoring of the fetal heart rate with the cardiotokograph and of the maternal pulse and blood pressure should take place.*

Catheter technique

A catheter technique has been used successfully but seems to be too complicated for routine use. The main problem is the displacement or even the removal of the catheter as a result of maternal motion.

Advocates of the catheter technique claim that the risks to the fetus are decreased. The ability to give fractional doses of the local anesthetic provides good analgesia with lower blood levels.

The use of an injection gun for paracervical blockade in obstetrics is a greatly debated matter, since this technique may lead to a rapid spread of the local anesthetic solution in all directions, including the direction of the uterus.

3.7. Dosage

10 ml local anesthetic solution, e.g., prilocaine 0.5%; bupivacaine 0.25%.

4. Special Complications

FIG 136.
(after Abouleish)
Complications of the paracervical block.

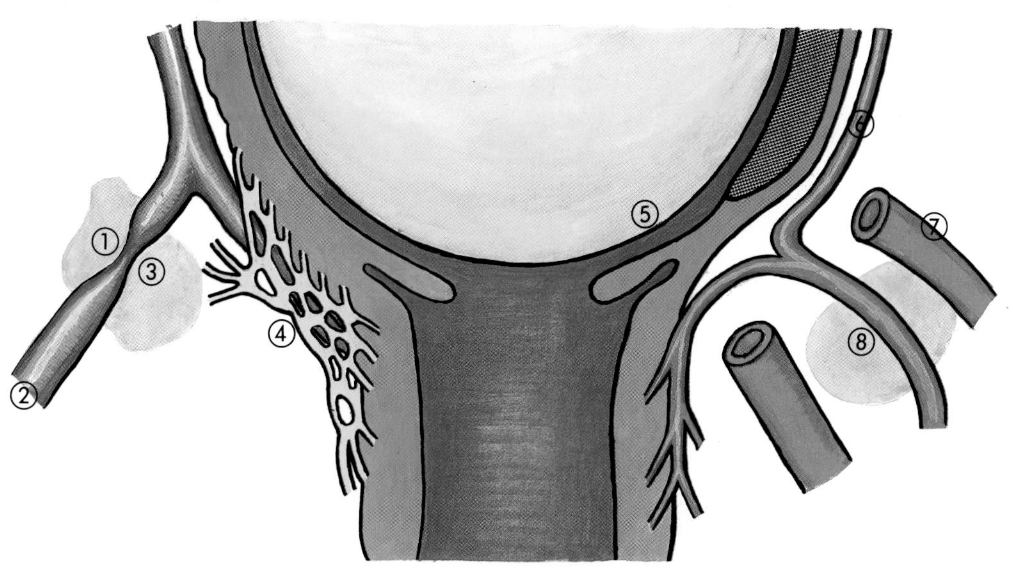

1. Mechanical compression
2. Hypotension
3. Vasoconstriction
   (e.g., epinephrine in the LAS)
4. Paracervical neural and vascular plexus
5. Injection into the head of the fetus
6. Injection into the uterine a.
7. Injection into the uterine v.
8. Diffusion of the local anesthetic solution into the uterine a.

4.1. Fetal and Neonatal Complications

Changes in fetal heart sounds on the cardiotokogram, e.g., bradycardias, tachycardias, variable and late deceleration.

The incidence of heart sound changes varies between 5 and 30% depending upon the local anesthetic used, the dose, and the user.

The effect of the local anesthetic on the fetus depends on the amount of the local anesthetic which passes through the placenta and on the resulting fetal blood level.

The initial bradycardia can be regarded as the direct effect of the local anesthetic, while a late deceleration is probably due to hypoxia.

Bradycardia, hypoxia, and acidosis lead to fetal hypotension and myocardial depression. A vicious circle is set up with a deteriorating fetal condition, where the

CNS effects depress the vasomotor center and increase hypotension. Depression of the cardiac accelerator center leads to bradycardia; depression of the higher inhibitory center leads to convulsions; depression of the respiratory center leads to hypoxia and acidosis.

The following complications lead to a rapid passage of the local anesthetic to the fetus:

a. The injection into the lateral vaginal vault is too deep.
   If the local anesthetic is injected only at a depth of 2–3 mm, the rapid absorption is delayed by 10 min.
b. Accidental injection into the lower uterine segment.
c. Intravenous or intraarterial injection.
d. Injection into a low-lying placenta.
e. Infusion of the local anesthetic solution via the uterine artery, directly into the intervillous space, and into the fetal circulation.
f. Individual differences in the rate of absorption of the local anesthetic depend on the maternal hemodynamics, e.g., arterial pressure, venous return from the paracervical space and its perfusion, the weight and functional capacity of the placenta.
g. Increased fetal sensitivity to the local anesthetic, e.g., in prematurity, "small-for-date-baby," preexisting fetal acidosis.
h. Direct injection into the fetal scalp, resulting in an intrauteirne or neonatal death.

Indirect effect of the local anesthetic solution on the fetus through the mother

a. Maternal aortocaval compression and effects of the local anesthetic in the lithotomy position after injection (after injection the mother must be placed into the left lateral position immediately).
b. Increased constriction of the uterine vessels by the addition of epinephrine to the anesthetic solution. Even without epinephrine, however, the local anesthetics have a vasoconstrictor effect. The use of epinephrine is controversial. Its advocates claim the advantage of increased duration and decreased absorption of the local anesthetic, with increased safety to the fetus. Its opponents point to the increase in fetal acid-base changes and fetal bradycardia related to the negative effect on uterine perfusion.

4.2. Maternal Complications

a. Intravascular injection.
Symptoms: Dizziness, tinnitus, convulsions.
Prevention: Injection without pressure on the vaginal vault decreases the likelihood of intravascular injection.

b. Injection in the vicinity of the sacral nerves leads to anesthesia of the lower extremities.

c. Bleeding in the vaginal vault with hematoma formation.

d. Hypotension. Rare, usually in combination with caval compression syndrome.

5. Indications

Labor pains in the middle and late first stage of labor. Cervix dilated 4–9 cm.
In gynecology: analgesia for cervical dilatation, e.g., diagnostic curettage, placement of IUD, intracavitary radium insertion.

6. Special Contraindications

No CTG
No chance for emergency cesarean section
Eclampsia
Diabetes mellitus
Twin pregnancy
Hypotension
Growth retardation
Fetal acidosis
Meconium-stained amniotic fluid and postmaturity
Rapid dilatation of less than 1 hr duration
Inexperience of the anesthesiologist, particularly ignorance of the complications

7. Advantages–Disadvantages

Advantages

The paracervical block is technically simple, and contrary to the other techniques, can be administered by the obstetrician with moderate experience.
The safety of the paracervical block depends on the skill and experience of the user with special reference to the ability to prevent and, if necessary, manage the complications.

Disadvantages

In 15–20% of the cases, there is only partial control of the pain of contractions and cervical dilatation.
The perineal pain is not affected. The many potential complications increase the danger of fetal morbidity and mortality.
In paracervical blockade, there is always a danger of fetal bradycardia, acidosis, and neonatal depression.

Because of the frequent fetal complications and the numerous reported fetal and neonatal deaths (2), the paracervical blockade has been abandoned by many obstetricians.

References

1. Abouleish E: Paracervical-block, in: *Pain control in Obstetrics.* Philadelphia–Toronto, JB Lippincott Co, 1977.
2. Finster M: Toxicity of local anesthetics in the fetus and the newborn, in Dudenhausen JW, Saling E, Schmidt E (Hrsg): *Perinatale Medizin,* Bd 6. Stuttgart, Thieme, 1975.
3. Jägerhorn, M: Paracervical block in Obstetrics. An improved injection method: A clinical and radiological study. *Acta Obstet Gynecol Scand* 1975; 54:9.
4. Teramo K: Effects of obstetrical paracervical blockade on the fetus. *Acta Obstet Gynecol Scand* 1971; (suppl) 16.
5. Thiery M, Vorman S: Paracervical block during labor. *Am J Obstet Gynecol* 1972; 113:988.

The Pudendal Block

H. Albrecht

1. Definition

Perineal anesthesia by blocking the pudendal nerve at the level of the ischial spine for the second stage of labor and for the expulsive pains.

The pain of distending the perineum by the descending fetal head is largely eliminated. The lower third of the vagina, the vulva, and the perineum are rendered pain-free. The levator ani muscle is not affected by the pudendal block. The pudendal block is the most frequently used technique in Europe to provide anesthesia for vaginal delivery. Smaller operative interventions, e.g., low forceps delivery, vacuum extraction, the repair of an episiotomy, or a perineal tear, can be performed painlessly under pudendal blockade.

2. Topographic Anatomy

The pudendal nerve originates from parts of the third and fourth sacral nerves in close relationship to the sacral plexus. The nerve accompanies the internal pudendal artery and ends as the dorsal nerve of the clitoris. Other branches include the perineal nerves which run in the ischiorectal fossa, branches to the external sphincter ani muscle, to the muscles of the perineum (transverse perineal muscle, bulbocavernosus muscle) and finally, the labial nerves going to the labia majora. The pudendal nerve runs between the sacrospinal ligament and the sacrotuberous ligament. For the purposes of the block, the pudendal nerve is sought at the level of the ischial spine.

3. Technique

3.1. Anesthesiologic Assessment

Careful anesthesiologic assessment including the identification of any contraindication.

Findings:

Cervical dilatation complete, leading point on the floor of the pelvis, strong, effective contractions.

3.2. Preparation

Intravenous cannula and infusion of a balanced electrolyte solution.
Ventilation equipment with O_2 connection, intubation equipment, atropine, sedative, succinylcholine, vasopressor, catecholamine.

3.3. Equipment

Set with a guide cannula, e.g., the IOWA TRUMPET
Needles for the injection
20 ml syringe with 20 ml of local anesthetic solution
The KOBACK needle and the guide cannula of Jung are also recommended

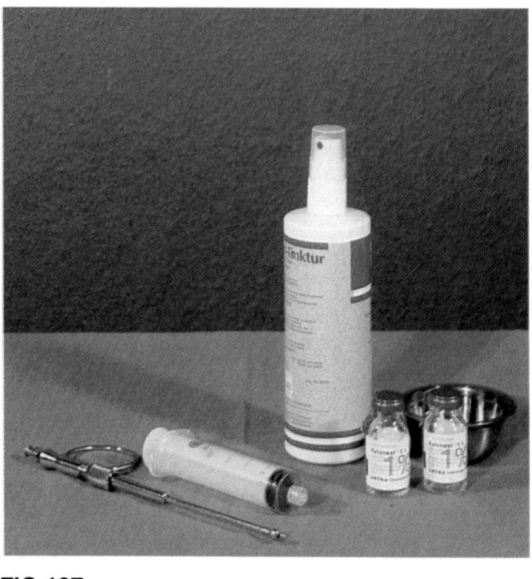

FIG 137.

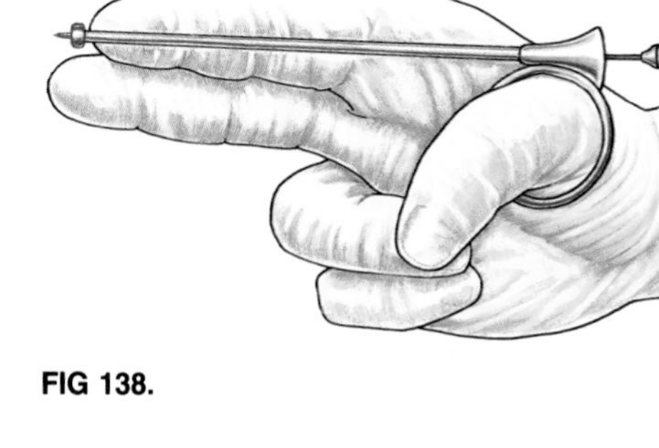

FIG 138.

3.4. Positioning

Supine in bed with the thighs flexed

3.5. Landmarks

The right and left ischial spines

3.6. Technical Procedure

Transvaginal pudendal anesthesia

The ischial spine is located with the index finger or the index and middle fingers. Introduction of the guide cannula into the vagina with two fingers (index and middle fingers, Fig 138); introduction of the injection needle and 20 ml syringe into the guide cannula. Puncture of the vaginal wall and the sacrospinal ligament, which is located beneath it, with gentle pressure approximately ½ cm below the ischial spine. The tip of the needle should be in the immediate vicinity of the pudendal nerve (Fig 139).

After aspiration, 10 ml of the local anesthetic solution are injected first on one side, and then in exactly the same way on the other side for a total of 20 ml.
The advantage of using a guide cannula: the pudendal block can be performed even if the leading point is very low and if there is considerable bearing down. Without the cannula, there is a danger of injuring the fetal head and the loosened vaginal wall. After 1–3 min following the injection, the lower third of the vagina, the vulva, and the perineum are anesthetized. In some cases, the pudendal blockade is not sufficient. To block the sensory branches of the ilioinguinal nerve and of

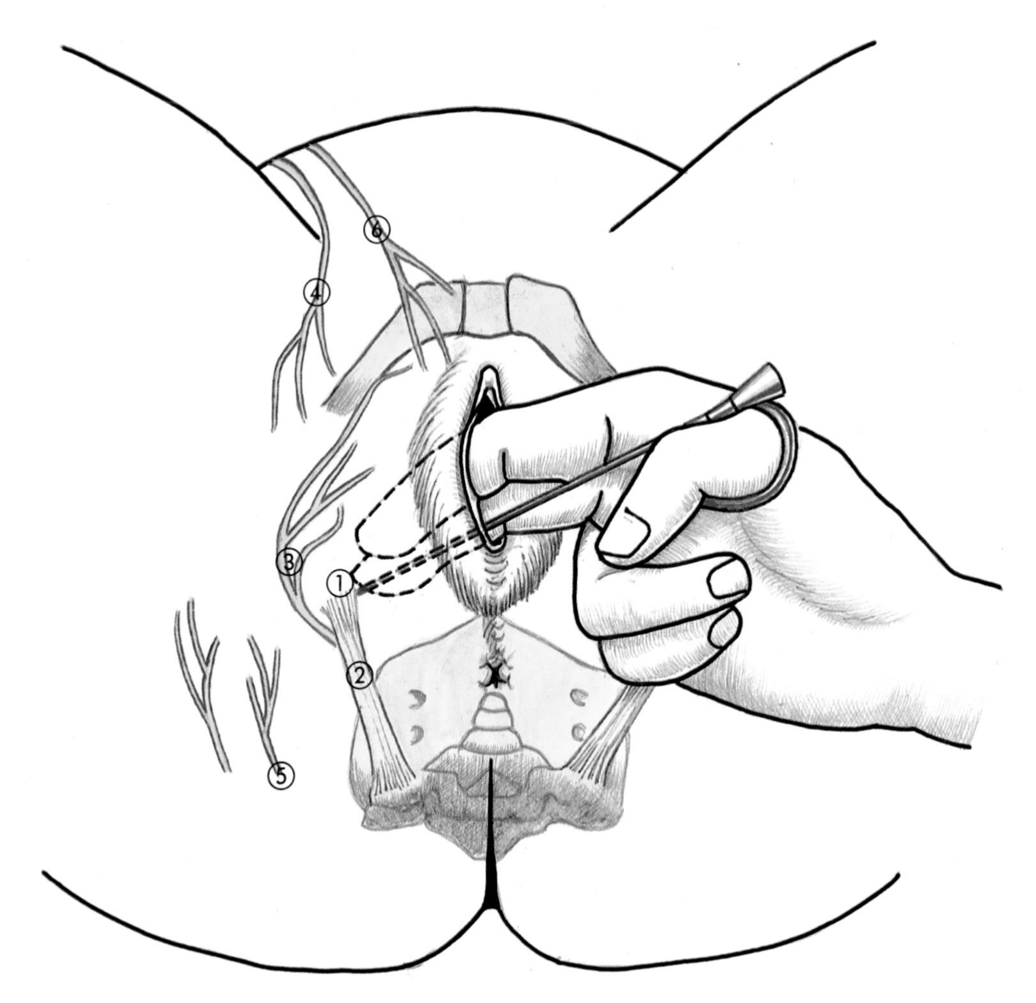

FIG 139.
(after Beck)
1. Ischial spine
2. Sacrospinalis ligament
3. Pudendal n.
4. Sensory branches of the genitofemoral n.
5. Sensory branches of the posterior femoral cutaneous n.
6. Sensory branches of the ilioinguinal n.

the genitofemoral nerve, which also supply the vulva with sensory fibers, the infiltration of the subcutaneous fat of the vulva is necessary (Fig 139). For this reason, it is advisable to test the extent of the pudendal block on the vulva and perineum with the tip of a needle, before the end of the birthing process.

Transcutaneous pudendal block

(Technically more difficult and not as reliable)

A 15 cm needle is directed towards the ischial spine, through the skin, 2–3 cm medially from the ischial tuberosity, in a line which leads from the anus to the tuberosity. The tip of the needle is guided and controlled by a finger in the vagina. The older percutaneous method has been largely abandoned in favor of the transvaginal method.

3.7. Dosage

2 × 10 ml local anesthetic solution, e.g., mepivacaine 1%, prilocaine 1%.

4. Special Complications

4.1. Fetal Complications

When used correctly, there is no danger of high blood levels in the newborn. Perinatal morbidity and mortality are not affected by the pudendal block.

4.2. Maternal Complications

Block of the sciatic nerve

In 5% (3) partial or complete block of the sciatic nerve with sensory and motor deficit in the lower extremities. These conditions disappear very rapidly.

Abscess formation

Possible if the rectum is perforated and an infection is seeded. The abscess is in the gluteal musculature, originating around the ischial spine, and invading the ischiorectal fossa (according to Meinrenken, the incidence is 0.06%).
Therapy: incision and drainage in the area between the ischial tuberosity and the anus.

Vaginal hematoma

Rare. Can occur when no pudendal block was administered. Disappears rapidly.

Maternal and fetal intoxication

Possible if a paracervical block was performed less than an hour earlier, if a large dose was administered, or if cumulatively the maximal permissible dose was exceeded (1).

5. Indications

The bearing down period of normally progressing spontaneous birth.

Particularly useful in premature delivery, since the pelvic floor is well relaxed, and the small fetal head can be protected well after a timely episiotomy. Stress-induced depresssion of the newborn can be avoided. In breech delivery the active participation of the mother is not affected.

Prophylactic outlet forceps delivery.

Light vacuum extraction.

6. Special Contraindications

Difficult operative vaginal delivery

7. Advantages–Disadvantages

Advantages

The pudendal block is an effective method to anesthetize the perineal area.
The method is simple and can be performed by the obstetrician with moderate experience.
The pain of dilatation in the expulsive stage is eliminated, and the analgesia of the perineum and muscle relaxation are usually satisfactory.

Properly done, the pudendal block has no deleterious effects on the mother, the fetus, or the newborn.
It is a good and popular method to provide painless completion of the birthing process, particularly in those pregnant women who wish to participate in natural childbirth, who refuse an epidural, or in whom an epidural is contraindicated.

Disadvantages

Effective only during the short expulsion stage.

References

1. Beck L: Geburtshilfe und Gynäkologie, in Killian: *Lokalanästhesie und Lokalanästhetika,* 2. Aufl Stuttgart, Thieme, 1973.
2. Beck L: *Geburtshilfliche Anästhesie und Analgesie.* Stuttgart, Thieme, 1968. (New edition in preparation.)
3. Meinrenken H, Rüter K, Stockhausen H: Transvaginale Leitungsanästhesie in ihrer praktischen Anwendung. *Gynäkologie* 1976; 9:193–198.

Pain Therapy

Sympathetic Blockade

U. Hankemeier

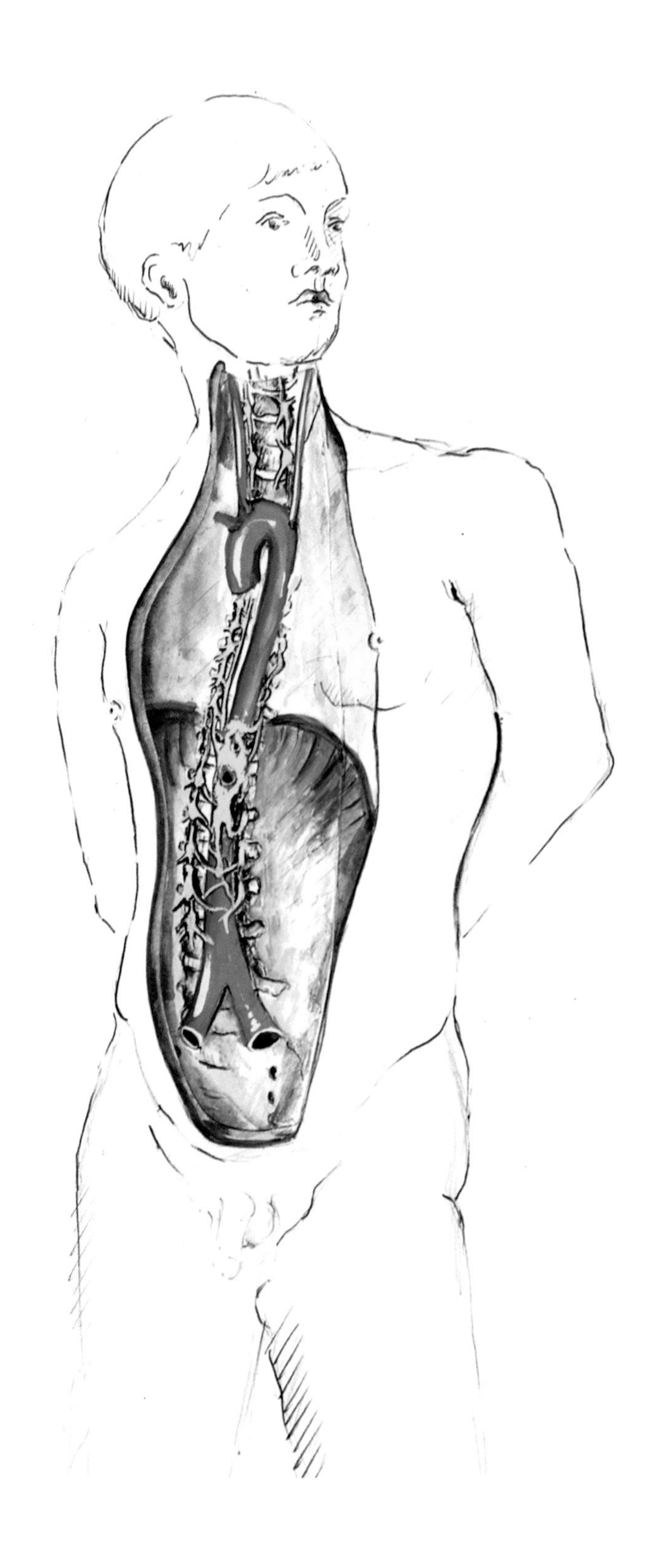

FIG 140.

I. Stellate ganglion block

1. Definition

Temporary interruption of the conduction of sympathetic impulses along the cervical sympathetic chain by local anesthetic solution.

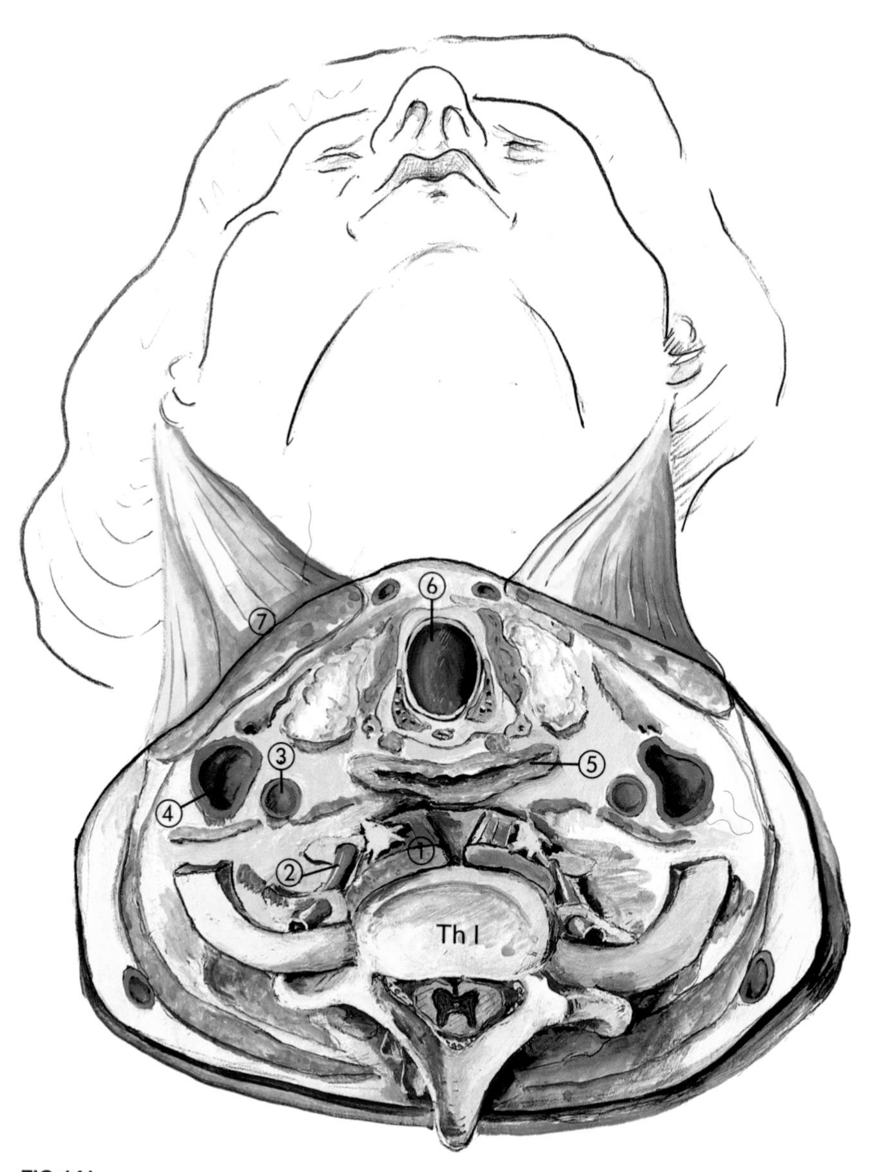

FIG 141.
1. Longus colli m.
2. Vertebral a.
3. Common carotid a.
4. Jugular v.
5. Hypopharynx
6. Larynx
7. Sternocleidomastoid m.

2. Topographic Anatomy

The cervical portion of the sympathetic chain lies on each side of the vertebral column, ventral to the vertebral artery and the transverse processes (separated from these by the longus colli muscle), somewhat medially and dorsally to the great vessels of the neck (common carotid artery, jugular vein), and lateral to the trachea and esophagus.

The stellate ganglion (cervicothoracic ganglion) is subject to great anatomic variations, and usually represents a fusion of the inferior cervical ganglion and the first thoracic ganglion of the sympathetic chain. In a craniocaudal direction, its length is approximately 2.5–3 cm, and it lies ventrally to the transverse processes of the 7th cervical and 1st thoracic vertebrae (Figs 141 and 143).

3. Technique

3.1. Anesthesiologic Assessment

Careful anesthesiologic assessment including the identification of any contraindication.

3.2. Preparation

IV infusion, O_2, atropine, sedative, catecholamine.

3.3. Equipment

Antiseptic solution
Sponges
Pillow
2 ml syringe
5 ml syringe
Needle for the skin wheal
3.5–4 (maybe 5) cm long 21 g needle for the block

3.4. Positioning

The patient is in the supine position with the pillow under the shoulders. The head is extended so that the chin and the sternum are at the same level (Fig 142).

3.5. Landmarks

Jugular fossa
Sternocleidomastoid muscle
Common carotid artery
Thyroid and cricoid cartilages
(Figs 143 and 144)

3.6. Technical Procedure

Skin prep. The patient must be instructed not to swallow or speak during the injection. The entry point is on the medial edge of the sternocleidomastoid muscle, at the level of the cricoid cartilage (in patients with a short neck, at the upper edge of the cricoid; in other patients, at the lower edge of the cricoid). After placing a skin wheal, the sternocleidomastoid m. is displaced laterally with two fingers. Pulsations of the common carotid artery should be readily felt at this time. The needle is introduced in a vertical-dorsal direction. At a depth of 2–3.5 cm, bony contact is made with the transverse process of C_6. (If no bony contact is made at this depth, the needle must be readjusted cranially or caudally.) The needle is withdrawn approximately 2 mm and, after careful aspiration in two planes (repeat several times during the injection), 5 ml of local anesthetic solution are injected.

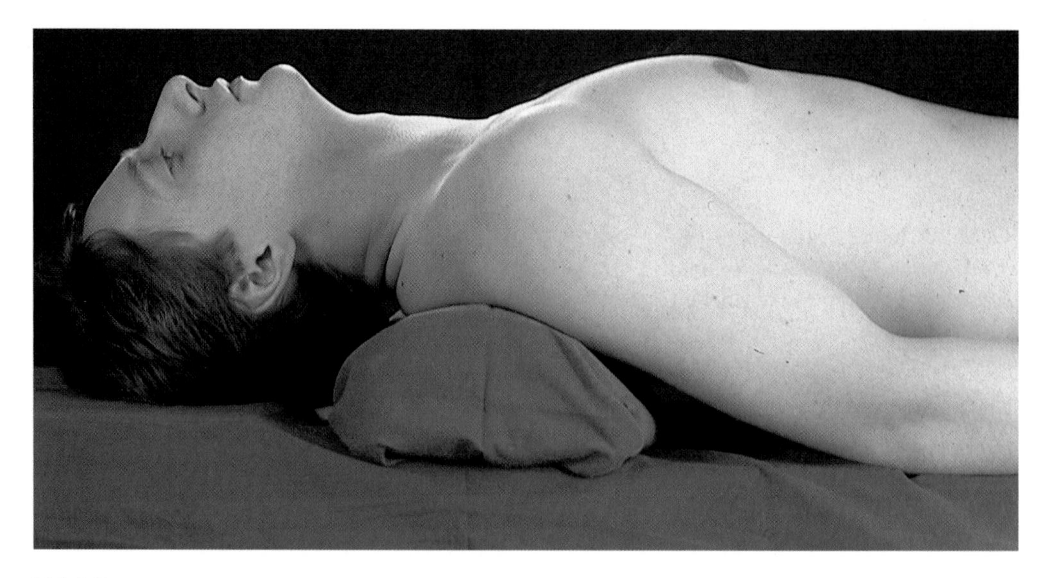

FIG 142.

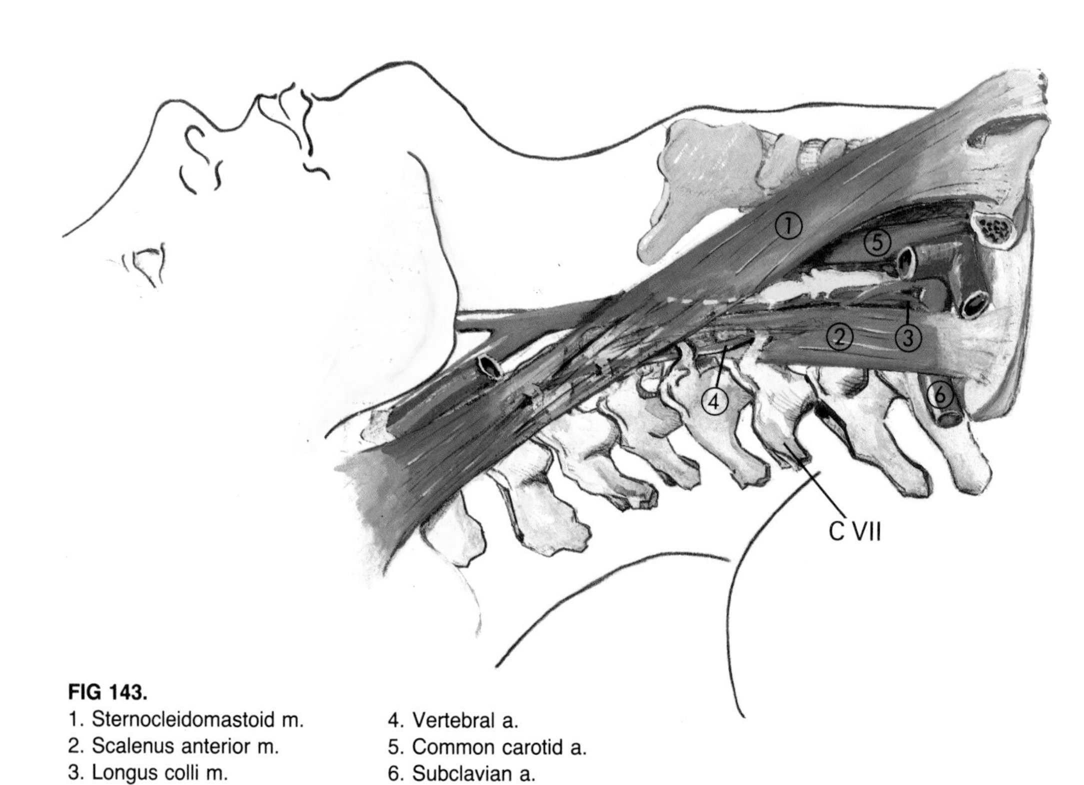

FIG 143.
1. Sternocleidomastoid m.
2. Scalenus anterior m.
3. Longus colli m.
4. Vertebral a.
5. Common carotid a.
6. Subclavian a.

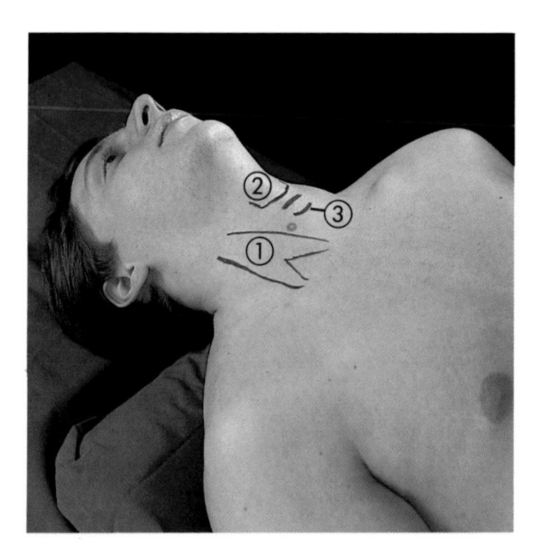

FIG 144.
1. Sternocleidomastoid m.
2. Thyroid cartilage
3. Cricoid cartilage
o = Point of entry

Subsequently, the patient's trunk is elevated.
If additional caudad spread of the local anesthetic is required, a volume of up to 10 ml must be administered.
The success rate is 80–90%.

3.7. Dosage

5 (–10) ml local anesthetic solution, e.g., mepivacaine 1%, bupivacaine 0.5%.

4. Special Side Effects and Complications

Side effects

(These are also signs of a successful block.)
Aside from Horner's Syndrome, the following side effects can be observed:

Increased tearing
Conjunctival injection
Swelling of the nasal mucosa
Temperature increase and anhydrosis on the arm and half the face

Complications

Hematoma, hoarseness, depression of the swallowing reflex (careful: danger of aspiration), and partial block of the brachial plexus. If the patient has been properly advised, these are of no significance.
Intravascular injection (particularly carotid and vertebral arteries).
High spinal anesthesia.
Pneumothorax is very rare if the above technique is followed.
To exclude the rare complication of a high epidural anesthesia, the patient must be observed for at least 20 min. Puncture of the esophagus (bitter taste during the injection) has a potential for a subsequent mediastinitis, and so mandates admission to the hospital for high-dose antibiotic therapy.

5. Indications

Thromboses, emboli, perfusion disturbances, and edema in the region of the arm and head (e.g., acute thrombosis of the central retinal artery and iatrogenic arterial spasm)
Reflex dystrophy
Acute hearing loss
Acute herpes zoster in the area innervated by the cervical sympathetic nerves
Hyperhydrosis
Chronic pain with, e.g. "burning" components

6. Special Contraindications

Contralateral pneumothorax
Severe conduction defects (e.g., 2nd degree A-V block)
Recent myocardial infarct

References

1. Moore DC: *Stellate Ganglion Block.* Springfield, Charles C. Thomas, 1954.

II. Celiac plexus block

1. Definition

Temporary (through local anesthetics) or permanent (through neurolytic substances) interruption of autonomic impulse transmission to the upper abdominal organs.

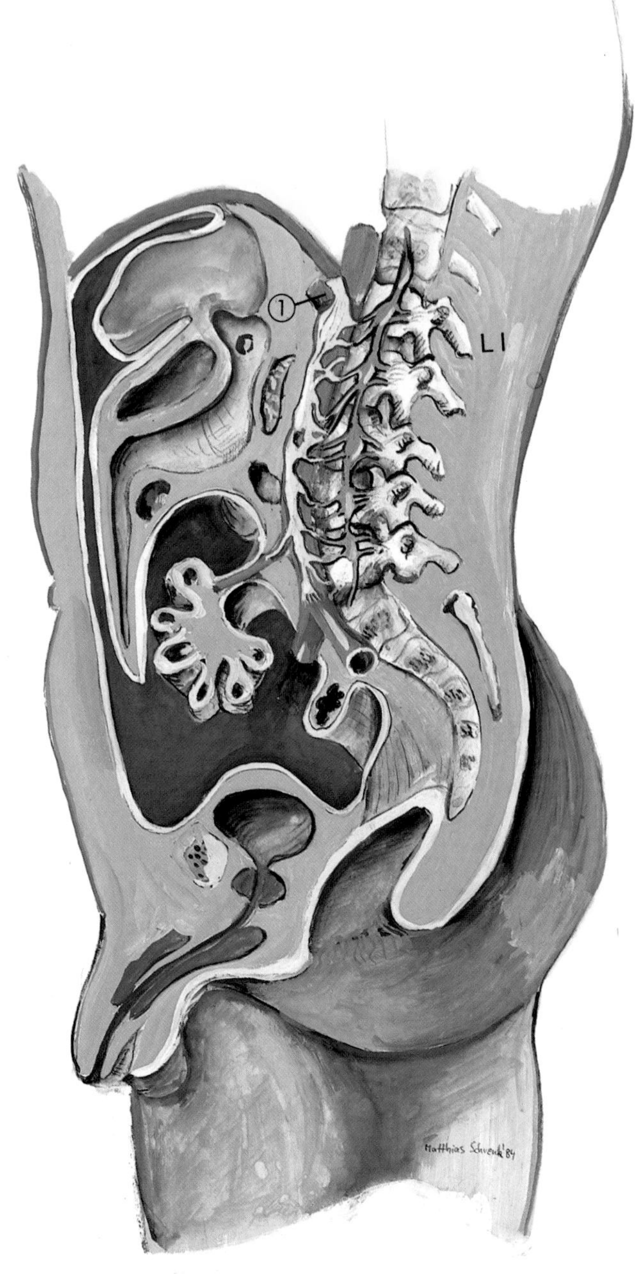

FIG 145.
1. Trunk of the celiac a.

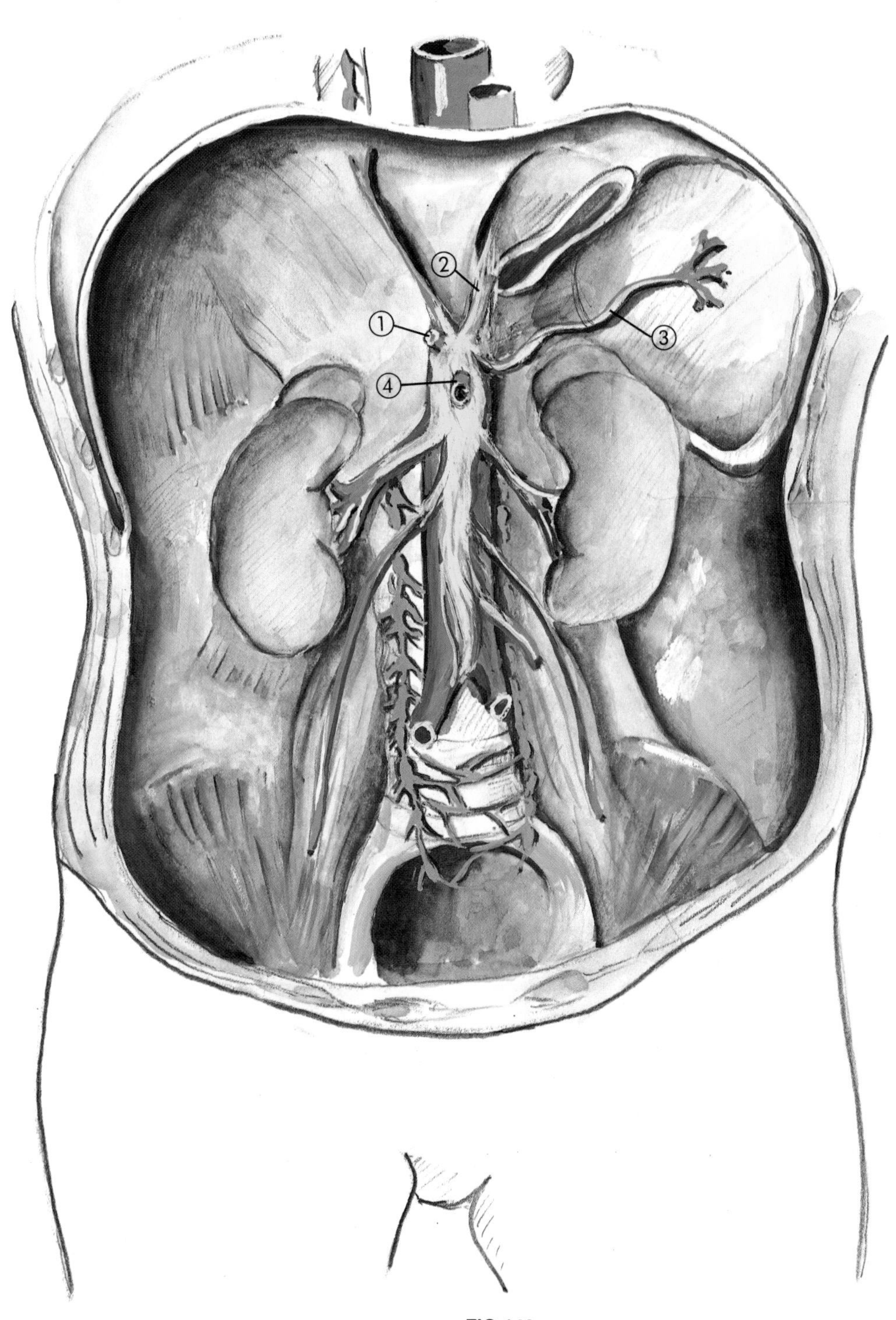

FIG 146.
1. Common hepatic a.
2. Left gastric a.
3. Splenic a.
4. Superior mesenteric a.

2. Topographic Anatomy

The paired celiac plexus lies ventral to the aorta about the level of the first lumbar vertebra (depending on size and extent, it may lie from the T_{12}–L_1 interspace to the middle of L_2) (Figs 145, 146, and 147).

3. Technique

3.1. Anesthesiologic Assessment

Careful anesthesiologic assessment including the identification of any contraindication.

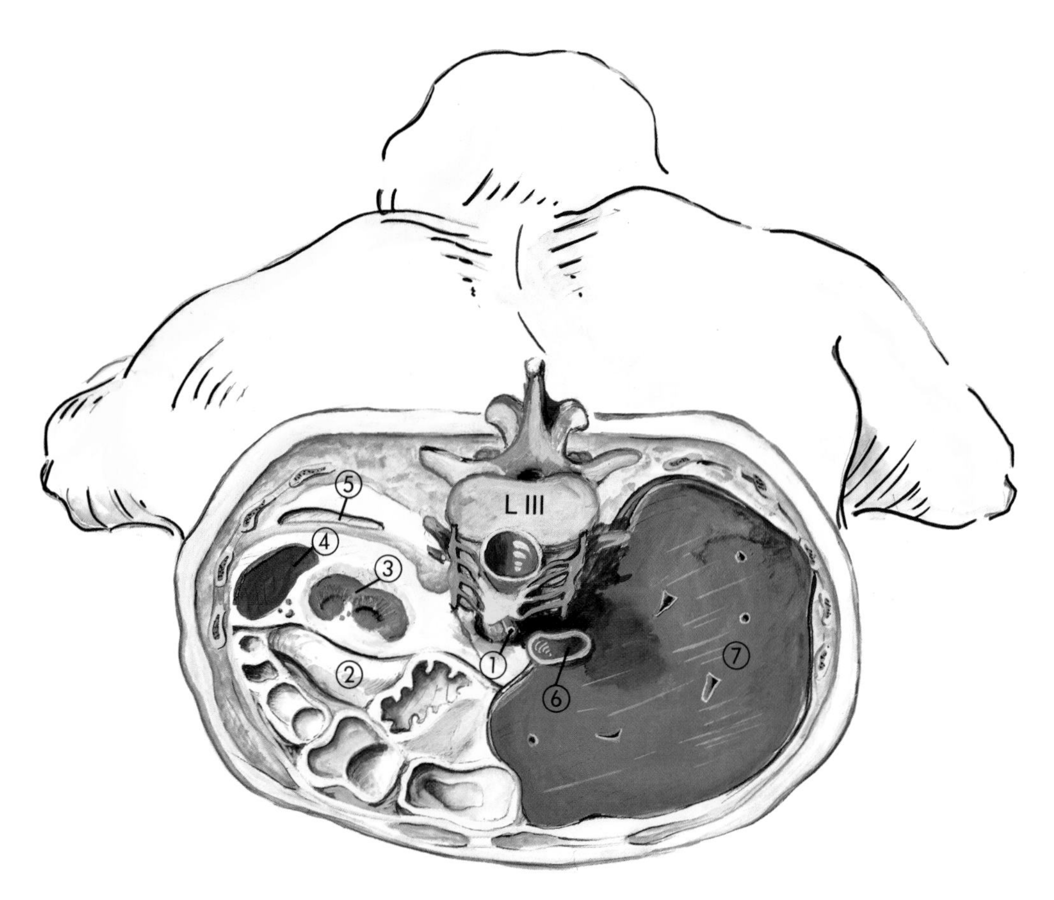

FIG 147.
1. Trunk of the celiac a.
2. Stomach
3. Kidney
4. Spleen
5. Phrenicostal sinus
6. Inferior vena cava
7. Liver

3.2. Preparation

Blood pressure measuring equipment, IV infusion, intubation equipment, O_2 supply, atropine, sedative, vasopressor, catecholamine, plasma expander.

3.3. Equipment

Antiseptic solution
Sponges
Pillow
Sterile towels
Sterile gloves
2 ml syringe
5 ml syringe
10 ml syringes
Needle for the skin wheal
12–15 long, firm 21 g needle for the block

3.4. Positioning

Unilateral celiac plexus block: lateral position (primarily painful side up), pillow under the flank (spinal column should be parallel to the top of the table), back slightly bent (Fig 148).
For bilateral block, the prone position is used.

3.5. Landmarks

Spinous processes of T_{12}, L_1, and L_2, 12th rib.

3.6. Technical Procedure

Preparation of the skin. The point of entry is 7–9 cm paravertebrally from the midline, directly below the 12th rib. After placing a skin wheal, a 12–15 cm long needle is advanced towards the body of L_1, ven-

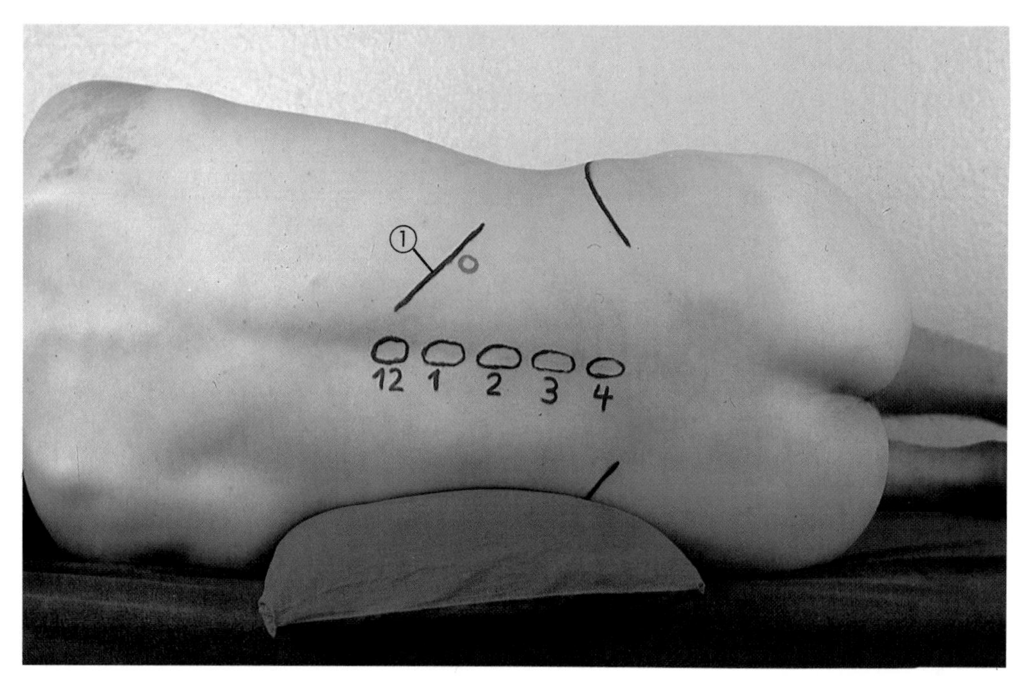

FIG 148.
1. 12th rib
o = Point of entry

trally, medially, and cranially (ventrally of the spinous processes of T_{12} and L_1). After bony contact is made, the needle is readjusted laterally so that it just barely clears the vertebral body. In blocks to the left side, the needle is advanced about 3 cm (careful: aorta!); in right-sided blocks, the needle is advanced about 4.5 cm. X-ray control with image intensifier: in the A-P projection, the tip of the needle lies at the upper two-thirds of L_1; in the lateral projection, the tip of the needle is about 2 cm ventrally from the spinal column. Administer 1–2 ml of a contrast medium to exclude malposition with certainty (Figs 149 and 150). After careful aspiration in two planes, the local anesthetic or neurolytic solution is injected.

In bilateral blockade in the prone position, the procedure is performed with two needles. It is advisable to place the needles so that the tips are separated in a craniocaudal direction (e.g., one needle at the upper third of L_1, and the other needle at the lower third of L_1).

The success rate is between 80–90%.

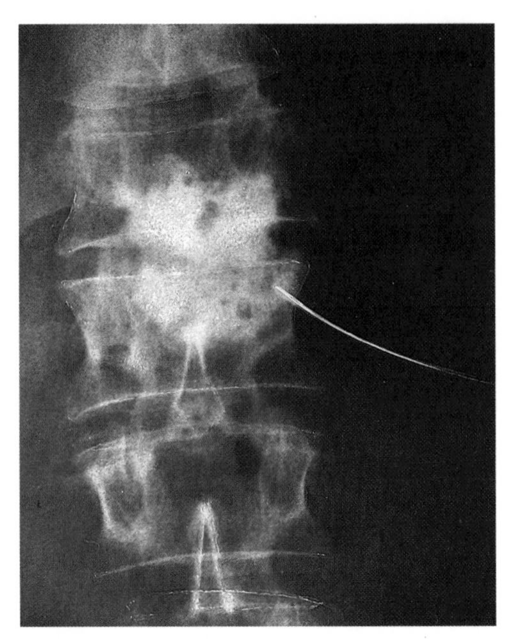

FIG 149.
Placement of the needle under x-ray control with contrast medium; a-p view (the bend in the needle is caused by changing the patient position after placement of the needle).

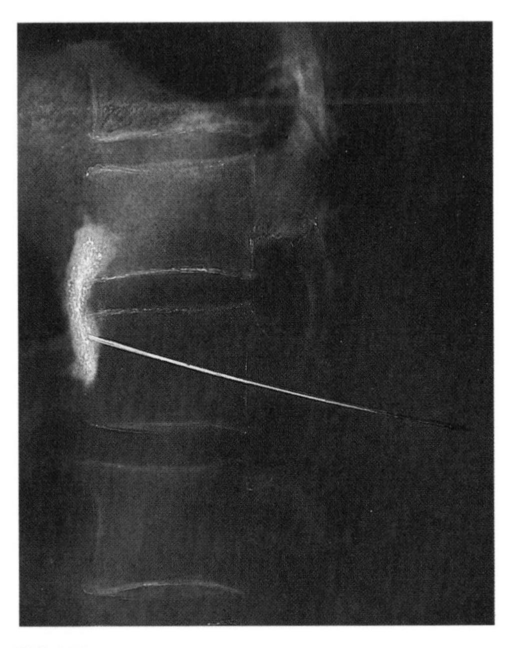

FIG 150.
Placement of the needle under x-ray control with contrast medium. Lateral view.

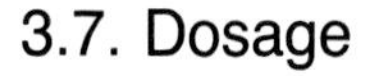

3.7. Dosage

Temporary block

40–50 ml local anesthetic solution, e.g., mepivacaine 0.5%; bupivacaine 0.2 to 0.25% (watch the maximum dose).

Permanent block

40–50 ml neurolytic solution (ethanol 50%, e.g., mixture of absolute alcohol and 1% mepivacaine).

4. Special Side Effects and Complications

Side effects

Feeling of warmth in the upper abdominal area (subjectively and objectively—simultaneous measure of success).
Burning pain during the administration of the neurolytic solution.
Usually only moderate hypotension.

Complications

Intravenous injection and/or injury to a major vessel (aorta, vena cava, celiac artery, renal artery).
Injury to other organs (pleura, peritoneum, kidney).

References

1. Kappis, M: Die Anästhesierung des Nervus splanchnicus. *Zentralbl Chir* 1918; 45:709–710.
2. Bridenbaugh LD, Moore DC, Campbell DD: Management of upper abdominal cancer pain. *JAMA* 1964; 190:877–880.
3. Moore DC, Bush WH, Burnett LL: Celiac plexus block with alcohol for cancer pain of the upper intraabdominal viscera; in Bonica JJ, Ventafridda V (eds): *Advances in Pain Research and Therapy,* vol 2. New York, Raven Press, 1979, pp 357–371.

5. Indications

With local anesthetic solutions

Chronic pain due to adhesions or chronic pancreatitis
For differential diagnostic evaluation of upper abdominal pain of uncertain etiology
As prognostic block in upper abdominal cancer pain

With neurolytic solution

Chronic pain in upper abdominal carcinoma or metastatic disease

6. Special Contraindications

Hypovolemia
Preterminal status (e.g., cachexia)
Severe narcotic addiction in cancer patients

III. Lumbar sympathetic blockade

1. Definition

Temporary (through local anesthetic solution) or permanent (through neurolytic solution) interruption of sympathetic impulse transmission over the lumbar sympathetic chain.

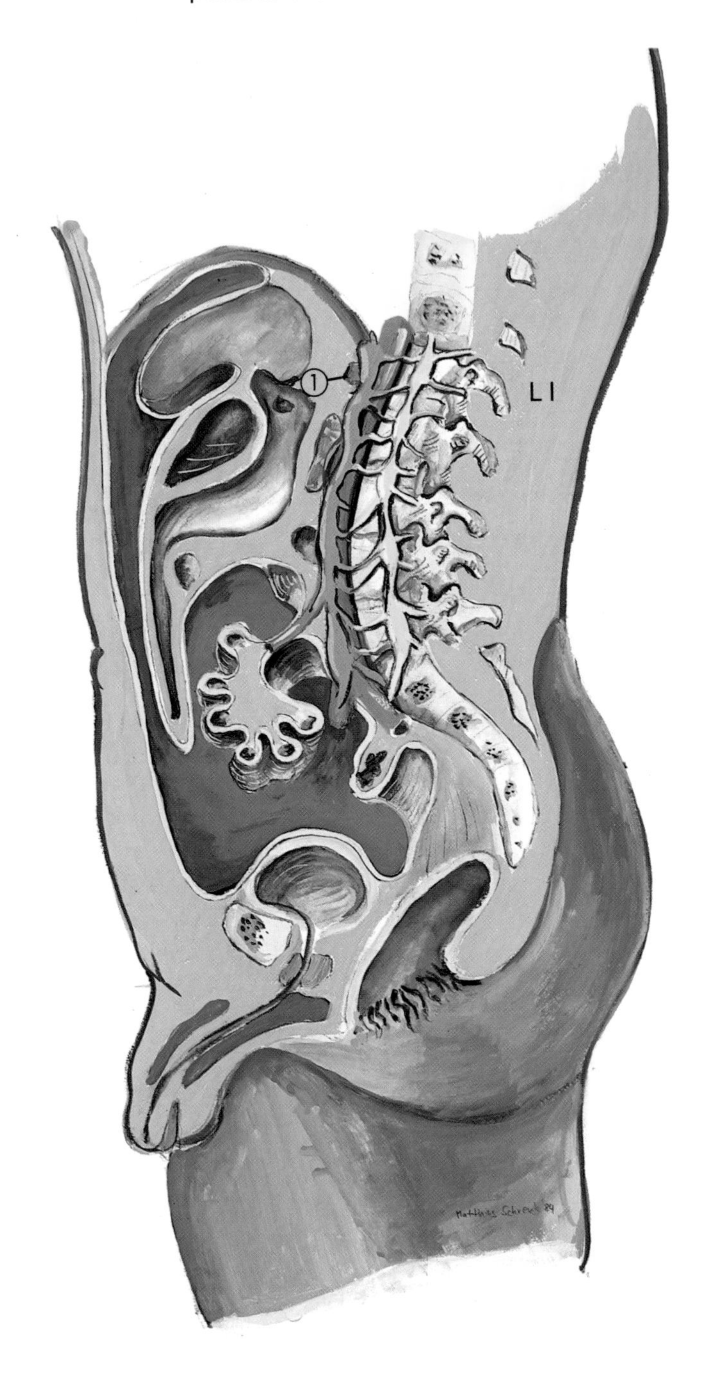

FIG 151.
Trunk of the celiac a.

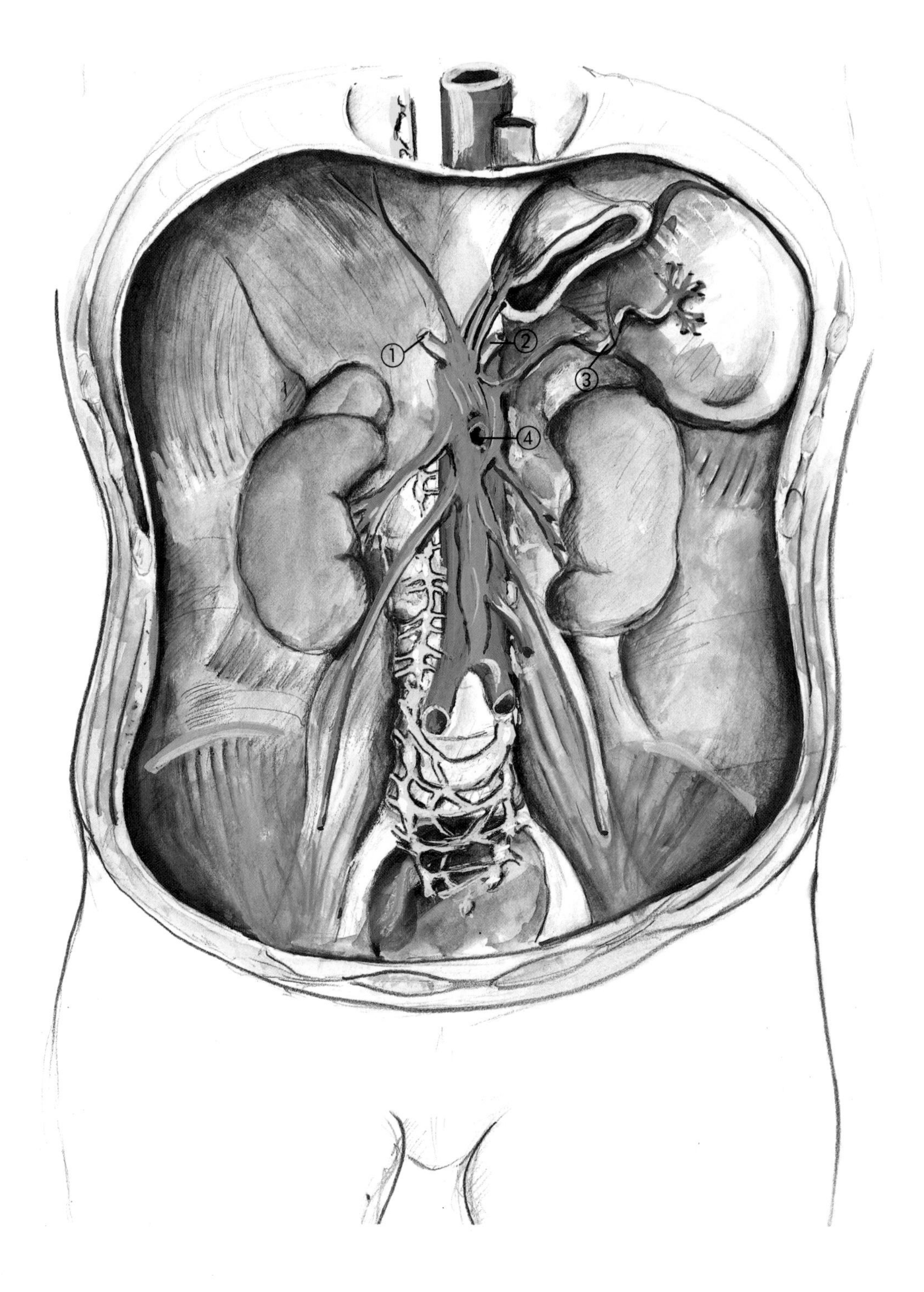

FIG 152.
1. Common hepatic a.
2. Left gastric a.
3. Splenic a.
4. Superior mesenteric a.

2. Topographic Anatomy

The chain and its ganglia lie in the lumbar region on the ventrolateral side of the spinal column inside a fascial sheath (between the psoas muscle and the vertebral column). Ventral to the chain lie the aorta and vena cava (Figs 151, 152, and 154).

3. Technique

3.1. Anesthesiologic Assessment

> Careful anesthesiologic assessment, including the identification of any contraindication; preliminary measurement of skin temperature, and psychogalvanic reflex.

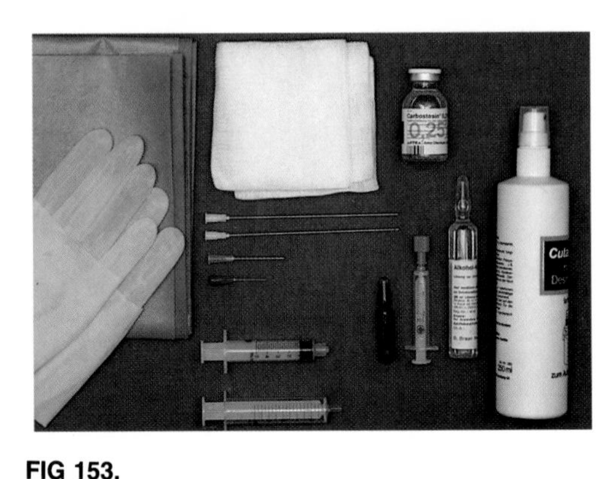

FIG 153.

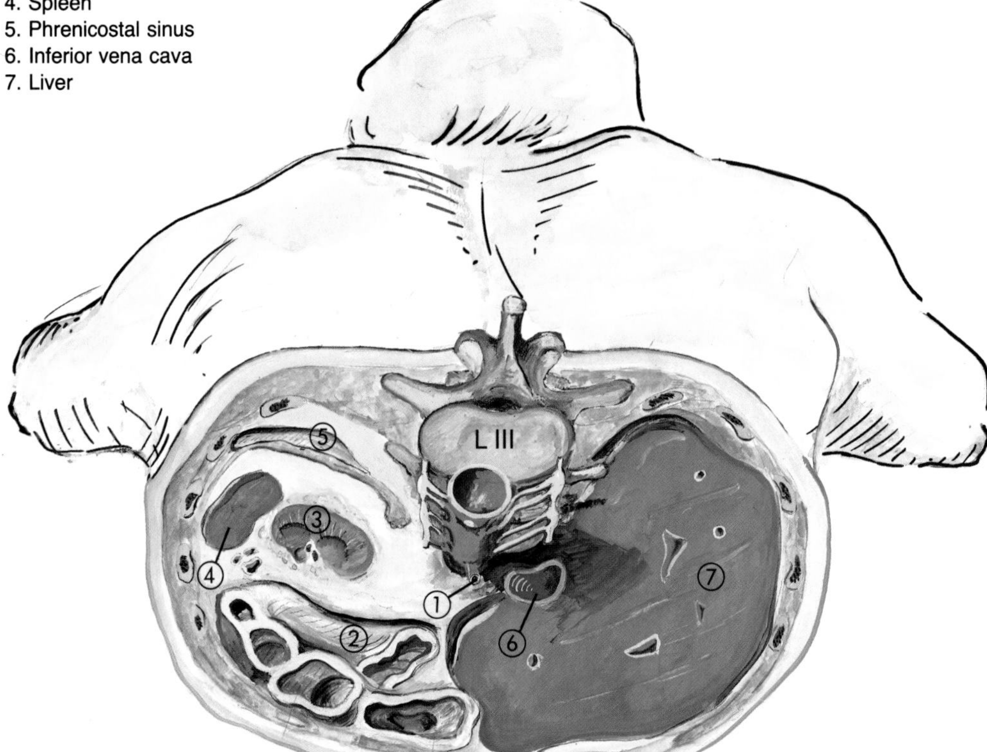

FIG 154.
1. Trunk of the celiac a.
2. Stomach
3. Kidney
4. Spleen
5. Phrenicostal sinus
6. Inferior vena cava
7. Liver

3.2. Preparation

IV infusion, intubation equipment. Ventilatory equipment, O_2 supply, atropine, sedative, vasopressor, and catecholamine.

3.3. Material

Antiseptic solution
Sponges
Sterile cloth
Sterile gloves
2 ml syringe
5 ml syringe
10 ml syringes
Needle for the skin wheal
12 cm long 21 g needle for the block (Fig 153)

3.4. Positioning

Lateral position, pillow under the flank (the spinal column should be parallel to the operating table), back slightly bent (Fig 158).

3.5. Landmarks

Spinous processes of the lumbar vertebrae, 12th rib, and iliac crest (Fig 155).

3.6. Technical Procedure

Preparation of the skin. The point of entry is 6–7 cm paravertebrally from the midline in the middle between the iliac crest and the 12th rib. After placing a skin

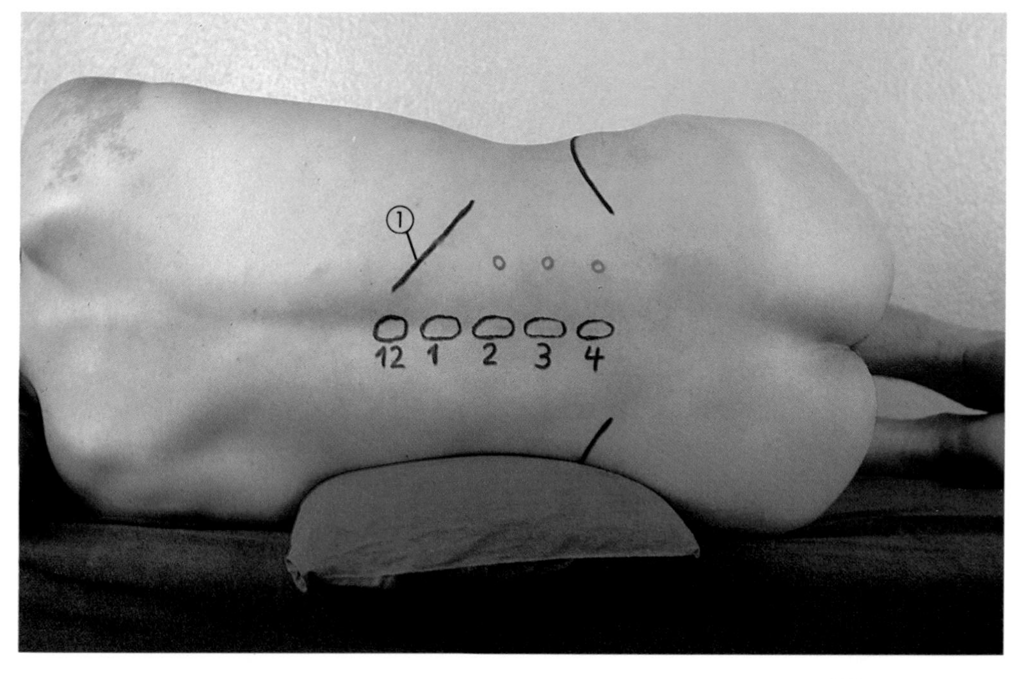

FIG 155.
1. 12th rib
o = Point of entry

wheal, a 12 cm long needle is advanced toward the body of L_2 in an approximately 80° medioventral direction. If bony contact is made at a depth of 2–3 cm (transverse process), the needle is redirected cranially or caudally. If sharp pain is triggered ("electric shock" pain radiating to the leg), due to irritation of a somatic nerve root, the direction of the needle must be adjusted cranially or caudally. When the needle makes contact with the body of L_2 at a depth of approximately 6–8 cm, the needle should be withdrawn 1–2 cm, and readjusted upwards so that it bypasses the body of L_1 laterally by approximately 1 cm. Careful aspiration in two planes. The injection of the local anesthetic solution should be achieved without any resistance.

For neurolytic blockade, it is recommended that two or three needles be introduced at the level of L_2–L_4, and x-ray control be maintained with image intensifier. The injection of contrast medium before neurolysis increases the accuracy of precise needle placement (Figs 156, 157, and 158).

For a temporary block, the introduction of one needle is sufficient. With this "blind" technique, the success rate is 80%. With x-ray and image intensifier control, the success rate should be near 100%.

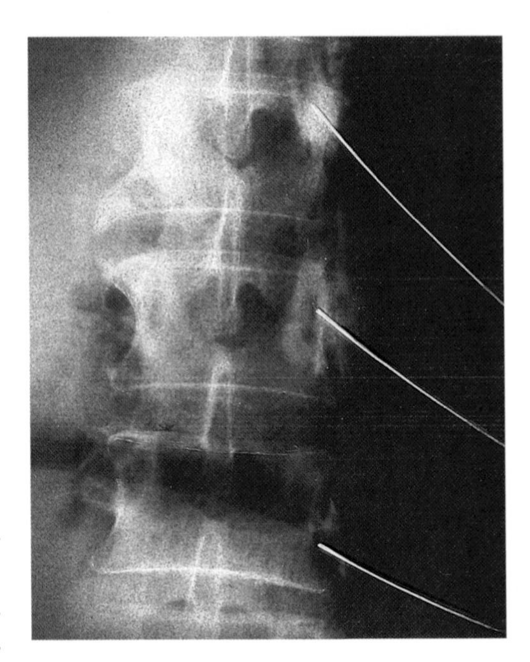

FIG 156.
Needle placement under x-ray control with contrast medium a-p view.

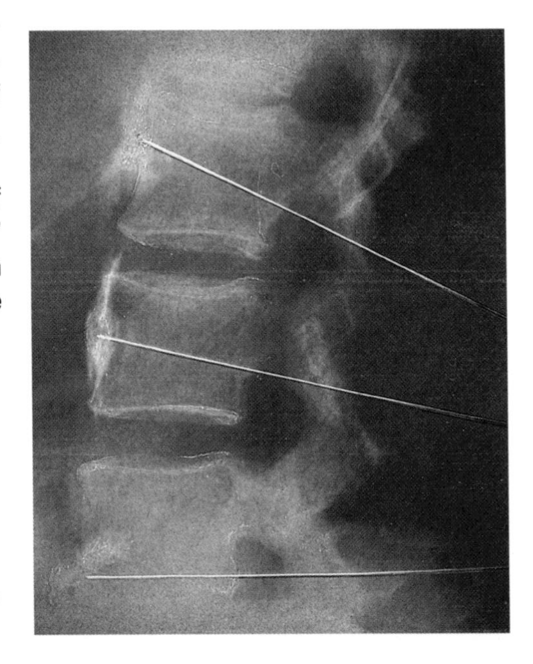

FIG 157.
Needle placement under x-ray control with contrast medium. Lateral view.
(The contrast medium injected through the caudal needle does not spread as expected.)

3.7. Dosage

Temporary block

10–15 ml local anesthetic solution, e.g., mepivacaine 1%; bupivacaine 0.25%.

Permanent block

1.5–2 ml neurolytic solution per needle, e.g., alcohol 95%.

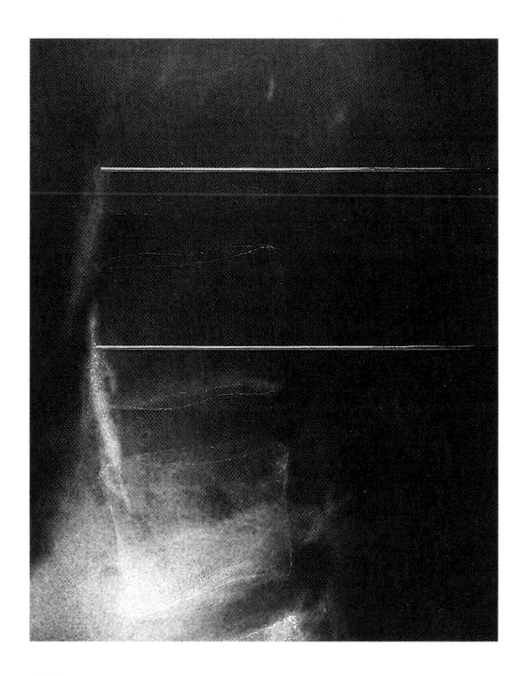

FIG 158.
Needle placement under x-ray control with contrast medium. Lateral view.
(The spread of the contrast medium, injected through the cranial needle, reveals incorrect placement into the psoas m.)

3.8. Assessment of the Block

Skin temperature

By measuring the surface skin temperature of both extremities, a comparison will determine the effectiveness of the block. The legs should be bare for at least 30 min.

Psychogalvanic reflex

To measure the psychogalvanic reflex (also known as the sympathogalvanic reflex), a multichannel ECG recorder is used. Two electrodes for each channel are attached to each foot (plantar and dorsal surface). The ground lead is attached to any place on the body surface.

The psychogalvanic reflex measures the changes in the electric skin resistance after blockade of the sympathetic fibers.
After a stimulus (e.g., loud clapping, light needle sticks), the side where the sympathetic fibers are blocked will show no deviation on the ECG strip as compared to the contralateral side.
A combination of skin temperature and psychogalvanic reflex measurement can be used to predict the likelihood of success of a planned neurolytic block, e.g., in patients with perfusion disturbances.

4. Special Side Effects and Complications

Side effects

Skin temperature elevation
Elimination of sweating
Partial block of paravertebral nerves

Complications

Intravascular (aorta, vena cava), peridural, or intrathecal injection
Injury to other organs (e.g., kidney)
Paresis and/or neuritis (with neurolytic solutions) in the region of the paravertebral nerves (e.g., genitofemoral nerve)

5. Indications

Thromboses, embolism, perfusion problems and edema in the lower extremities
Reflex dystrophies
Phantom pain
Chronic pain with, e.g., "burning" components

6. Special Contraindications

None

Blocks in the Area of the Head

Th. Flöter

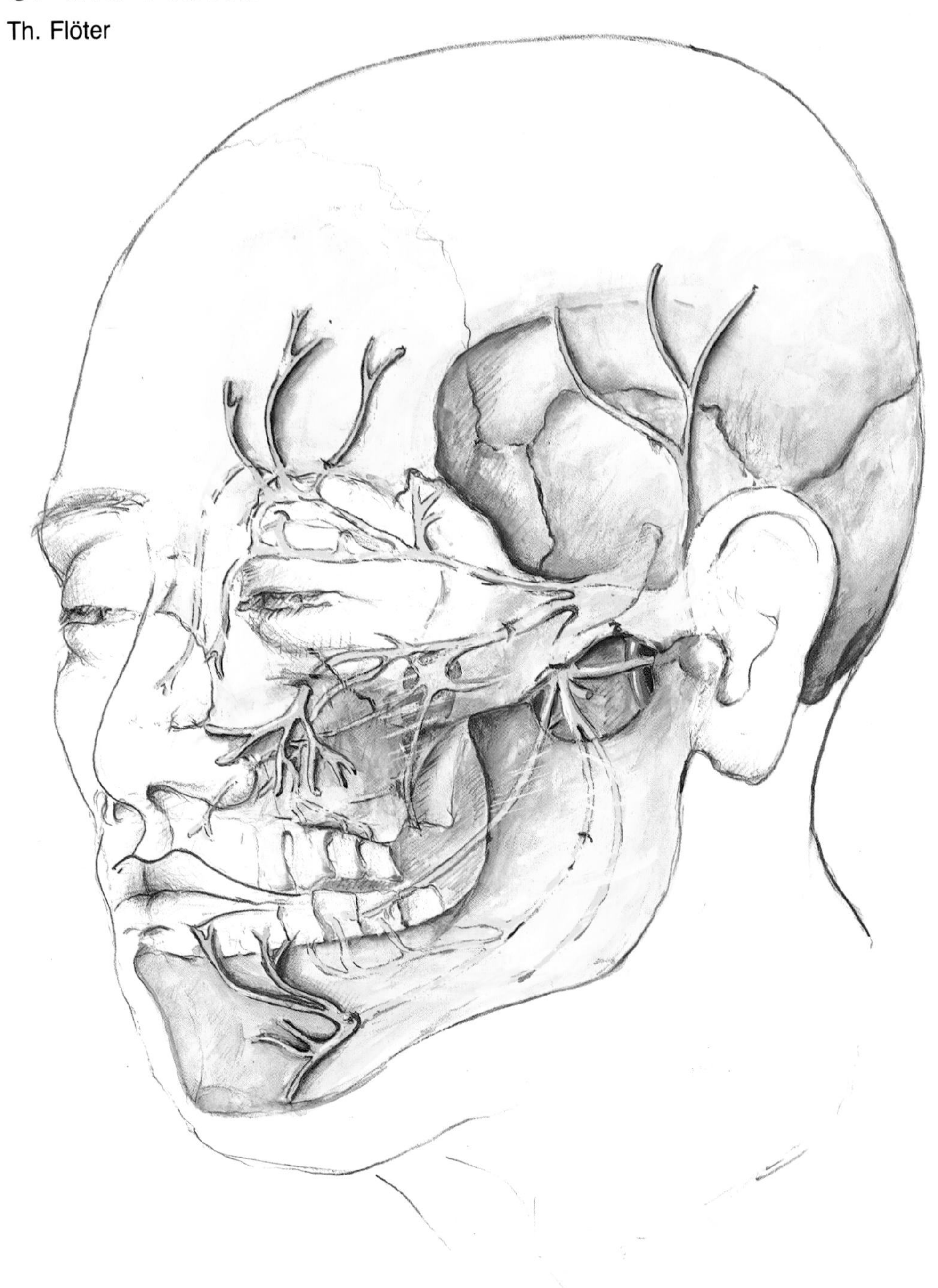

FIG 159.
Distribution of the branches of the trigeminal n.

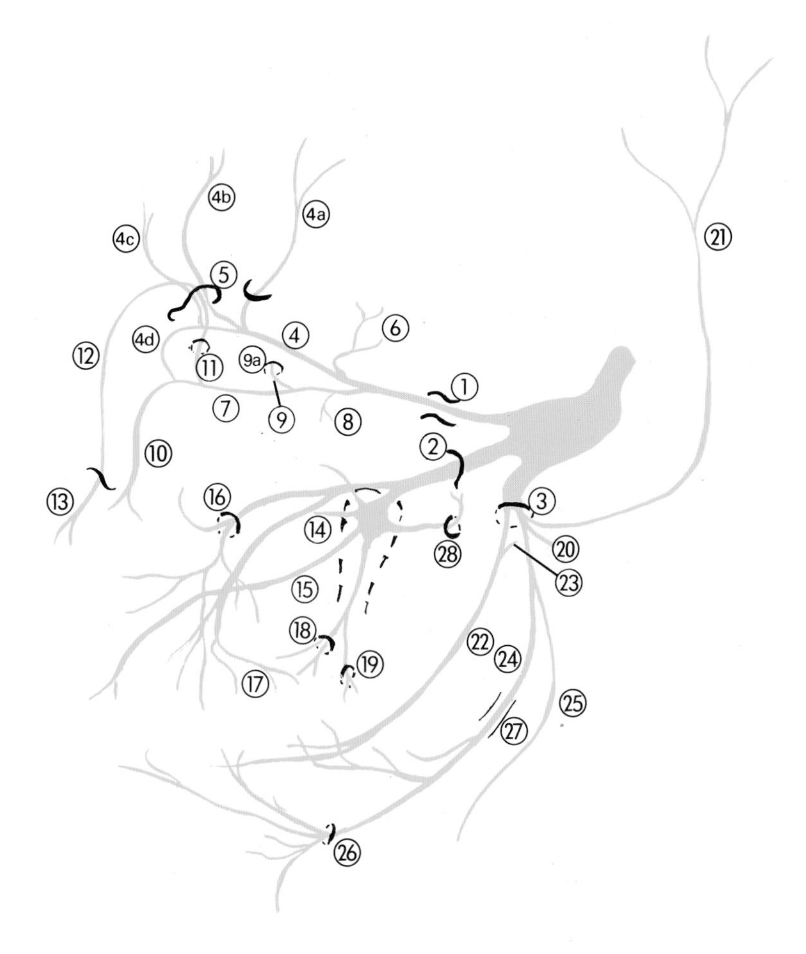

FIG 160.
Distribution of the branches of the trigeminal n.

1. Superior orbital fissure (ophthalmic n.)
2. Round canal (maxillary n.)
3. Foramen ovale (mandibular n.)
4. Frontal n.
   a. Right lateral supraorbital n.
   b. Right medial supraorbital n.
   c. Supratrochlear n.
   d. Anastomosis with the infratrochlear n.
5. Supraorbital incisura
6. Lacrimal n.
7. Nasociliary n.
8. Ciliary nn.
9. Posterior ethmoidal n.
   a. Posterior ethmoid foramen
10. Infratrochlear n.
11. Anterior ethmoidal n.
12. Anterior nasal branches
13. Right external nasal n.

Maxillary n.

14. Posterior nasal branches
15. Nasopalatine n.
16. Infraorbital foramen (infraorbital n.)
17. Dental plexus
18. Greater palatine foramen (greater palatine n.)
19. Lesser palatine foramen (lesser palatine n.)

Mandibular n.

20. Masseter n.
21. Auriculotemporal n.
22. Lingual n.
23. Chordatympany (originates from the facial n. and forms an anastomosis at this site)
24. Mandibular alveolar n.
25. Myohyoid n.
26. Mental foramen (mental n.)
27. Mandibular canal
28. Nerve of the pterygoid canal

Anatomy

The trigeminal nerve (5th cranial n.) supplies most of the face with sensory fibers. The small motor component of this mixed nerve supplies the muscles of mastication. The ganglion for the sensory portion, the gasserian, or semilunar ganglion, is located on the floor of the middle cranial fossa. It is here that the nerve divides into its three main branches: the ophthalmic nerve, the maxillary nerve, and the mandibular nerve.

The *ophthalmic n.* emerges through the superior orbital fissure into the orbit and divides here into three branches: the lacrimal n., the nasociliary n., and the frontal n., with its two terminal branches, the *supraorbital n.* and the *supratrochlear n.*

The *maxillary n.* passes through the foramen rotundum into the pterygopalatine fossa. Here it divides into the zygomatic n., the posterior nasal nerves, the palatinus major n. and the *infraorbital n.,* which proceeds anteriorly on the floor of the orbit, gives off branches to the teeth of the maxilla, and emerges through the infraorbital foramen.

The *pterygopalatine ganglion* lies in the pterygopalatine fossa medially and caudally to the maxillary n. It contains sensory, parasympathetic, and sympathetic fibers. The pterygopalatine fossa is a triangular space, located between the maxilla and pterygoid process of the sphenoid bone, in the upper part of the infratemporal fossa. In addition to the maxillary n. and the pterygopalatine ganglion, this space also contains the maxillary artery and vein.

The *mandibular n.* contains the motor fibers for the muscles of mastication. The most important sensory branches are the auriculotemporal n., the lingual n., the inferior alveolar n., and the mental n., which emerges through the mental foramen to innervate the lower lip and chin.

The dorsal branch of the second cervical nerve is primarily a sensory nerve. One of its components, the *major occipital n.,* perforates the tendinous insertion of the trapezius muscle, approximately 3 cm laterally to the middle of the linea nuchae, and supplies the medial portion of the skin on the back of the head between the nape and the top of the head. The *minor occipital n.* (from C_2 and C_3) supplies the lateral parts of the back of the head and the upper part of the external ear. Its point of emergence is directly behind and above the mastoid process.

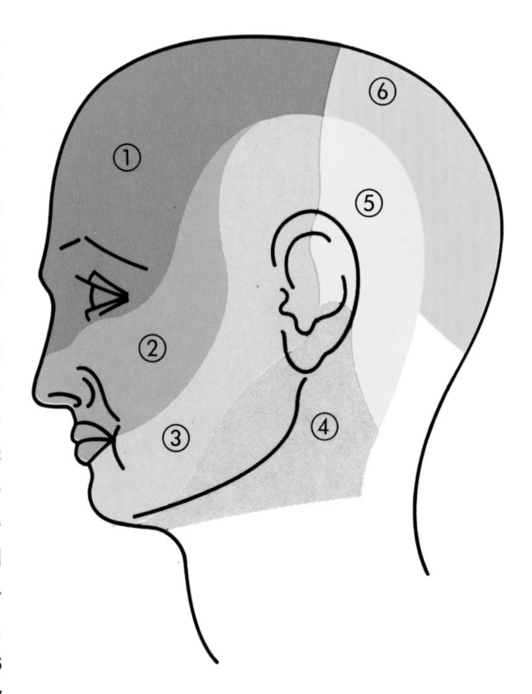

FIG 161.
Areas of analgesia in the area of the head:
1. Ophthalmic n.
2. Maxillary n.
3. Mandibular n.
4. Greater auricular n.
5. Lesser occipital n.
6. Greater occipital n.

I. The supraorbital and supratrochlear nerves

1. Definition

Blockade of the terminal branches of the ophthalmic nerve at the superior edge of the orbit.

2. Topographic Anatomy

The supraorbital nerve leaves the orbit with a medial and a lateral branch, at the junction of the middle third and the inner third of the superior edge of the orbit. The supratrochlear nerve emerges at the medial superior corner of the orbit. These nerves provide sensory innervation to the forehead.

3. Technique

3.1. Anesthesiologic Assessment

Careful anesthesiologic assessment including the identification of any contraindication.

3.2. Preparation

The emergency equipment must be tested to assure its proper functioning.

3.3. Equipment

Cleansing equipment
2 ml syringe
Short, thin 25 g needle (2–3 cm long)

3.4. Positioning

Patient in the supine position

3.5. Landmarks

Supraorbital nerve

Palpation of the supraorbital foramen and the supraorbital incisura, approximately 2.5 cm from the sagittal plane on the superior edge of the orbit.

Supratrochlear nerve

Palpation of the superior interior orbital corner (the root of the nose).

3.6. Technical Procedure

The supraorbital nerve

Introduction of the needle to the supraorbital foramen. It is not necessary to elicit paresthesias. When bony contact is made, the local anesthetic solution is injected (Fig 162).

The supratrochlear nerve

Entry at the superior, medial corner of the orbit until bony contact is made (Fig 163).

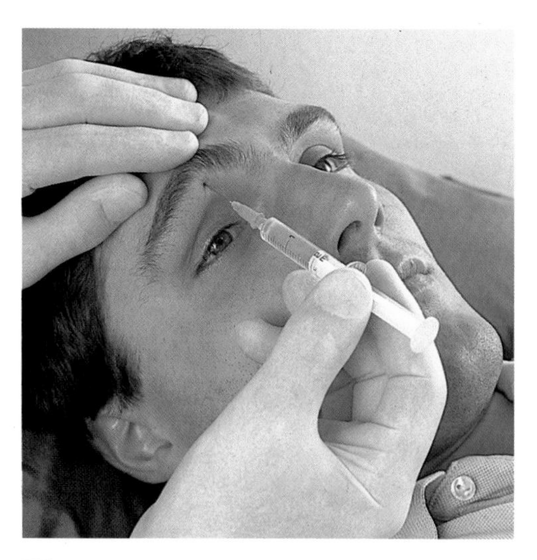

FIG 162.
Block of the supraorbital n.

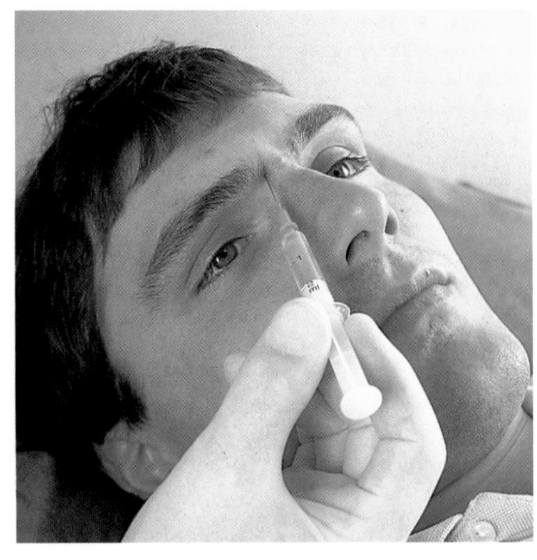

FIG 163.
Block of the supratrochlear n.

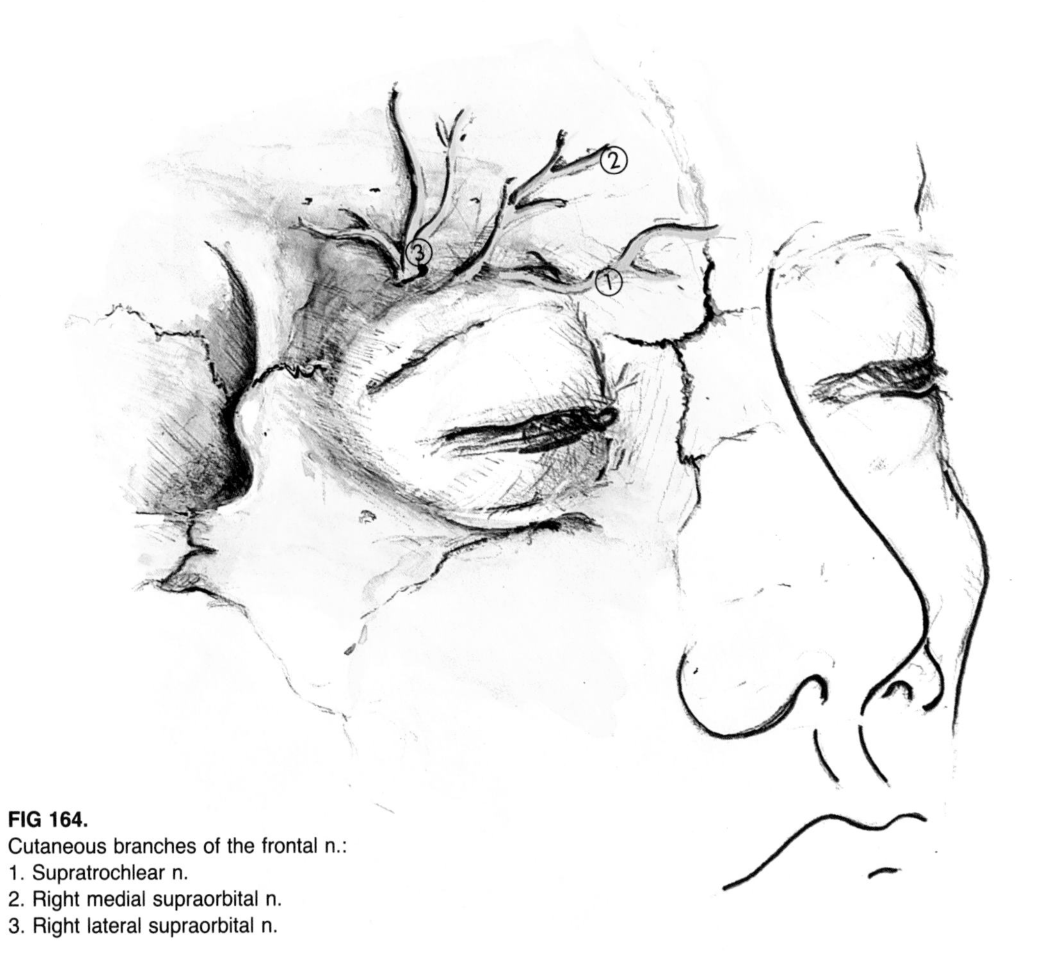

FIG 164.
Cutaneous branches of the frontal n.:
1. Supratrochlear n.
2. Right medial supraorbital n.
3. Right lateral supraorbital n.

3.7. Dosage

0.5–1 ml local anesthetic solution for each nerve, e.g., prilocaine 0.5%, mepivacaine 0.5%; bupivacaine 0.25%.

4. Special Complications

Bleeding, hematoma formation on the face; hence, pressure is indicated for a sufficiently long period of time.
Because of the danger of vascular injury and nerve compression, the injection should not be made into the supraorbital foramen.

5. Indications

Trigeminal neuralgia of the first branch, particularly for the differential diagnosis of the trigger points.
Postoperative and posttraumatic pain.
Pain due to inflammatory or neoplastic origin in the orbit, the frontal sinus, and the ethmoid sinus.

6. Special Contraindications

None

II. The maxillary nerve and the pterygopalatine ganglion

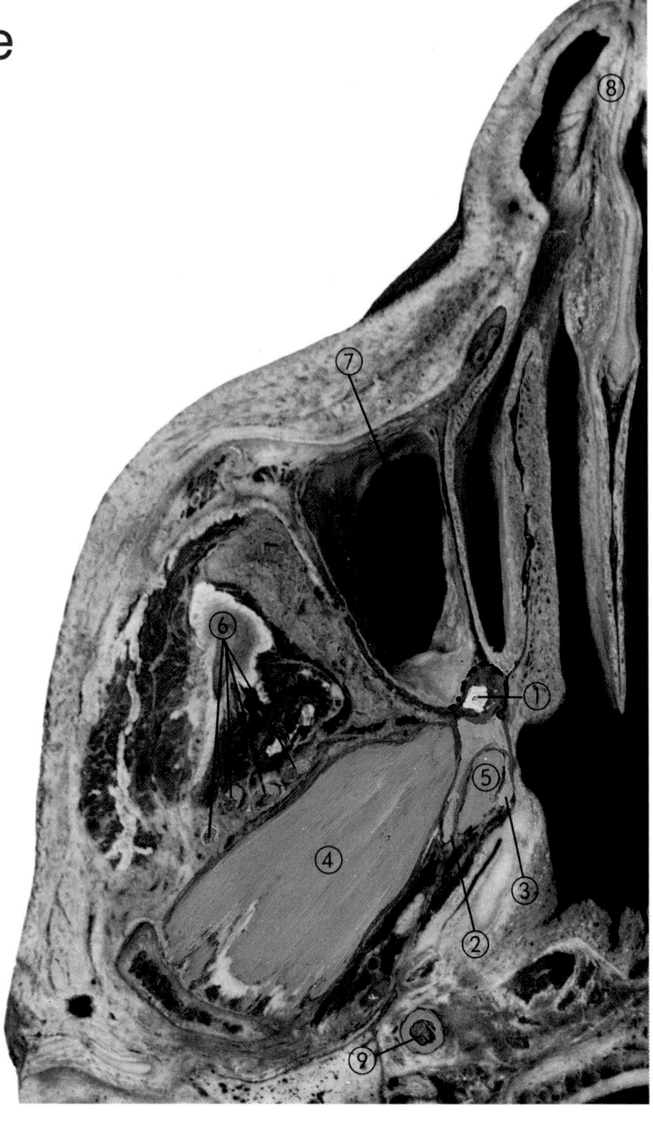

FIG 165.
Horizontal section at the level of the pterygopalatine fossa
1. Pterygopalatine ganglion
2. Lateral lamina of the pterygoid process
3. Medial lamina of the pterygoid process
4. Lateral pterygoid m.
5. Medial pterygoid m.
6. Vascular plexus
7. Maxillary sinus
8. Nasal septum
9. Carotid a.

1. Definition

Blockade of the second principal branch of the trigeminal nerve and of the pterygopalatine ganglion in the pterygopalatine fossa.

2. Topographic Anatomy

The pterygopalatine fossa is a triangular space between the pterygoid process of the sphenoid bone, and the maxilla in the upper part of the infratemporal fossa. It contains the maxillary nerve, the pterygopalatine ganglion, the maxillary artery and vein, and some fatty tissue. The nerve and the ganglion are responsible for the sensory and autonomic innervation of the mid-face and of the mid-area of the head (Figs 165 and 166).

3. Technique

3.1. Anesthesiologic Assessment

Careful anesthesiologic assessment including the identification of any contraindication.

3.2. Preparation

The emergency equipment must be tested to assure its proper functioning.

3.3. Equipment

Skin prep equipment
5 ml syringe
8 cm long, fine 22 g needle

3.4. Positioning

Patient in the supine position with the head turned to the contralateral side

3.5. Landmarks

Palpation of the middle of the zygomatic arch and the mandibular notch, between the coronoid and condylar processes. Slow opening and closing of the mouth facilitates the palpation.

3.6. Technical Procedure

Puncture is made vertically to the plane of the skin through the middle of the mandibular notch, directly below the midpoint of the zygomatic arch. At a depth of approximately 4 cm, the tip of the needle makes contact with the lateral lamina of the pterygoid process. The needle is withdrawn into the subcutaneous tissue and is readjusted, so that it can be introduced with the tip 1 cm further anteriorly and 1 cm further superiorly from the first bony contact. If the needle cannot be introduced to this depth, the tip is probably impinging again on the pterygoid process or on the maxilla. The direction of the needle must be readjusted once more. Paresthesias are frequently elicited in the area served by the maxillary nerve, but these are of no significance to the success of the block (Fig 167).

3.7. Dosage

2–3 ml of the local anesthetic solution, e.g., prilocaine 0.5%, mepivacaine 0.5%; bupivacaine 0.25%.
This amount of local anesthetic solution anesthetizes both the pterygopalatine ganglion and the maxillary nerve. When only 0.5–1 ml local anesthetic solution is used, it is possible to selectively anesthetize the pterygopalatine ganglion alone.

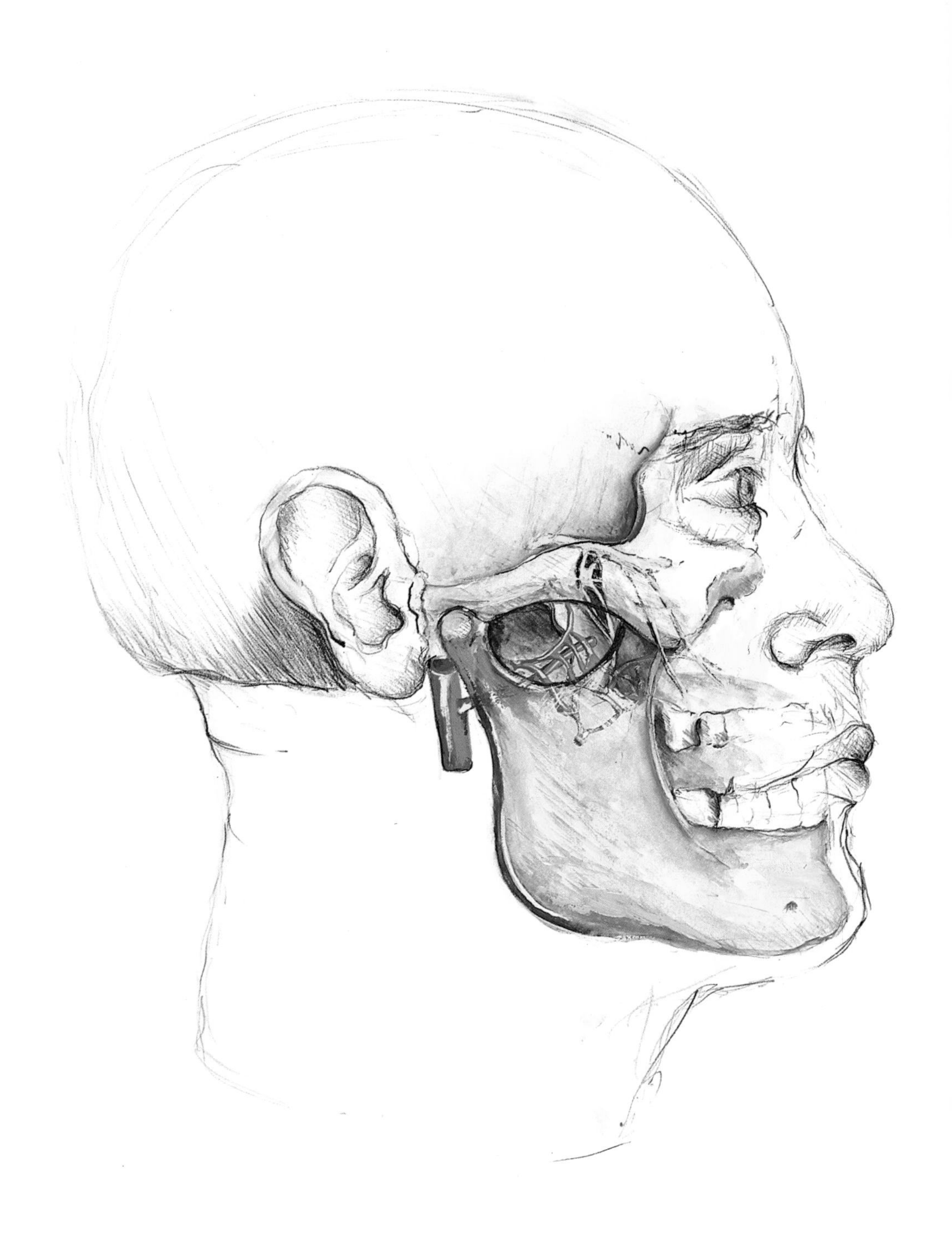

FIG 166.
The pterygopalatine ganglion and sensory branches of the maxillary n. with the adjacent vascular plexus in the pterygopalatine fossa.

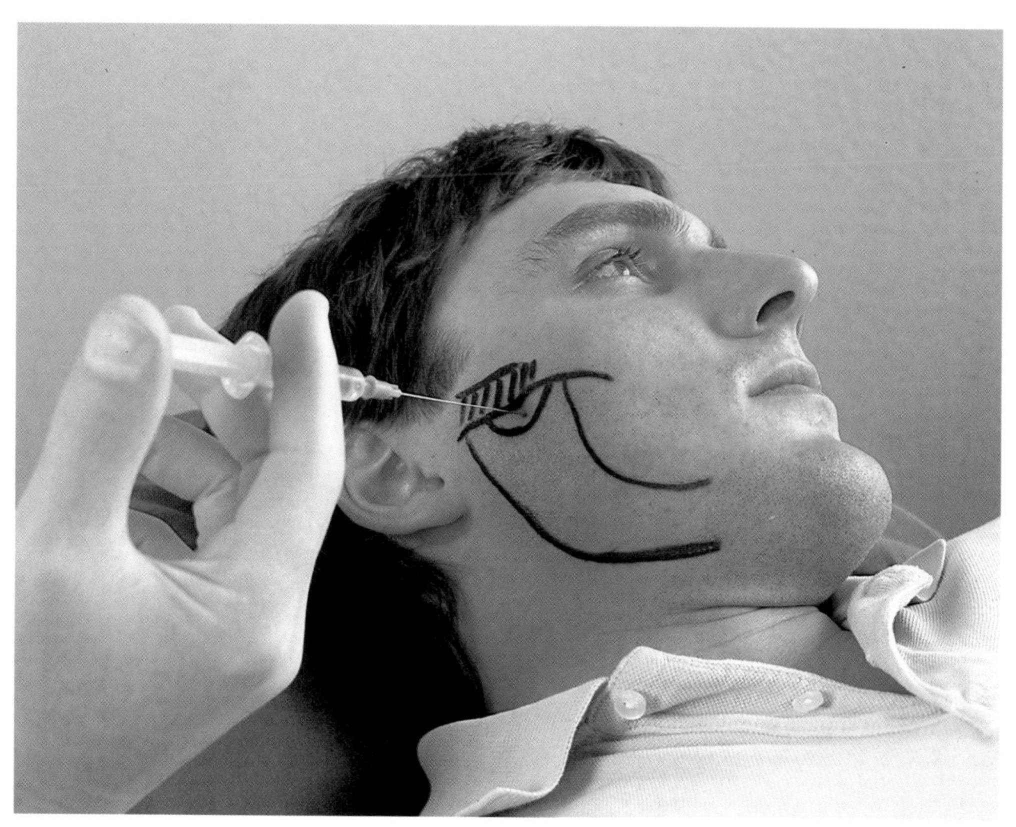

FIG 167.

4. Special Complications

Hemorrhage due to an injury to the maxillary artery
Subarachnoid injection

5. Indications

Trigeminal neuralgia of the second branch (the most common form)
Pain of maxillary neoplasm
Postoperative pain (maxillary sinus or teeth)
Atypical facial neuralgia
Acute herpes zoster in the area of the trigeminal nerve
Cluster headaches

6. Special Contraindications

Bleeding tendency

III. The infraorbital nerve

1. Definition

Blockade of the terminal branches of the maxillary artery.

2. Topographic Anatomy

The infraorbital nerve emerges through the infraorbital foramen, approximately 1 cm below the middle of the inferior edge of the orbit. The nerve provides sensory innervation to the lower eye lid, to the lateral wall of the nose, and to the upper lip (Fig 170).

3. Technique

3.1. Anesthesiologic Assessment

Careful anesthesiologic assessment including the identification of any contraindication.

3.2. Preparation

The emergency equipment must be tested to assure its proper functioning.

3.3. Equipment

Skin prep equipment
2 ml syringe
Short, fine 25 g needle (2–3 cm long)
A lighted spatula is helpful

3.4. Positioning

Patient in the supine position

3.5. Landmarks

Palpation of the infraorbital foramen and the pulsations of the neurovascular bundle, 1 cm below the middle of the lower edge of the orbit.

3.6. Technical Procedure

Introduction of the needle just below the area of palpation. The cannula is advanced cranially until bony contact is made (Fig 168).
If the intraoral approach is used, the needle is introduced in the upper labial fold over the canine tooth in the direction of the infraorbital foramen until bony contact is made. This approach is more elegant and less painful for the patient than the external approach (Fig 169).

3.7. Dosage

0.5–2 ml of the local anesthetic solution, e.g., prilocaine 0.5%, mepivacaine 0.5%; bupivacaine 0.25%.

4. Special Complications

Vascular injury and facial hematoma formation
Mechanical injury to the nerve during injection into the infraorbital foramen

5. Indications

Trigeminal neuralgia of the second branch
Differential diagnosis of the trigger zones
Postoperative, posttraumatic, or postinflammatory pain in the area of the maxilla

6. Special Contraindications

None

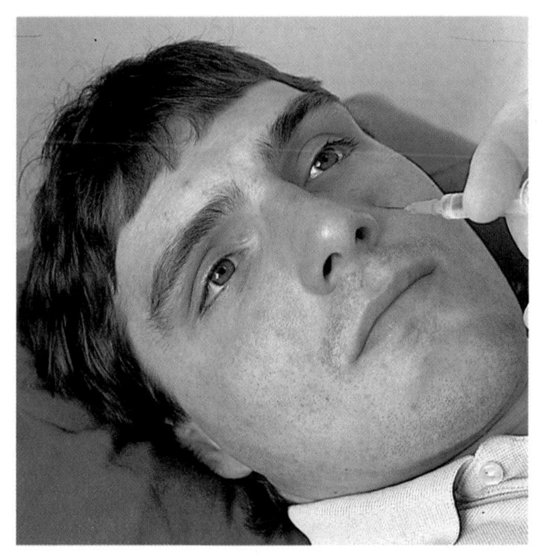

FIG 168.

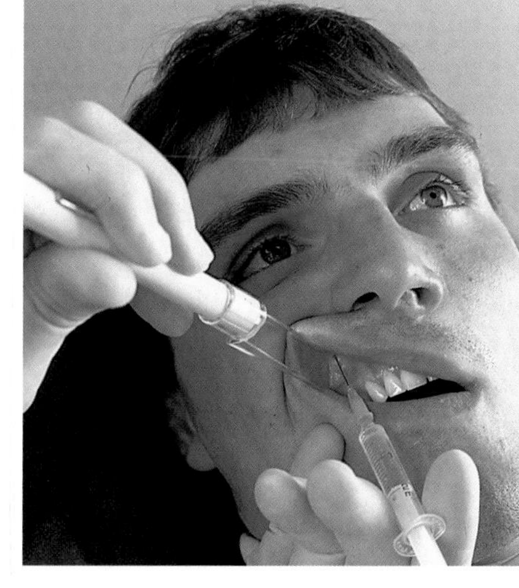

FIG 169.

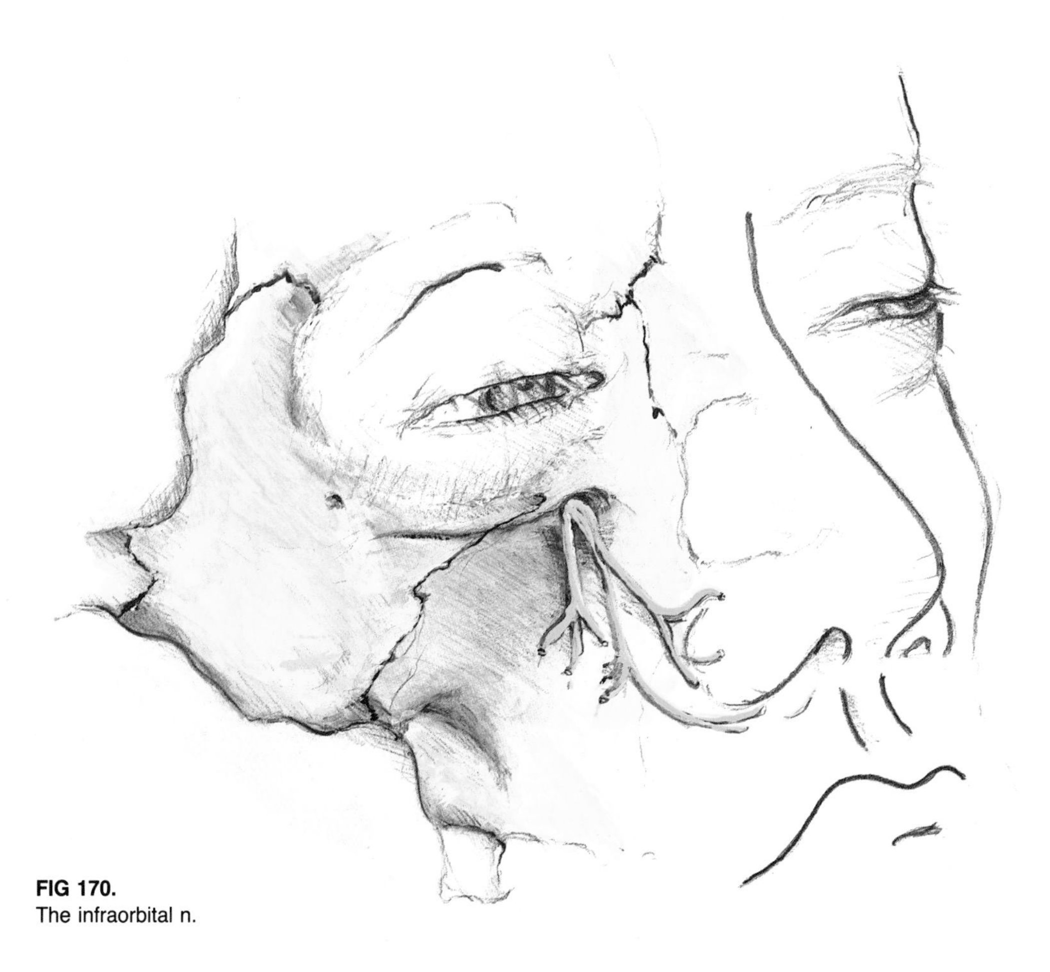

FIG 170.
The infraorbital n.

IV. The mental nerve

1. Definition

Blockade of one of the sensory terminal branches of the mandibular nerve.

2. Topographic Anatomy

The mental nerve is a branch of the inferior alveolar nerve, and emerges from the mental foramen at the level of the second premolar. It provides sensory innervation to the skin, to the mucosa of the lower lip, and to the chin (Fig 174).

3. Technique

3.1. Anesthesiologic Assessment

Careful anesthesiologic assessment including the identification of any contraindication.

3.2. Preparation

The emergency equipment must be tested to assure its proper functioning.

3.3. Equipment

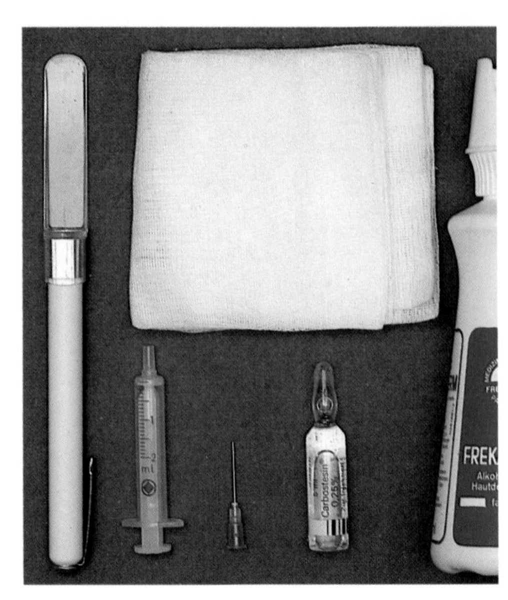

FIG 171.

Skin prep equipment
2 ml syringe
Short, fine 25 g needle (2–3 cm long)
A lighted spatula is helpful

3.4. Positioning

Patient in the supine position

3.5. Landmarks

Palpation of the mental foramen and the pulsations of the neurovascular bundle directly behind the first premolar.

3.6. Technical Procedure

Injection from the outside with the needle introduced at an angle in the direction of the palpated mental foramen (Fig 172). Using the *intraoral technique,* the entry point is in the lower labial fold, next to the first premolar (Fig 173).

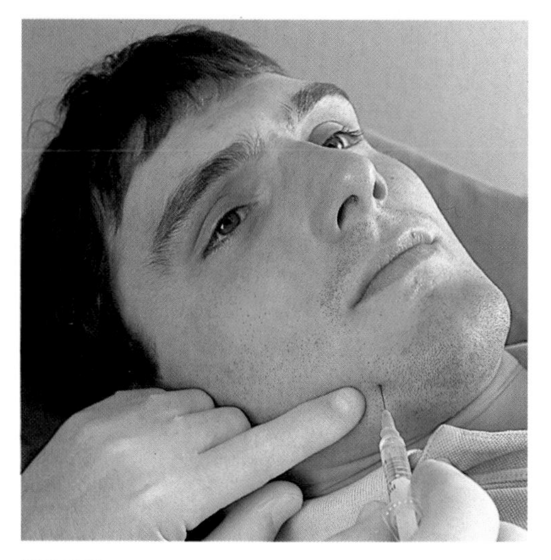
FIG 172.

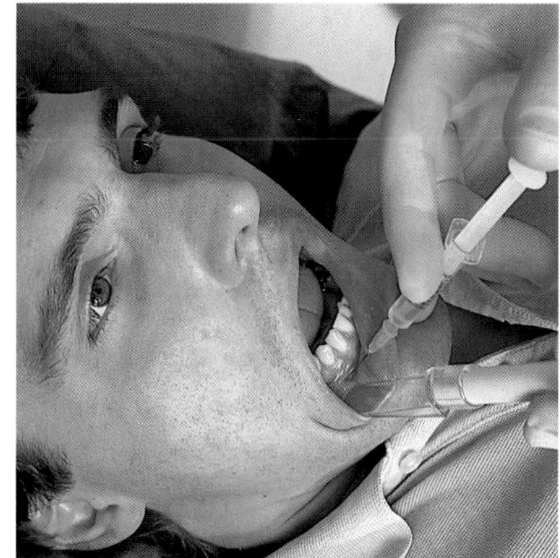
FIG 173.

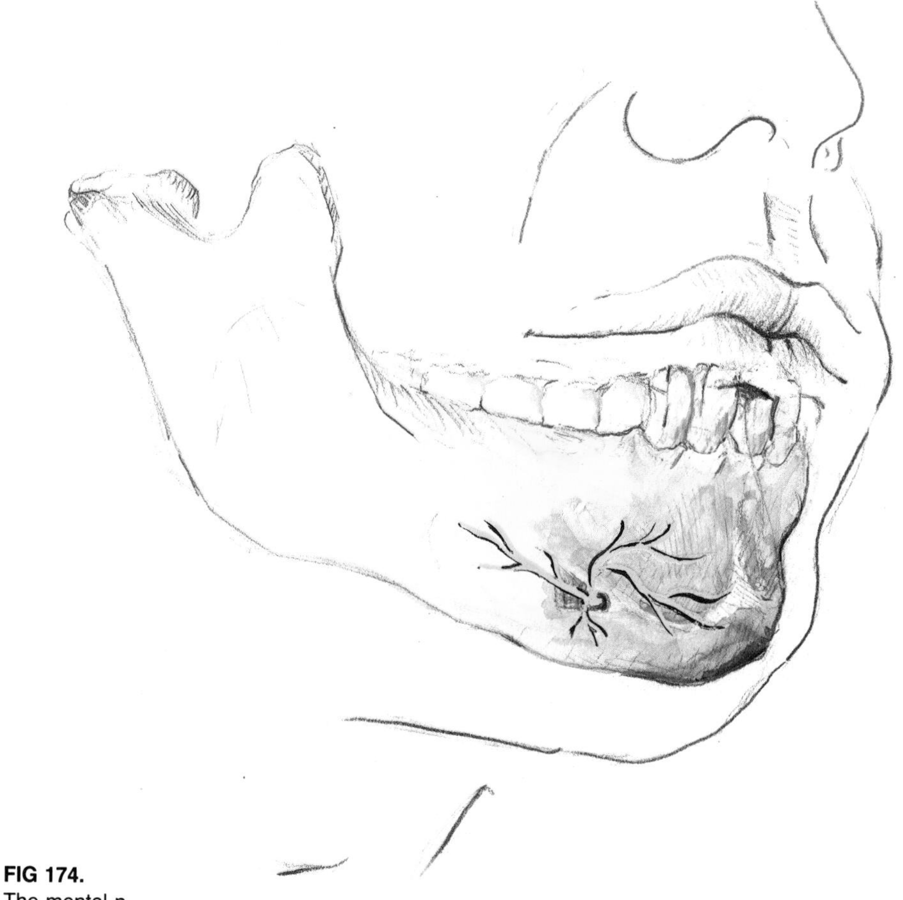
FIG 174.
The mental n.

3.7. Dosage

0.5–2 ml local anesthetic solution, e.g., prilocaine 0.5%, mepivacaine 0.5%; bupivacaine 0.25%.

4. Special Complications

Bleeding, due to vascular injury; hence, pressure is required after the injection.
Injury to the nerve or pressure injury due to injection into the bony canal.

5. Indications

Trigeminal neuralgia of the third branch.
Differential diagnosis of the trigger points.
Pain originating in the incisors, canines, or first premolars.

6. Special Contraindications

None

V. The occipital nerves

1. Definition

Blockade of the occipitalis major and minor nerves, where they emerge from the muscles of the neck.

2. Topographic Anatomy

The occipitalis major nerve perforates the muscles of the neck 3 cm laterally from the occipital protuberance, at the level of the linea nuchae. It lies directly medially from the occipital artery, which is readily palpable at this point. The occipitalis minor nerve is approximately 2.5 cm lateral to this point, and is found directly above and behind the mastoid process (Fig 176).

3. Technique

3.1. Anesthesiologic Assessment

Careful anesthesiologic assessment including the identification of any contraindication.

3.2. Preparation

The emergency equipment must be tested to assure its proper functioning.

3.3. Equipment

Skin prep equipment
10 ml syringe
Short, fine 22–25 g needle (2–3 cm long)

3.4. Positioning

The patient is in the prone or sitting position.

3.5. Landmarks

Palpation of linea nuchae, the occipital artery, and the mastoid process.

3.6. Technical Procedure

Entry with the needle vertically to the skin, directly at the exit point of the nerve (Fig 175).

3.7. Dosage

2–10 ml local anesthetic solution, e.g., prilocaine 0.5%, mepivacaine 0.5%; bupivacaine 0.25%.

4. Special Complications

When the injection is made, only after definite bony contact has been established is there no danger of a suboccipital or intrathecal injection.
Due to the vicinity of vessels, a hematoma is always a possibility.

5. Indications

The so-called occipital neuralgias, i.e., painful conditions in the region of the upper cervical nerves due to irritation of the nerve roots, through degenerative spinal column changes or muscular tension.
The same type of pain is also noted in neoplasms of the posterior cranial fossa. A differential diagnosis *must* be made.
To achieve good results, it is frequently necessary to identify the myofascial trigger points and to anesthetize them as well.

6. Special Contraindications

None

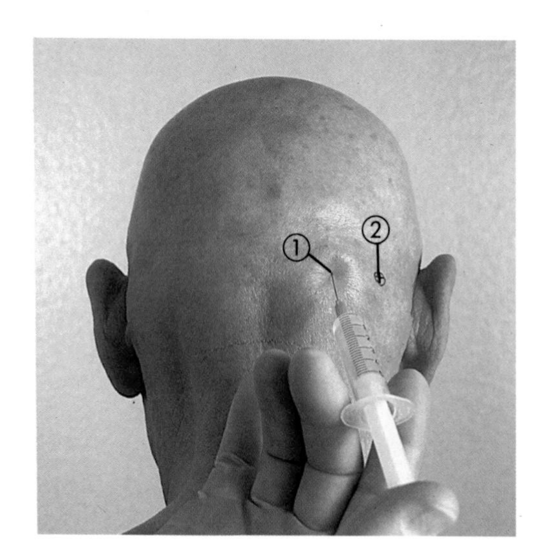

FIG 175.
Points of entry:
1. Block of the greater occipital n.
2. Block of the lesser occipital n.

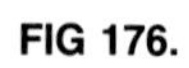

FIG 176.
1. Greater occipital n.
2. Lesser occipital n.

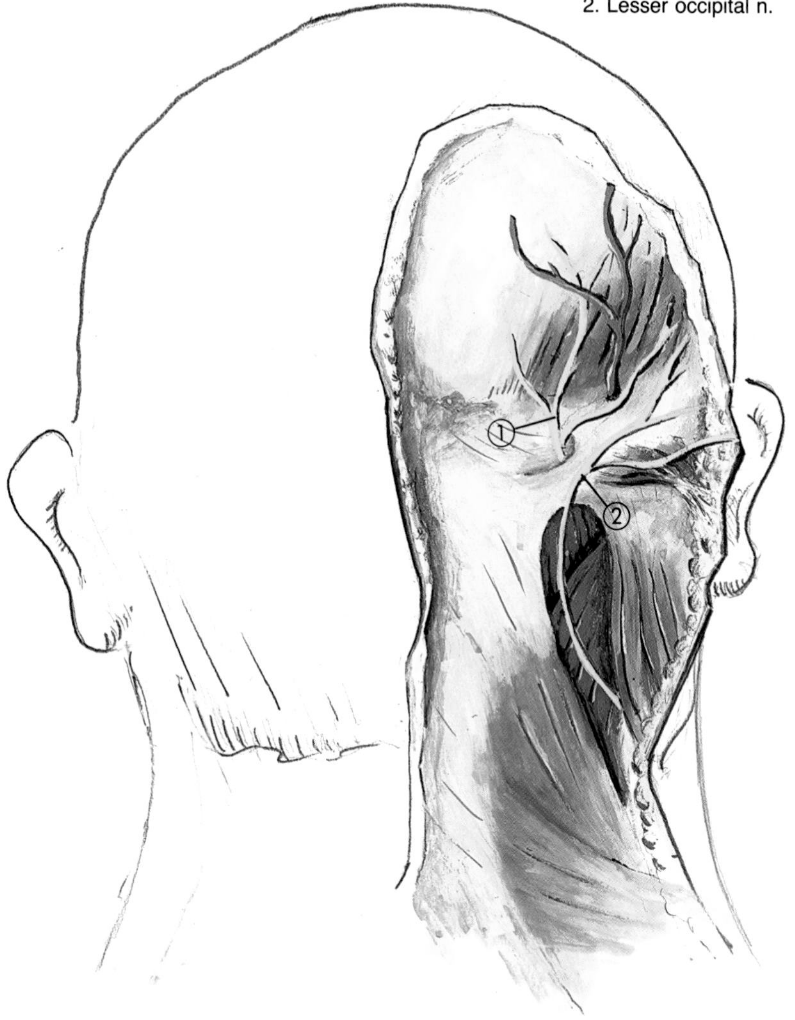

VI. The myofascial trigger points

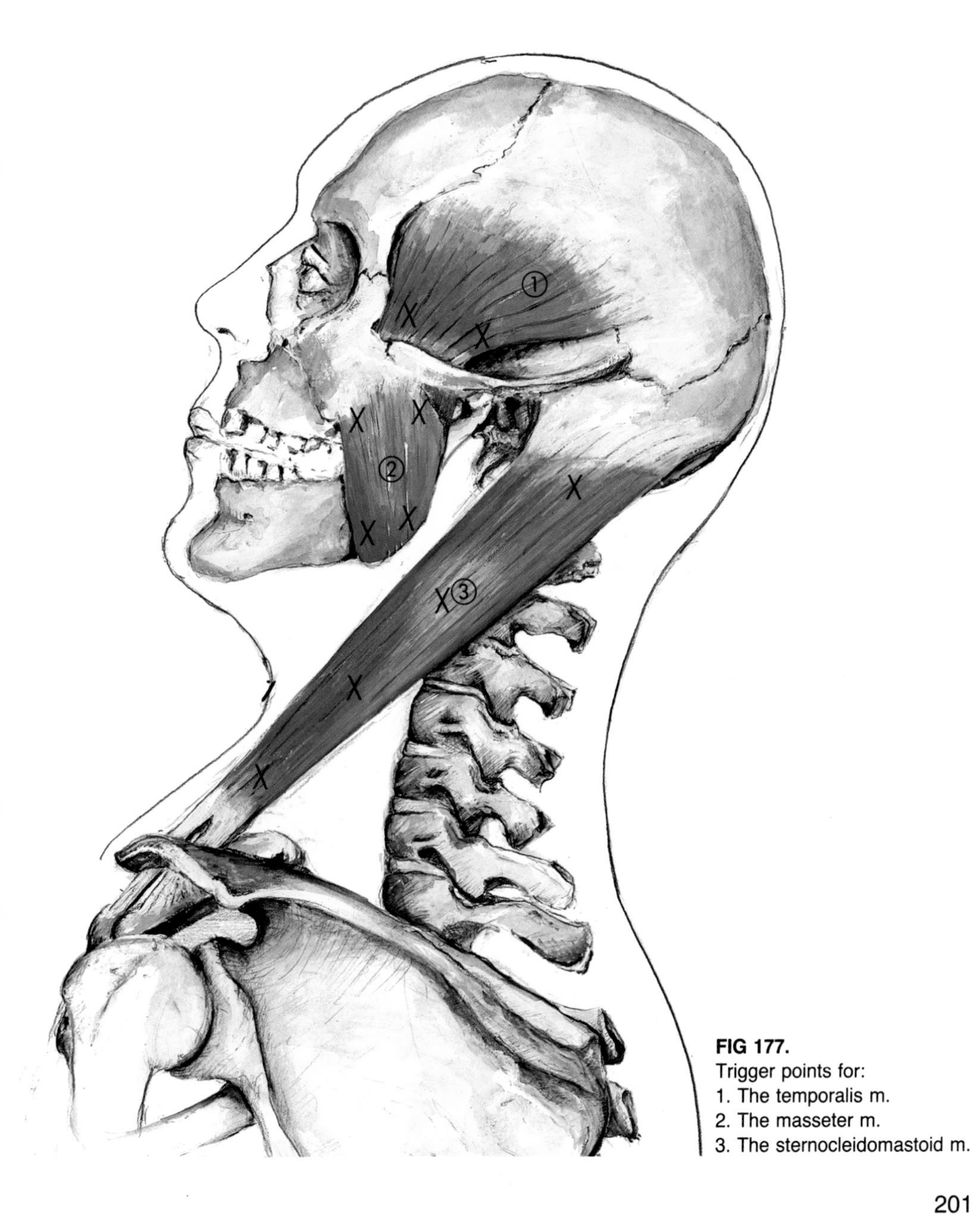

FIG 177.
Trigger points for:
1. The temporalis m.
2. The masseter m.
3. The sternocleidomastoid m.

1. Definition

The myofascial trigger points are hypersensitive, palpably firm sites in a weakened, contracted muscle or its fascia. They are sensitive to touch and can initiate pain and autonomic disturbances in a large and nonsegmental area (referred pain).

2. Topographic Anatomy

In the area of the head, face, and neck, trigger points can occur in practically any muscle. They are most frequently found in the following muscles: trapezius m., semispinalis capitis m., splenius capitis m., occipitofrontalis m., and the short, suboccipital muscles. Not infrequently, the muscles of the neck, the muscles of mastication, and the muscles of facial expression are also involved. Localization is accomplished by palpation and observing the radiation of the pain. The cooperation of the patient is desirable (Figs 177 and 178).

3. Technique

3.1. Anesthesiologic Assessment

Careful anesthesiologic assessment including the identification of any contraindication.

3.2. Preparation

The emergency equipment must be tested to assure its proper functioning.

3.3. Equipment

Skin prep equipment
2 ml syringe
Medium length, fine, 25 g needle (3–5 cm long)

3.4. Positioning

Depending on the site, either supine, prone, or sitting

3.5. Landmarks

Precise palpation of the belly of the muscle, the edge of the muscle, and the tendinous attachments.

3.6. Technical Procedure

Precise, accurate palpation and identification of the point of maximal pain. Careful inspection of the topography, prior to injection. Injection into or around the trigger point (Fig 178).

3.7. Dosage

0.1–1 ml of the local anesthetic solution for each trigger point, e.g., prilocaine 0.5%, mepivacaine 0.5%; bupivacaine 0.25%.

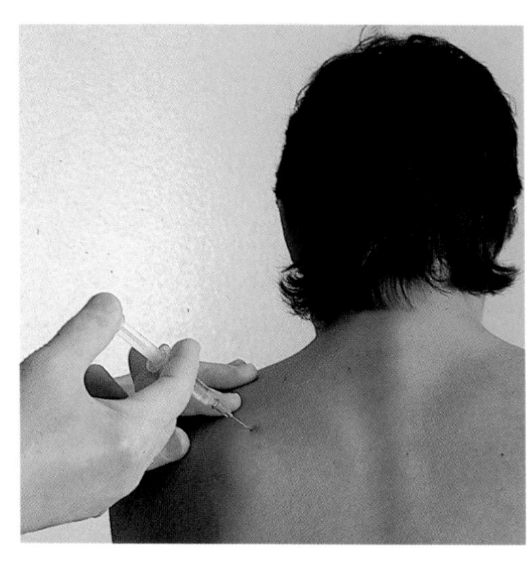

FIG 178.
Infiltration of the trigger point; levator scapulae m.

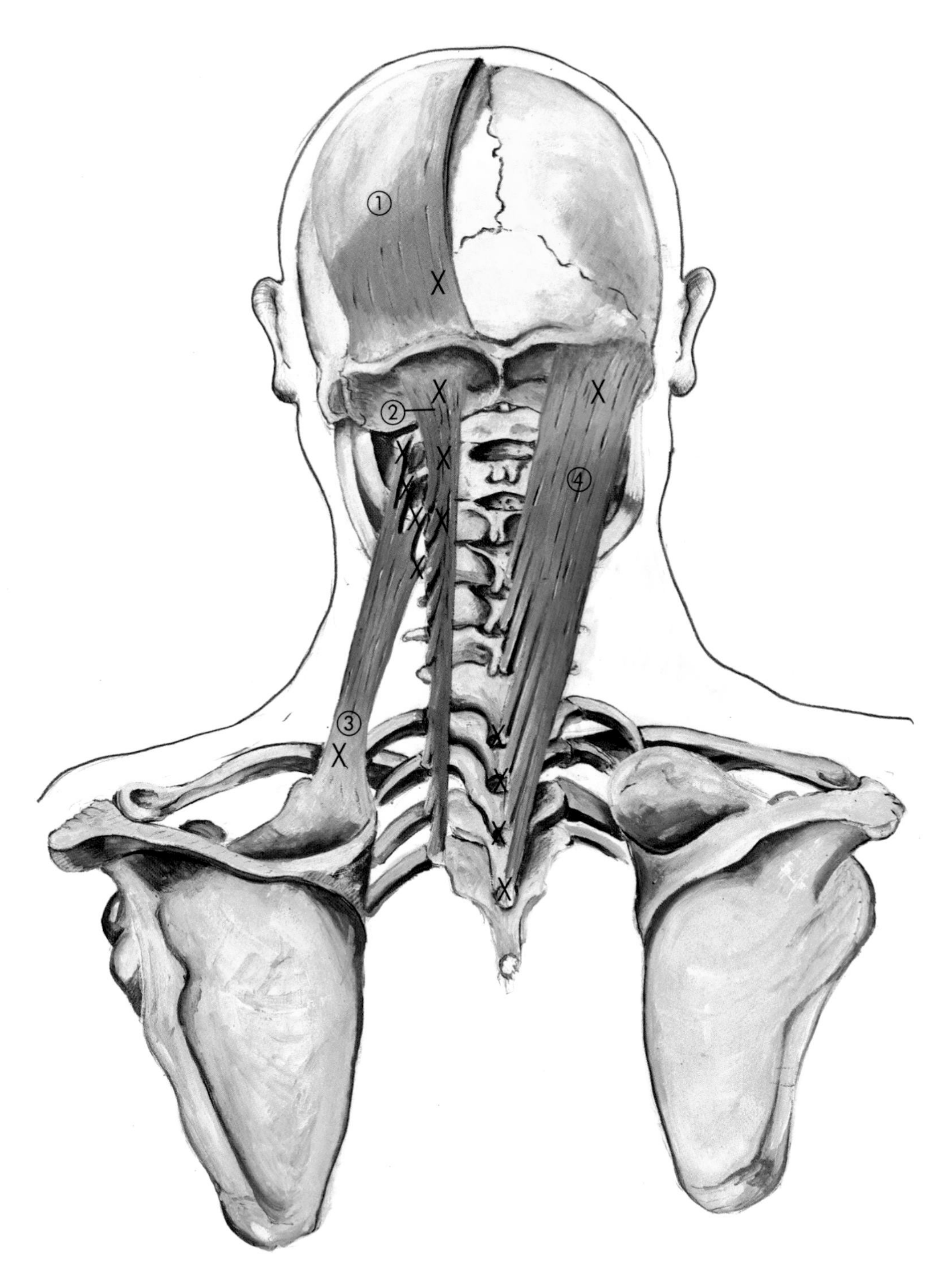

FIG 179.
Trigger points for:
1. The occipitofrontal m. (occipital part)
2. The semispinalis capitis m.
3. The levator scapulae m.
4. The splenius capitis m.

4. Special Complications

In the cervical region, there is a danger of intravascular or intrathecal injection. When the anesthesia wears off, pain may be accentuated after the first few treatments.

5. Indications

Myofascial pain syndromes
Trigger points participate in almost all painful conditions in the area of the head, face, and neck

6. Special Contraindications

None

References

1. Auberger HG: *Regionale Schmerztherapie.* Stuttgart, Thieme, 1971.
2. Bonica JJ: *The Management of Pain.* Philadelphia, Lea and Febiger, 1954.
3. Travell JG, Simons DG: *Myofascial Pain and Dysfunction.* Baltimore-London, Williams and Wilkins, 1983.

Intercostal Block

H. Kreuscher

1. Definition

Temporary (local anesthetic solution) or permanent (neurolytic solution) *interruption* of sensory, motor and autonomic impulse conduction along one or more thoracic spinal nerves.

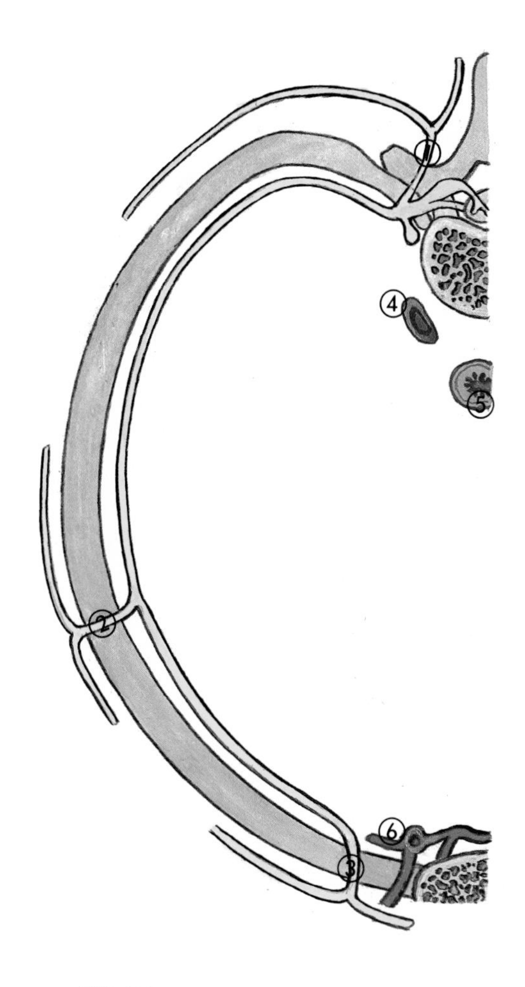

FIG 180
(after Tondury)
1. Dorsal branch of the spinalis n.
2. Lateral cutaneous branch of the spinal n.
3. Anterior cutaneous branch of the spinal n.
4. Azygos v.
5. Esophagus
6. Internal thoracic a.

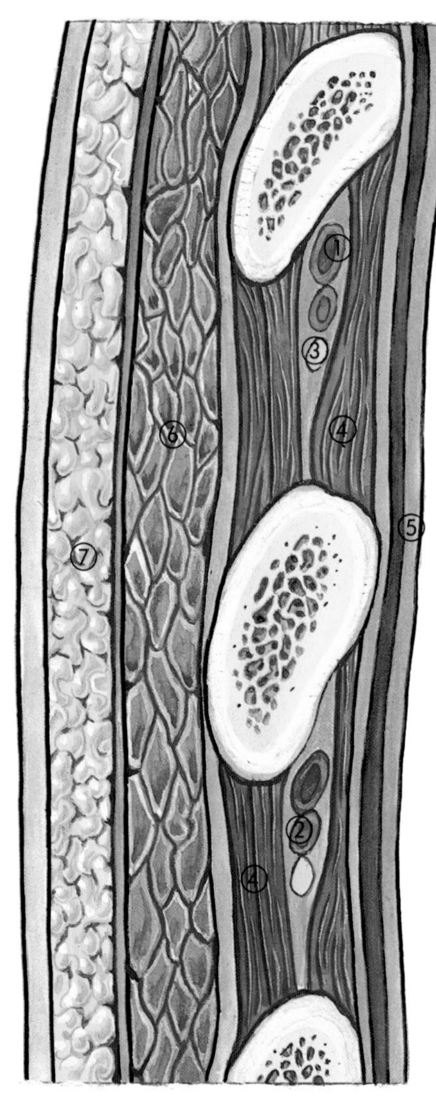

FIG 181
(after Tondury)
Schematic cross section through two intercostal spaces in the area of the posterior axillary line.

1. Intercostal v.
2. Intercostal a.
3. Intercostal n.
4. Intercostal m.
5. Parietal pleura
6. Pectoralis major m.
7. Subcutaneous layer

FIG 182
(after Spalteholtz)
Line C = Posterior axillary line
Line D = Anterior axillary line
(o = Points of entry)

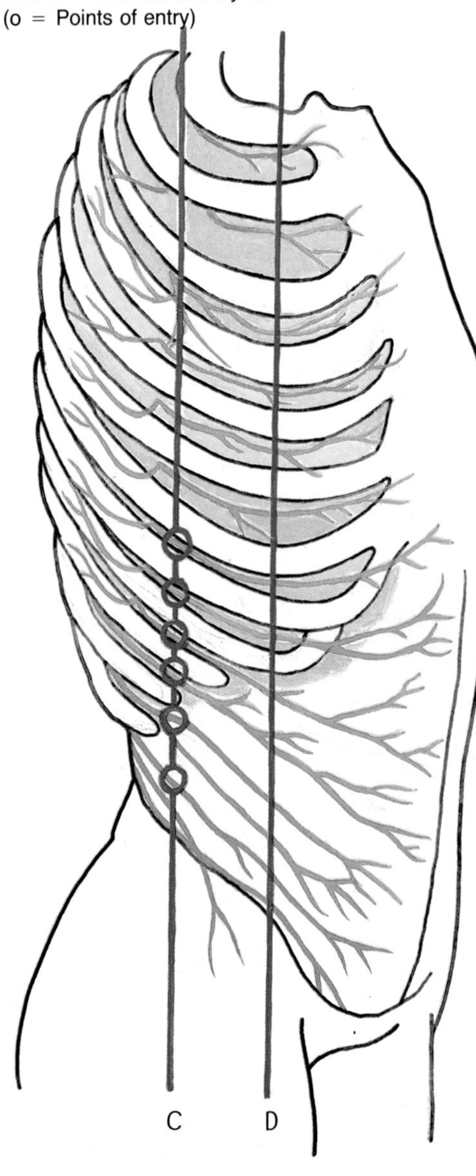

2. Topographic Anatomy

Directly distal to the spinal ganglia, the thoracic spinal nerves give off the white and gray *rami communicantes* of the sympathetic system, which go to or come from the particular ganglion of the sympathetic chain.

Distal to the rami communicantes, the nerve trunk divides into the *dorsal branch* and the *ventral branch.* The *dorsal branch* supplies the skin of the back, the muscles of the back, and the periosteum of the vertebrae through its lateral and medial branches.

The *ventral branch* follows the rib into the costal sulcus, into the dorsal thoracic region and between the two lamina of the intercostal muscles in the intercostal space, and into the lateral and ventral portion of the thorax (Fig 181). The ventral branches each give off a lateral cutaneous branch, the 1st to the 5th in the posterior axillary line, and the 6th to 12th in the anterior axillary line (Fig 182).

The lateral cutaneous branches of the 7th to 12th intercostal nerves participate in the sensory and motor innervation of the anterior abdominal wall (skin, muscles, parietal peritoneum).

3. Technique

The *topographic anatomy* of the thoracic spinal nerves lends itself—according to the extent of the block required—to the following techniques:

A. Blockade of the thoracic *spinal roots* (paravertebral block)

B. Blockade of the *dorsal branch*

C. Blockade of the *ventral branch* at the *angle of the rib*

D. Blockade of the *ventral branch in the posterior axillary line* (dorsolateral intercostal block)

E. Blockade of the *anterior branch in the anterior axillary line* (anterolateral intercostal block)

F. *Parasternal* intercostal blockade

3.1. Anesthesiologic Assessment

Careful anesthesiologic assessment including the identification of any contraindication. Pulmonary function testing before a multiple segment block or a bilateral block, particularly if neurolytic agents are to be used.

3.2. Preparation

Intubation equipment, ventilation equipment, oxygen connection, intravenous infusion in high risk patients. Atropine, sedative, succinylcholine, vasopressor, catecholamine.

A. Paravertebral blockade

Effect

Elimination of sensory, motor, and autonomic impulse conduction along a thoracic spinal nerve.

3.3. Equipment

Sterile gloves
Antiseptic solution
Sponges
Drapes
Flat, firm pillow
Small needle for the skin wheal
8–10 cm long short bevel needle
5 ml syringe
2 ml syringe
Small cup for the anesthetic solution

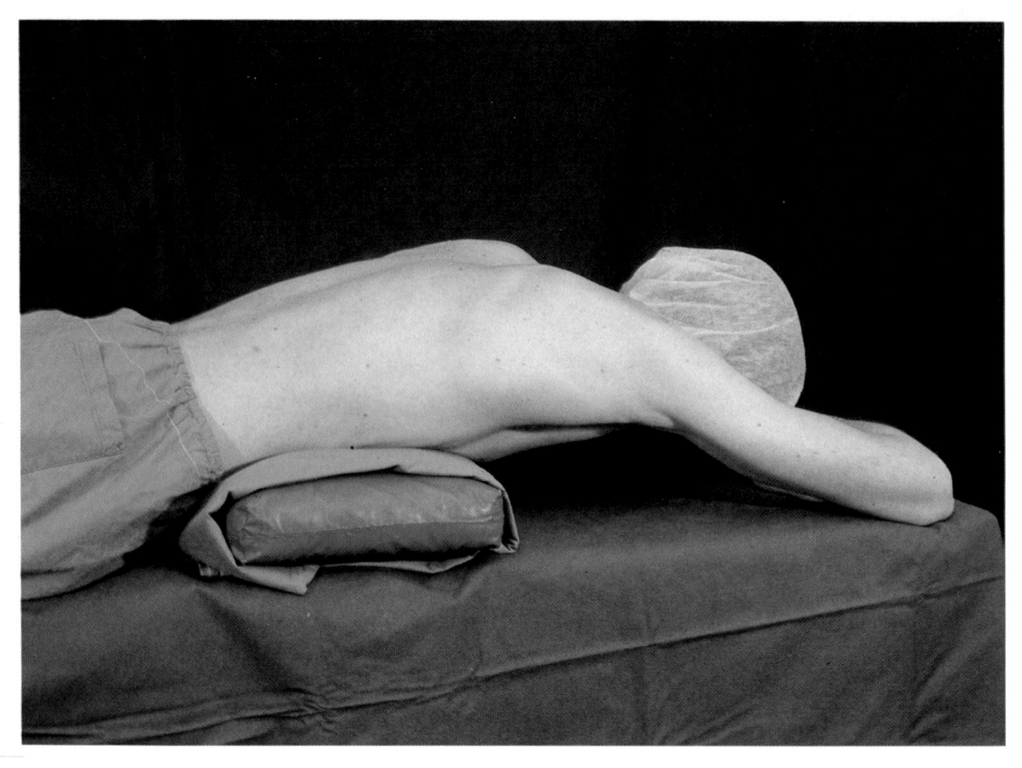

FIG 183.

FIG 184.

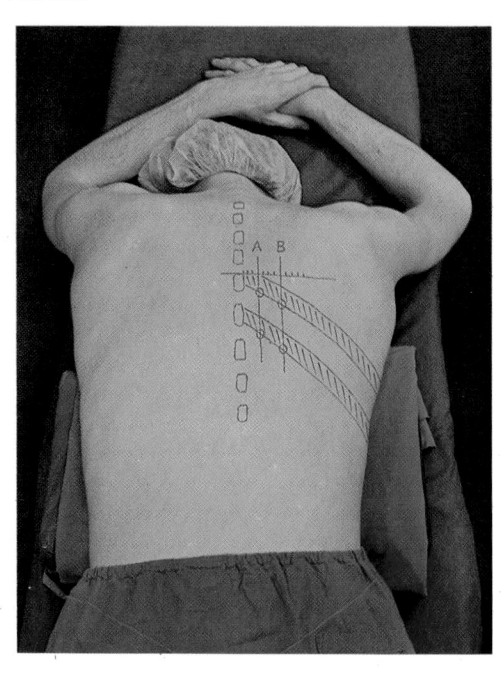

3.4. Positioning

Prone position. Enhancement of the thoracic kyphosis with a flat, hard pillow. The arms are extended over the head so that the scapulae are pulled laterally (Fig 183).

3.5. Landmarks

The upper edge of the spinous process is marked with a horizontal line. Three cm laterally (line A) and 3 cm caudally from this point is the site of entry for the block of the spinal nerve, one segment below the level to which the spinous process belongs (Fig 184).

3.6. Technical Procedure

Degreasing, disinfection, and sterile draping of the area of injection. The point of entry is identified and a skin wheal is raised. An 8–10 cm long, short bevel needle, with a 5 ml syringe attached, is advanced vertically, until bony contact is made (transverse process). The needle is withdrawn and readjusted at 80° caudally. The needle is again advanced and the tip is placed 2–2.5 cm beyond the transverse process. If the tip of the needle is placed accurately and is in contact with the spinal ganglion, paresthesias will be elicited. Even in the absence of paresthesias, if the needle tip is within a few millimeters of the ganglion, a good block can be obtained, thanks to the diffusing ability of the local anesthetic solution. In the aspiration test, watch for CSF as well as blood, since the dura occasionally forms an outpouching as far as the spinal ganglion. If the needle tip is too far medial, dural puncture can occur.

3.7. Dosage

Temporary blockade

5–8 ml local anesthetic solution for each segment, e.g., etiodocaine 1% or bupivacaine 0.5%.

Permanent blockade

E.g., 2–3 ml 95% ethylalcohol, or 3 ml 10% ammonium sulfate, or 5–6 ml 8% phenol in water.

The permanent block can be very painful, and may have to be administered under general anesthesia. When ammonium sulfate is used, it is advisable to dilute a 20% solution with an equal volume of 2% mepivacaine.

B. *Blockade of the dorsal branch*

Effect

Anesthesia of the skin over the spinous process, and of the periosteum of the vertebra.

3.3. Equipment

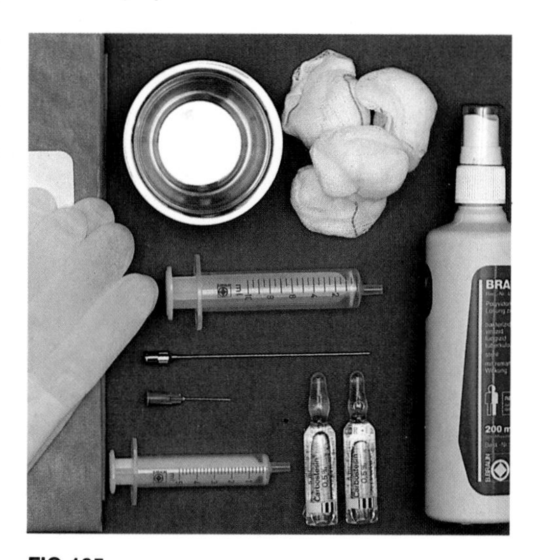

FIG 185.

Sterile gloves
Antiseptic solution
Sponges
Drapes
Small needle for the skin wheal
4–8 cm long needle
10 ml syringe
2 ml syringe
Small cup for the local anesthetic solution

3.4. Positioning

Sitting (Fig 186) or prone (Fig 183)

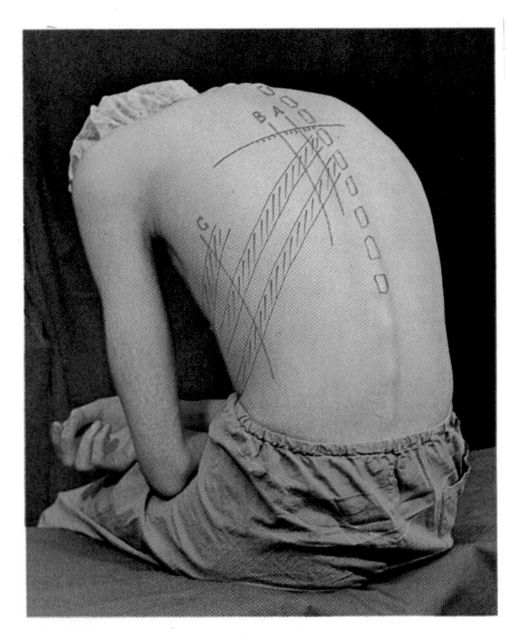

FIG 186.
The feet are placed on a stool.

3.5. Landmarks

The middle of the spinous process is marked with a horizontal line. The injection site is one finger's breadth (2 cm) lateral to the midspinal line, where it meets the above mentioned horizontal line.

3.6. Technical Procedure

Degreasing, disinfection, and draping of the area of the injection. After placing a skin wheal, a 5–8 cm long needle with a 10 ml syringe attached is advanced at a 90° angle to the skin, until the trapezius fascia is reached (2–3 cm). While advancing the needle slowly, the anesthetic solution is administered into the muscle to a depth of 5–6 cm.

3.7. Dosage

8–10 ml local anesthetic solution for each segment, e.g., etidocaine 1% or bupivacaine 0.5%.

C. Blockade of the ventral branch at the angle of the rib

Effect

Blockade of the intercostal nerve distal to the start of the dorsal branch. Segmental anesthesia of the skin on the lateral and anterior thoracic wall. Motor blockade of the intercostal nerves. Below the 7th intercostal nerve, there is a simultaneous motor blockade of the abdominal muscles, and a sensory blockade of the skin and peritoneum of the abdominal wall.

3.3. Equipment

Sterile gloves
Antiseptic solution
Sponges
Drapes
Needle, 5 cm long, 21 g
Needle, 25 g for the skin wheal
5 ml syringe
2 ml syringe
Small cup for the anesthetic solution

3.4. Positioning

Sitting (Fig 186) or prone (Fig 183)

3.5. Landmarks

The costal angle is, on the average, 7 cm from the midline (line B). The site of injection is where the B line crosses the palpable inferior edge of the rib (Fig 184).

3.6. Technical Procedure

Degreasing, disinfection, and draping of the area of the injection. After placing a skin wheal, a 5 cm long, 21 g needle, with a 5 ml syringe attached, is introduced. The needle is advanced at a 90° angle to the skin until bony contact is made (rib). The needle is slightly withdrawn, readjusted caudally, and advanced slowly until it just passes the inferior margin of the rib. The tip of the needle is now elevated so that it approaches the sulcus of the rib. Care must be taken to keep the tip of the needle in the immediate vicinity of the rib. Aspiration test must be performed.

3.7. Dosage

Temporary blockade

3 ml of the local anesthetic solution for each segment, e.g., etidocaine 1%, bupivacaine 0.5%.

Permanent blockade

2–3 ml 95% ethyl alcohol, or 2–3 ml 10% ammonium sulfate solution.
The administration of the neurolytic substances is very painful, so prior analgesia with a small amount (1–2 ml) of local anesthetic solution is recommended. When ammonium sulfate is used, it is recommended that the 10% solution be obtained by mixing equal amounts of 20% ammonium sulfate and 2% mepivacaine solution. When more than one segment is to be blocked with a neurolytic solution, consideration should be given to the performance of the block under general anesthesia.

D. Blockade of the ventral branch in the posterior axillary line (dorsolateral intercostal block)

Effect

Same as the block at the costal angle.

3.3. Equipment

Sterile gloves
Antiseptic solution
Sponges
Drapes
Flat pillow
25 g needle for the skin wheal
21 g needle
2 ml syringe
5 ml syringe
Small cup for the local anesthetic solution

3.4. Positioning

Supine position (Fig 187). The body is slightly tilted to the contralateral side by the insertion of a small, hard pillow. The arm on the side to be blocked is abducted beyond the horizontal line, and the hand is placed under the nape of the neck.

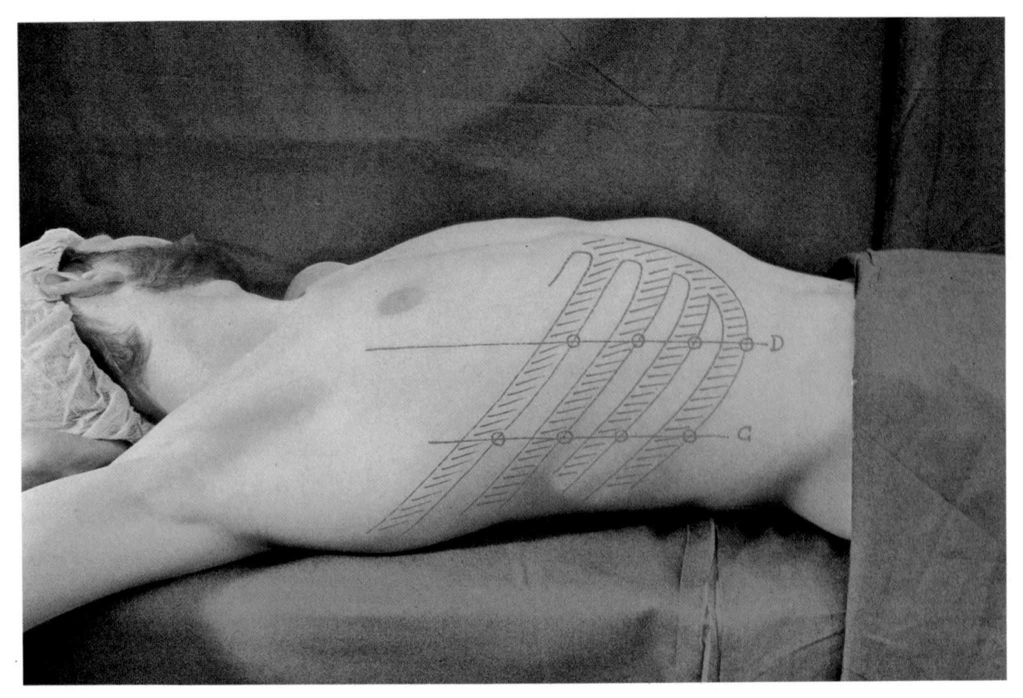

FIG 187.

3.5. Landmarks

Intersection of the posterior axillary line (Line C), with the inferior margin of the rib (Fig 187).

3.6. Technical Procedure

Degreasing, disinfection, and draping of the area of injection. After placement of the skin wheal, a 21 g short bevel needle, with a 5 ml syringe attached, is advanced in the direction of the lower third of the rib to be blocked until bony contact is made. The needle is slightly withdrawn and readjusted caudally, and advanced 2–3 mm to just below the inferior margin of the rib. Since the intercostal nerve still lies in the sulcus of the rib at this level, the tip of the needle must be adjusted sharply cranially, and advanced another 1–2 mm.

3.7. Dosage

Temporary blockade

3 ml local anesthetic solution for each segment, to be blocked, e.g., etidocaine 1% or bupivacaine 0.5%.

Permanent blockade

2–3 ml 95% ethyl alcohol or 2–3 ml 10% ammonium sulfate solution. When ammonium sulfate is to be used, it is recommended that the 10% solution be obtained by mixing equal amounts of a 20% ammonium sulfate solution and a 2% mepivacaine solution.

E. *Blockade of the ventral branch in the anterior axillary line (anterolateral intercostal block)*

Effect

Segmental anesthesia of the skin and motor blockade of the pertinent intercostal muscles (the abdominal wall is not blocked).

3.3. Equipment

Sterile gloves
Antiseptic solution
Sponges
Drapes
21 g needle
5 ml syringe
Small cup for the local anesthetic solution

3.4. Positioning

Prone position

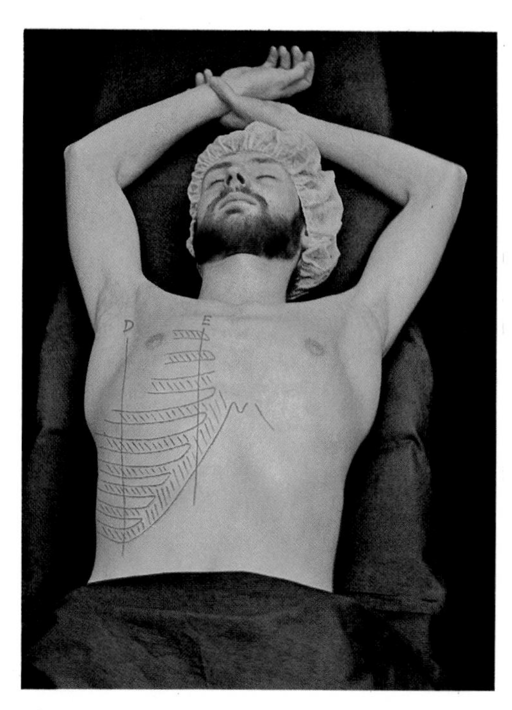

FIG 188.

3.5. Landmarks

Intersection of the anterior axillary line and the inferior margin of the rib to be blocked.

3.6. Technical Procedure

Degreasing, disinfection, and draping of the area of the injection. Using a 21 g needle with a 5 ml syringe attached, the inferior margin of the rib is approached. When bony contact is made, the tip of the needle is sharply depressed caudally, and advanced about 5 mm (middle of the intercostal space; in this area, the intercostal nerve lies between the adjacent ribs and between the leaves of the internal and external intercostal muscles).

3.7. Dosage

3–5 ml local anesthetic solution for each segment to be blocked, e.g., etidocaine 1% or bupivacaine 0.5%.

F. *Parasternal intercostal blockade*

Effect

Analgesia of the skin over the sternum, and of the periosteum of the sternum.

3.3. Equipment

Sterile gloves
Antiseptic solution
Sponges
Drapes
21 or 23 g needle
5 ml syringe

3.4. Positioning

Supine position (Fig 188)

3.5. Landmarks

Approximately 3 cm laterally from the edge of the sternum (line E). Intersection of line E and the middle of the intercostal space of the ribs to be blocked.

3.6. Technical Procedure

Degreasing, disinfection, and draping of the area of the injection. Puncture of the intercostal space using a short bevel 21 or 23 g needle with a 5 ml syringe attached.

3.7. Dosage

3–5 ml local anesthetic solution for each segment to be blocked, e.g., etidocaine 1% or bupivacaine 0.5%.

4. Special Complications

Puncture of the pleura with ensuing pneumothorax
Danger of local anesthetic overdose if multiple segments are blocked
Bleeding into the intercostal space or into the pleural space (hemothorax)

5. Indications

Temporary blockade

Postoperative or posttraumatic pain therapy (e.g., after upper abdominal surgery, after rib or sternum fracture)

Permanent blockade

Control of pain in rib metastases, herpes zoster, or intercostal neuralgia

6. Special Contraindications

None

References

1. Hay RC: Intercostal nerve block in 4333 patients. Indications, technique and complications. *Anesth Analg Curr Res* 1962; 41:11.
2. Hollmén A, Saukkonen J: Zur postoperativen Schmerzausschaltung nach Oberbauchoperationen. Narkotika, Interkostalblockade und Epiduralanästhesie und deren Einfluss auf die Atmung. *Anästhesist* 1969; 18:298.

The Management of Acute and Chronic Pain with Neural Blockade

H. Kreuscher

"Divinum est sedare dolorem" (Galen)
"It is divine to allay pain"

The following pages will present some general principles on the use of regional anesthesia techniques in the treatment of acute pain problems. As far as the actual performance of the individual blocks is concerned, the reader is referred to the corresponding chapters.

Through a blockade of the peripheral nerves or through spinal and epidural blocks, the centripetal conduction of nociceptive stimuli can be temporarily or permanently interrupted. In painful conditions which are due to disturbances in the blood supply, perfusion can be improved by blocking the appropriate sympathetic nerves. Depending on the purpose we can distinguish:

—diagnostic or differential blocks, and
—therapeutic blocks

Temporary blocks are performed with long acting local anesthetic agents (e.g., bupivacaine). For permanent blocks, neurolytic substances are used (e.g., 96% ethyl alcohol, 10% ammonium sulfate, or 6–8% phenol). Before a neurolytic substance is administered for a permanent block, it is absolutely mandatory that the patient's informed, written consent be obtained after a thorough and careful explanation of the effects, side effects, and hazards of the particular block. It is desirable also from this point of view to perform a temporary block on the patient, anesthetizing the same area which would be covered by the permanent blockade. This allows both the physician and the patient to evaluate the effects that a permanent interruption of the sensory and motor pathways may have in the specific sensory or motor distribution. It is also recommended that permanent blocks be performed under x-ray control of the needle position and of the spread of a test dose of radiographic contrast medium. If possible, a permanent x-ray record should be made of the procedure for purposes of documentation.

1. The Treatment of Painful Conditions in the Thoracic Area

Peripheral, spinal, or epidural blocks are particularly suitable for the decrease, elimination, or prevention of postoperative pain. These techniques not only promote the psychophysical comfort of the patient, but also eliminate the stress-induced negative effects on vital functions, and the splinting or other guarding due to pain (e.g., respiration).

Another option for pain control in this area is offered by a continuous epidural anesthetic (see "Thoracic epidural anesthesia," p. 122).

The treatment of an acute herpes zoster should consist of an immediate paravertebral block of the affected segments. This can shorten the course of the disease, significantly reduce the pain, and avoid postherpetic pain, which may be very resistant to therapy (see p. 12). Bupivacaine 0.5% is the drug of choice. The blocks must be performed twice each day.

1.1. Acute Pain in the Area of the Thorax

The incisional pain of lateral thoracotomies which adversely affects respiration can be largely eliminated for 4–5 hours by an intercostal block with bupivacaine 0.5%. Blockade of the ventral branches of the intercostal nerves is performed at the angle of the ribs, but centrally to the dorsal end of the incision. Blocking three segments is usually sufficient, with the incision lying at the level of the middle block. The injection should be performed as soon as the skin is closed, and before the patient's position is changed on the operating table. The block must be repeated when the pain returns (see "Blockade of the ventral branch at the angle of the rib," p. 210). After a sternotomy, a bilateral parasternal block is performed (see "Parasternal intercostal block," p. 213). The segments that must be blocked depend on the length of the sternum, i.e., intercostal nerves 1–6. These blocks are also performed immediately after the skin is closed and must be repeated, should the pain return.

1.2. Chronic Pain in the Thoracic Area

Chronic postherpetic pain can persist for years. Initially, it can be treated with temporary blocks. This will prove that the painful condition can be alleviated by the interruption of the nervous impulses along these mixed nerves. When, after repeated blocks, the freedom from pain persists for the expected duration of the anesthetic (4–6 hours), serious consideration can be given to the use of a neurolytic agent.

Metastatic malignant lesions in the thoracic spine can cause both local pain and/or segmental radiating pain, if there is compression of the vertebrae. The vertebral bodies and their periosteum receive their sensory innervation from the dorsal branches of the spinal nerves. A bilateral, temporary block provides freedom from pain for 4–6 hours (see "Blockade of the dorsal branch," p. 209). This procedure is most appropriate for otherwise painful diagnostic (radiologic) manipulations, for therapeutic procedures (radiation therapy, the application of a cast), or for transporting the patient, since it can be administered rapidly and with relatively minor inconvenience. Because of the extensive branching of these nerves, this technique cannot be used with a neurolytic substance. Epidural narcotic administration through an epidural catheter has proven very satisfactory (see "Thoracic epidural anesthesia," p. 122). This technique can be used in the nonhospitalized patient. In these cases, it is very important to fixate the catheter very carefully and to protect the epidural space from infections. Fixation can be accomplished readily by using a special transparent plastic adhesive strip over the entry point of the catheter, which is looped once at this point in order to increase the length under the adhesive strip (Figs 189 and 190).

The prevention of infection is accomplished by applying a small amount of an antiseptic ointment at the site of entry, by using a bacterial filter, and by observing the strictest aseptic technique during the placement of the catheter and during the injections. The free end of the catheter is placed along the spinal column to the shoulder, and is fixated along its entire length by a flexible, adhesive plastic strip.

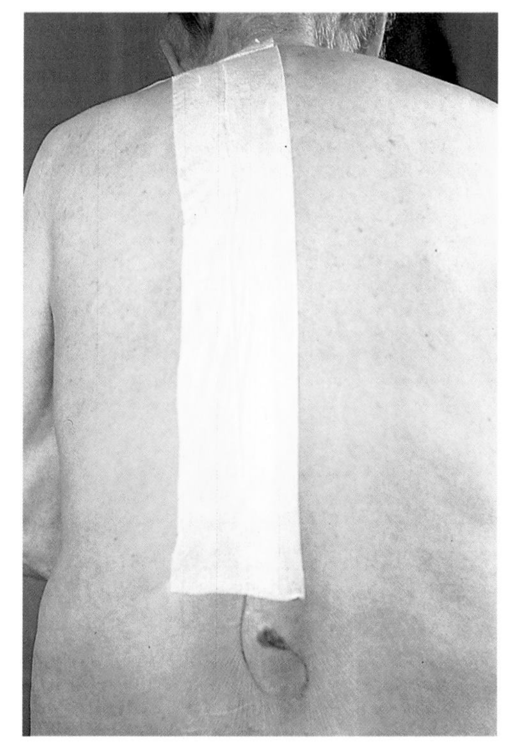

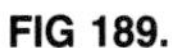

FIG 189.

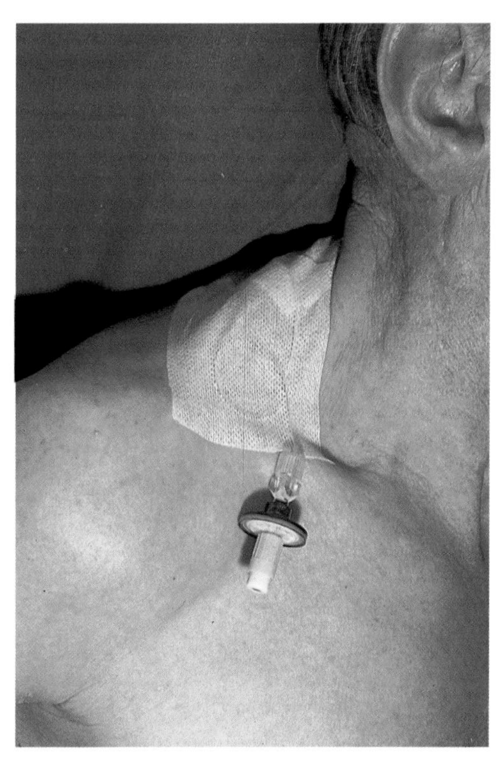

FIG 190.

To achieve narcotic epidural anesthesia, use:

- 20 mg morphine hydrochloride in 50 ml 0.9% NaCl solution, corresponding to 0.4 mg morphine per ml, or
- 0.3 mg buprenorphine in 20 ml 0.9% NaCl solution, corresponding to 0.015 mg buprenorphine per ml

Of these solutions, 6–10 ml are injected through the catheter in the morning and in the evening at predetermined times, independent of whether or not there is pain. If necessary, a third injection can be given in the middle of the day. Depending on circumstances, the patient or a member of the family can be taught to perform the injections. If this is not possible, the attending physician (nurse) must assume this responsibility.

2. The Therapy of Painful Conditions in the Abdominal Area

2.1. Acute Pain in the Area of the Abdomen

In this area consideration must also be given first to the management of postoperative pain. Nociceptive signals from the abdominal skin, the fascia of the abdominal wall, and the peritoneum are carried by the lateral cutaneous branches of the 6th–12th intercostal nerves. The temporary blockade of these intercostal nerves at the level of the posterior axillary line (see *Block of the ventral branch in the posterior axillary line,* p. 211) eliminates painful sensations for several hours, and eliminates or sharply reduces the need for potent analgetics.

Abdominal pain can be managed for longer periods of time with epidural local anesthetic or opiate administration. It is therefore recommended that an epidural catheter be placed prior to major abdominal surgery, and that a bupivacaine or etidocaine anesthetic be established. This is then followed by general endotracheal anesthesia. In most cases, the further administration of analgetics and muscle relaxants is unnecessary. The amount of inhalation anesthesia used can also be significantly reduced. In the postoperative period, effective anesthesia can be maintained by the administration of a 0.25–0.375% bupivacaine solution through the epidural catheter. This procedure will also enhance intestinal motility by providing a sympathetic blockade.

2.2. Chronic Pain in the Abdominal Area

As a rule, these are caused by malignant neoplasms and/or metastatic malignancies.

Chronic pain in the upper and midabdomen can be well controlled temporarily or permanently with a celiac plexus block (see "Celiac plexus block," p. 172).

3. Pain Originating in the Vertebrae

The most frequent acute and chronically painful conditions are due to changes in the area of the spinal column and the other structures responsible for the upright position. Other than metastases to the vertebrae (see p. 12), segmental pain or discomfort—e.g., hypo-, hyper-, or paresthesias—are caused by poor posture of the spinal column, and by degenerative changes of the vertebrae, their articulations, and the intervertebral discs. Poor position or degenerative changes in the cervical spine frequently lead to headache syndromes, particularly pains in the back of the head and the nape of the neck, at times accompanied by a cap-like spread as far as the forehead.

The immediate causes of the pain are spasms and tensions in the static musculature of the neck, caused by splinting or malpositioning of the support apparatus. There can also be compression of the spinal roots in the area of the intervertebral foramina. This compression is caused by spurs on the vertebral bodies (particularly on the uncinate process), or by a protrusion of the intervertebral disc.

Severe compression of the roots, with sensory and/or motor loss, requires early neurosurgical intervention. All other cases require primarily an effective elimination of the pain by blocks in the area of the spinal cord. This can be done only after careful orthopedic, neurologic, and roentgenologic investigation. A rational therapeutic strategy is of great importance: first, lasting and complete freedom from pain must be achieved, so that the pain-induced malposition of the spinal column and the ensuing muscular dystonia can be relieved. Once the pain is precisely identified, a variety of blocks can be used. It is important that all physical means measures such as massage, gymnastics, and baths be strictly avoided. The local application of heat may be permitted. This principle of therapy will break the vicious cycle of pain generating pain.

3.1. Headaches Originating in the Area of the Vertebrae

In most cases, these are typical neuralgiform pains, unilateral or bilateral, in the sensory area of the major and minor occipital nerves. A block of the occipitalis major with 3–5 ml of a 0.5% bupivacaine solution stops the pain immediately and for several hours (see "The occipital nerves," p. 199). These blocks must be repeated daily so that the poor posture of the cervical spine, which is both caused by pain and causes pain, can be eliminated. Once the block has eliminated the pain, the frequently present myogelosis of the cervical and shoulder muscles can be treated with careful massage after the application of heat (infrared radiations, heat packs), and thus contribute to the success of the therapy.

3.2. Pain in the Thorax and the Abdomen Originating in the Vertebrae

The management of this pain is accomplished with the techniques described in sections 1.2. and 2.

3.3. Pain in the Area of the Lumbar Spine and Lower Extremity Originating in the Vertebrae

The etiology of painful conditions in this area is usually found in degenerative changes in the bones and ligaments of the lumbar spine and the pelvis and/or in postural abnormalities. Distinction must be made between the pain which originates in the dynamic structures, i.e., muscles, the articulations of the spinal column, the periosteum in the area of tendinous insertion, and the pain which originates through mechanical pressure on the spinal nerves. Frequently, both types of pain are found simultaneously. The principles of therapy are the complete elimination of the pain, and the relaxation (immobilization) of the patient.

The immediate disappearance of the pain can be accomplished by caudal epidural anesthesia (see "Caudal anesthesia," p. 126) or, even better, through a continuous lumbar epidural anesthesia with 0.25–0.375% bupivacaine (see "Lumbar epidural anesthesia," p. 111).

In addition to the elimination of pain, careful positioning of the patient with protrusions of the discs has been found to be particularly helpful. This positioning entails the use of a hospital bed, where the patient can rest with the knees drawn up. This will eliminate the exaggerated lumbar lordosis, and will increase the size of the intervertebral foramina. If there are persistent hypo-, hyper- or paresthesias and in every case of motor loss, neurosurgical intervention is indicated. Similar to the thoracic spine procedure (see section 1.2), the sensory input into the individual lumbar vertebrae can be eliminated by a temporary blockade of the dorsal branches of the spinal nerves. Epidural opiate analgesia is also an effective method of pain control, particularly cancer pain, in the lumbar spine area.

4. The Myofascial Syndrome

This painful syndrome usually appears suddenly, and is frequently triggered by thermal (cold) or mechanical stimuli. There is rarely any pathophysiologic foundation. The presence of a trigger point is characteristic. Digital pressure on the trigger point produces or aggravates the typical pain. If the trigger point is "needled" as in acupuncture, or injected with a local anesthetic solution, the pain is eliminated. One must assume that there is a self-perpetuating pain cycle. The trigger points are occasionally found in muscles, tendons, ligaments, or even in scars. The effectiveness of a field block is very great, so that the search for trigger points is very rewarding. Frequently, the trigger points are at the site of the well known acupuncture sites. (See "Myofascial trigger points," p. 201.)

5. The Treatment of Painful Conditions or Disease Entities Due to Circulatory Disturbances, with Blocks of the Sympathetic Nervous System

5.1. Acute Hearing Loss

Acute, mostly unilateral, hearing loss is usually associated with tinnitus, i.e., an adventitious buzzing or ringing in the ear. It is assumed to be the consequence of a local perfusion defect in the inner ear. The early, preferably immediate, therapy with a stellate ganglion block (see "The stellate ganglion," p. 168) has a surprisingly and pleasingly high success rate when compared to conventional drug therapy. The stellate ganglion block must be repeated daily. In general, ten consecutive stellate ganglion blocks are performed. Drug therapy designed to improve circulation should be instituted simultaneously.

5.2. Causalgia, Sudeck's Reflex Dystrophy, Raynaud's Disease, Arteriosclerotic Perfusion Disturbances

These are all disease entities for which there is no more effective single conservative therapy than sympathetic blockade. The techniques used are stellate ganglion blocks for diseases of the upper extremity, and lumbar sympathetic chain blocks for diseases of the lower extremity. The indications and the likelihood of therapeutic results of a sympathetic block can be tested by examining the psychogalvanic reflex (PGR) (see "Sympathetic blocks," p. 183). This test will also serve to establish the presence of a sympathetic block.

The presence of a PGR should be determined before the performance of the sympathetic block. A negative, i.e., nonmeasurable PGR raises serious questions about the potential benefits of a sympathetic block. On the other hand, the absence of the PGR after the administration of a sympathetic block is objective evidence of the effectiveness of the block.

In perfusion disturbances of the lower extremity, a permanent lumbar sympathetic block at the level of L_1–L_3 with alcohol gives results similar to surgical lumbar sympathectomy, with less effort and less risk (see "Lumbar sympathetics," p. 178).

6. The Management of Intractable Pain with a Permanent Intrathecal Alcohol Block (Chemical Rhizolysis)

The chronic, intractable pain associated particularly with advanced and metastatic, malignant neoplasms can be eliminated or alleviated by a chemical rhizolysis of the dorsal spinal roots. This form of therapy should be considered for those pain problems which are in the sensory area of the thoracic, lumbar, or sacral spinal segments. Alcohol 96% or phenol 8% in glycerin can be used as neurolytic substances. Dogliotti (1931) was the first to use intrathecal alcohol to eliminate the dorsal roots, and thus to interrupt the afferent sensory impulses. The duration of the intrathecal block is highly variable, and may last from 6 weeks to 6 months, and even for 24 months. Alcohol rhizolysis tends to be more permanent than the phenol-glycerin block. The danger of a permanent motor block is minimal if the technique is used properly (see "Spinal anesthesia," p. 96), but it does exist and must be included in the discussion with the patient. Depending on the level of the blocked segments, urinary and fecal retention, as well as incontinence are possible. In most cases, these complications disappear in 1–2 months (2).

References

1. Cousins MJ, Bridenbaugh PO (eds): *Neural Blockade,* Philadelphia–Toronto, JB Lippincott Co, 1980.
2. Gerbershagen HU, Baar HA, Kreuscher H: Langzeitnervenblockaden zur Behandlung schwerer Schmerzzustände. I. Die intrathekale Injektion von Neurolytika. *Der Anästhesist* 1972; 21:112–121.
3. Gerbershagen HU: Methodik der Spinalblockade mit Neurolytika, in Killian H (Hrsg): *Lokalanästhesie und Lokalanästhetika,* 2. Aufl. Stuttgart, Thieme, 1973.
4. Zimmermann M: Schmerz und Schmerztherapie: Neue Konzepte aus der Grundlagenforschung (I). *Klinik Journal* 1983; 11:23–32.

References

1. Ahnefeld FW, Bergmann H, Burri C, Dick W, Halmagyi M, Hossli G, Rügheimer E: Lokalanasthesie in: *Klinische Anästhesiologie und Intensivtherapie,* Band 18. Berlin–Heidelberg–New York, Springer, 1978.
2. Bromage R: *Epidural Analgesia.* Philadelphia–London–Toronto, WB Saunders Co, 1978.
3. Covino BG, Vasallo HG: *Local Anesthetics. Mechanisms of Action and Clinical Use.* New York–San Francisco–London, Grune and Stratton, 1976.
4. De Jong: *Local Anesthetics,* ed 2. Springfield, Charles C. Thomas, 1977.
5. Killian H (Hrsg): *Lokalanästhesie und Lokalanästhetika,* 2. Aufl. Stuttgart, Thieme, 1973.
6. Moore DC: *Regional Block,* ed 4. Springfield, Charles C. Thomas, 1965.
7. Nolte H, Meyer J (Hrsg): *Die rückenmarksnahen Anästhesien.* Stuttgart, Thieme, 1972.
8. Strasser K: *Lumbale Periduralanästhesie in der Geburtshilfe.* München–Wien–Baltimore, Urban & Schwarzenberg, 1980.

Index

C

D

E

F

G

H

I

K

L

M

N

O

P

R

S

T

U

V

W

Bruce & Mary Hausauer
2019 Southland Lane
New London, Wis 54961

Ped Caudal

0.175 % Marcaine c̄ Epi.
(3 ml NaCl / 7 ml 0.5 % Mar. c̄ Epi
per 10 cc)

Give 0.8 - 1.0 ml per Kg / wt.

Post Epid. Dosing

1) 0.25% Bupivacaine 2 cc PF
Astramorph 2 cc
Epineph 0.05 mg
PF. NS q.s.
= 10 ml thru cath

Ankle block

15 cc — 2% Xylo
5 cc — .75 % Marcaine